ANIMAL MODELS
OF OCULAR DISEASES

ANIMAL MODELS OF OCULAR DISEASES

Edited by

KHALID F. TABBARA, M.D.

and

ROBERT M. CELLO, V.M.D.

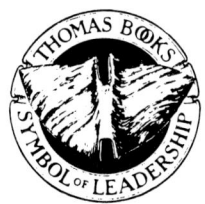

CHARLES C THOMAS • PUBLISHER
Springfield • Illinois • U.S.A.

Published and Distributed Throughout the World by
CHARLES C THOMAS • PUBLISHER
2600 South First Street
Springfield, Illinois 62717

This book is protected by copyright. No part of it may be reproduced in any manner without written permission from the publisher.

© *1984 by* CHARLES C THOMAS • PUBLISHER
ISBN 0-398-04890-8
Library of Congress Catalog Card Number: 83-5028

With THOMAS BOOKS *careful attention is given to all details of manufacturing and design. It is the Publisher's desire to present books that are satisfactory as to their physical qualities and artistic possibilities and appropriate for their particular use.* THOMAS BOOKS *will be true to those laws of quality that assure a good name and good will.*

Printed in the United States of America
SC-R-3

Library of Congress Cataloging in Publication Data
Main entry under title:

Animal models of ocular diseases.

   Presentations from a seminar held at Lake Tahoe, Sept. 11-13, 1982, sponsored by the Alta California Eye Research Foundation.
   Bibliography: p.
   Includes index.
   1. Eye—Diseases and defects—Animal models—Congresses. I. Tabbara, Khalid F.   II. Cello, Robert M. III. Alta California Eye Research Foundation. [DNLM: 1. Ophthalmology—Congresses.   2. Disease models, Animal—Congresses.   WW 100 A598 1982]
RE48.A55   1983   617.7′027   83-5028
ISBN 0-398-04890-8

PARTICIPANTS IN THE ALTA/TAHOE SEMINAR

Gary Barth, M.D.: Postdoctoral Research Fellow, Francis I. Proctor Foundation, University of California, San Francisco, California.

Kathleen L. Boldy, V.M.D.: Resident in Ophthalmology, Verterinary Teaching Hospital, University of California, Davis, California.

Robert P. Burns, M.D.: Professor and Chairman, Department of Ophthalmology, University of Missouri, Columbia, Missouri.

Robert Cello, V.M.D.: Professor, Veterinary Medicine, Vice Chancellor for Academic Affairs, University of California, Davis, California.

Vincent P. deLuise, M.D.: Postdoctoral Research Fellow (1981–1982), Francis I. Proctor Foundation, University of California, San Francisco, California.

Joseph A. Eliason, M.D.: Assistant Professor, Department of Surgery, Division of Ophthalmology, Stanford University Medical Center, Stanford, California.

Mitchell H. Friedlaender, M.D.: Associate Research Ophthalmologist, Clinical Associate Professor of Ophthalmology, Francis I. Proctor Foundation, University of California, San Francisco, California.

David Fuerst, M.D.: Postdoctoral Research Fellow, Francis I. Proctor Foundation, University of California, San Francisco, California.

Careen Yen-Lowder, M.D., Ph.D.: Postdoctoral Research Fellow, Francis I. Proctor Foundation, University of California, San Francisco, California.

Raga Malaty, M.D., Ph.D.: Assistant Research Microbiologist, Francis I. Proctor Foundation, University of California, San Francisco, California.

John C. Merriam, M.D.: Postdoctoral Research Fellow, Francis I. Proctor Foundation, University of California, San Francisco, California.

Joseph P. Metcalf, M.D.: Associate Research Cell Biologist, Department of Optometry, University of California, Berkeley, California.

J. Fraser Muirhead, M.D., F.R.C.S.C. (C): Associate Clinical Professor of Ophthalmology, University of California, San Francisco, California.

G. Richard O'Connor, M.D.: Professor of Ophthalmology; Director, Francis I. Proctor Foundation, University of California, San Francisco, California.

Jang O. Oh, M.D., Ph.D.: Research Microbiologist, Francis I. Proctor Foundation, University of California, San Francisco, California.

Masao Okumoto, M.A.: Specialist in Microbiology, Francis I. Proctor Foundation, University of California, San Francisco, California.

H. Bruce Ostler, M.D.: Research Ophthalmologist, Francis I. Proctor Foundation, Clinical Professor of Ophthalmology; Research Associate, Microbiology, University of California, San Francisco, California

Eduardo P. Penna, M.D.: Postdoctoral Research Fellow, Francis I. Proctor Foundation, University of California, San Francisco, California.

James T. Rosenbaum, M.D.: Assistant Professor of Medicine, Department of Medicine, University of California, San Francisco, California (San Francisco General Hospital).

Alan M. Roth, M.D.: Professor of Ophthalmology and Pathology; Vice Chairman of Ophthalmology, School of Medicine, University of California, Davis, California.

Gilbert Smolin, M.D.: Clinical Professor and Research Ophthalmologist, Francis I. Proctor Foundation, University of California, San Francisco, California.

Joseph S. Spinelli, D.V.M.: Director, Animal Care Facility; Associate Clinical Professor of Veterinary Medicine, University of California, San Francisco, California.

E. Lee Stock, M.D.: Director, Cornea and External Eye Disease Laboratory, Northwestern University Medical School, Chicago, Illinois.

Khalid F. Tabbara, M.D.: Associate Professor of Ophthalmology; Director, Heintz Laboratory, Francis I. Proctor Foundation, University of California, San Francisco, California.

Phillips Thygeson, M.D.: Professor Emeritus, Department of Ophthalmology; Research Ophthalmologist, Francis I. Proctor Foundation, University of California, San Francisco, California.

Robert M. Webb, M.D.: Postdoctoral Research Fellow, Francis I. Proctor Foundation, University of California, San Francisco, California.

Leigh West-Hyde, V.D.M.: Lecturer, Section of Ophthalmology, Department of Surgery, School of Veterinary Medicine, University of California, San Francisco, California.

Ira G. Wong, M.D.: Research Associate, Francis I. Proctor Foundation, University of California, San Francisco, California.

PREFACE

The Alta California Eye Research Foundation, principal sponsor of the three-day research seminar that this book summarizes, was founded in 1969 in San Francisco. Its purposes, as stated in the founding documents, are to foster eye research through educational programs and financial contributions, to promote the dissemination of new knowledge about diseases of the eye through publications, and to facilitate the training of scientists interested in pursuing ophthalmic research, particularly at the graduate level.

Located in San Francisco near the main buildings of the University of California's Medical Center, the Alta California Eye Research Foundation has fulfilled most of its goals through the support of educational and investigative activities at the Francis I. Proctor Foundation for Research in Ophthalmology, one of the so-called Organized Research Units of the University. It has made yearly financial contributions to the Proctor Foundation and has underwritten the latter's efforts to promote yearly seminars on some aspect of ophthalmic research. These seminars, usually held in mid-September at the home of Dr. and Mrs. Phillips Thygeson at Lake Tahoe, have been arranged in collaboration with Dr. Robert Cello of the Division of Ophthalmology of the University of California's Veterinary Teaching Hospital at Davis. Topics of mutual interest to the Davis group and to investigators at the Proctor Foundation are usually selected a year in advance, and at this time guest speakers of scientific prominence are also invited from various medical institutions and veterinary centers throughout the United States. Most of the seminars have dealt with external ocular diseases, with special emphasis on the microbial and immunologic aspects of these diseases. Where naturally occurring animal models of a given human ocular disease exist, much useful information can be learned about the natural course of a disease, its epidemiology, and its response to various forms of therapy. For example, NZB/NZW F_1 mice are subject to the spontaneous lupuslike syndrome complicated by keratoconjunctivitis sicca. When the lacrimal glands of the affected mice are examined histologically, cellular infiltrations exactly analogous to those seen in human cases of keratoconjunctivitis sicca are seen. Recent studies have shown that restriction of saturated fats in the diet of the NZB/NZW mice ameliorates the pathologic changes that occur in the lacrimal glands. These investigations may eventually provide insight into the pathogenesis of the disease and lead the way to a therapeutic approach to human disease that had not been previously recognized.

This book, *Animal Models of Ocular Disease*, is the fourth formal publication to come out of the Lake Tahoe seminars. Others include *Herpetic Diseases of the Eye*, published as a supplement to *Survey of Ophthalmology* in 1976, *Immunologic Diseases of the Mucous Membranes* (Masson & Co., 1980), and *Antimicrobial Therapy of Ocular Diseases* (Masson & Co., in press). The present volume takes a special look at infectious, immunologic, and neoplastic diseases that affect the eyes of man and various animals. It examines the suitability of certain animal models in terms of reproducibility of the disease, hereditary factors that influence it, and environmental factors that might affect it.

With regard to the environment under which the various experiments described in this book were performed, the contributors were acutely aware of the need for humane treatment of the animals involved in these studies, and there was considerable discussion of this matter. Each institution represented at the symposium was registered with the United States Department of Agriculture under the provisions of the Animal Welfare Act, and each had filed a written assurance with the United States Department of Health and Human Services stating that it was committed to comply with that department's *Principles for the Use of Animals*. In brief, those principles are as follows:

- Projects or activities involving live, warm-blooded animals and the procurement of living animal tissues for biomedical activities must be performed by, or under the immediate supervision of, a scientist qualified in the scientific area under study.
- The housing, care, and feeding of all laboratory animals must be supervised by a properly qualified veterinarian or other scientist competent in such matters.
- The intent of the project or activity should be such as to yield fruitful results for the good of society, and not be random and unnecessary in nature.
- The project or activity should be so conducted as to avoid all unnecessary suffering and injury to the subject animal.
- If any aspect of the project or activity is likely to cause greater discomfort than that attending anesthetization, the subject animals must be rendered incapable of perceiving the pain prior to its possible onset and must be maintained in that condition until the threat of pain is ended. The only exception to this guideline should be in those cases where anesthesia would defeat the purpose of the project; such exceptions must be specifically approved and supervised by the principal investigator.

- If it is necessary to sacrifice a laboratory animal, the subject animal must be killed in a humane manner in such a way as to insure immediate death in accordance with procedures approved by the institutional committee. *No animal shall be discarded until death is certain.*
- Postexperiment care of subject animals must be such as to minimize discomfort, in accordance with acceptable practice in veterinary medicine.
- Standards for the construction and use of housing, service, and surgical facilities should be consistent with the recommendations in the DHEW publication, "Guide for Care and Use of Laboratory Animals," Fourth Edition, or as otherwise required by the U.S. Department of Agriculture regulations established under the terms of the Animal Welfare Act.

With regard to the above, I would draw the attention of all readers to the presentation of Joseph Spinelli, D.V.M., Director of the Vivarium of the University of California at San Francisco, which is to be found in this volume. The contributors to this book subscribe *in toto* to the need for supervision of all animal observations and experiments by qualified veterinarians, and we feel, furthermore, that this is one of the important messages of this book: consult a qualified veterinarian before you begin any experiment.

The reader should find this book an important source of references concerning existing animal models of ocular diseases. Although many of the chapters begin with a historical review of the particular model or disease under discussion, every attempt has been made to present an up-to-date compilation of facts, based on the most recent pertinent literature. Certainly one may use these presentations as a starting place for future investigations in any case, and that was another important goal of this publication: to stimulate further research into eye diseases shared by man and animals.

The editors of *Animal Models of Ocular Disease* join me in thanking Mr. King Kryger of the Proctor Foundation for the invaluable assistance that he has given us in the preparation of the finished manuscript. We also wish to thank Charles C Thomas, Publisher for assistance and advice with regard to the actual production of the book.

G. Richard O'Connor, M.D.
President, Alta California
Eye Research Foundation

CONTENTS

Page

Chapter

Preface
    G. Richard O'Connor vii
1. The Selection of Animal Models for Scientific Investigations
    Joseph S. Spinelli, D.V.M. 3

SECTION I – INFECTIOUS DISEASES

2. The Rabbit Model of Herpetic Keratitis
    John C. Merriam, M.D. 23
3. Herpes Simplex Retinochoroiditis in Newborn Rabbits
    Jang O. Oh, M.D., Ph.D. 39
4. Herpetic Keratitis in Normal and Athymic Mice
    Joseph P. Metcalf, M.D. 53
5. Models of Chlamydial Conjunctivitis in Nonhuman Primates
    Phillips Thygeson, M.D. 63
6. Chlamydial Infections in Cats
    Kathleen L. Boldy, V.M.D. 71
7. Chlamydial Conjunctivitis in the Guinea Pig
    Raga Malaty, M.D., Ph.D. 79
8. Ocular Toxoplasmosis
    Eduardo P. Penna, M.D. 87
9. Experimental Models of Toxoplasmosis
    G. Richard O'Connor, M.D. 97
10. The Nine-Banded Armadillo (*Dasypus Novemcincutus* L.)
    as a Model for Leprosy (Hansen's Disease)
    H. Bruce Ostler, M.D. 105
11. Antibiotics in the Treatment of
    Experimental Bacterial Endophthalmitis
    Careen Yen-Lowder, M.D., Ph.D. 111

12. Ocular Listeriosis
    Masao Okumoto, M.A. 121
13. Animal Models of Bacterial Corneal Ulcers
    Gary Barth, M.D. 129
14. Experimental Bacterial Endophthalmitis
    Ira G. Wong, M.D. 137

SECTION II — NEOPLASTIC DISEASES

15. Ocular Findings in Cutaneous Malignant Melanomas in Swine
    Robert P. Burns, M.D., et al. 145
16. Immunotherapy for Rabbit Lid Papillomas
    Gilbert Smolin, M.D., et al. 167
17. Bovine Ocular Squamous Cell Carcinoma
    Leigh West-Hyde, V.M.D. 173

SECTION III — METABOLIC AND MISCELLANEOUS DISORDERS

18. Oval Corneal Opacities in Beagles: An Animal Model of
    Schnyder's Crystalline Dystrophy 183
    Alan M. Roth, M.D., et al.
19. Animal Models of Corneal Vascularization
    Joseph A. Eliason, M.D. 201
20. Tyrosinemia in Mink
    David Fuerst, M.D. 207
21. Taurine Deficiency in Cats
    Leigh West-Hyde, V.M.D. 215
22. Animal Models of Band Keratopathy
    J. Fraser Muirhead, M.D., F.R.C.S. (C).
    and Laura Tomazzoli-Gerosa, M.D. 221

SECTION IV — IMMUNOLOGIC DISORDERS

23. NZB/NZW F_1 Hybrid Mice:
    An Animal Model of Sjögren's Syndrome
    Vincent P. deLuise, M.D. and Khalid F. Tabbara, M.D. 237
24. Endotoxin-Induced Uveitis in Rats
    James T. Rosenbaum, M.D. 247
25. Canine Systemic Lupus Erythematosus
    Robert M. Webb, M.D. 255

26. Contact Hypersensitivity in Guinea Pigs
    Mitchell H. Friedlaender, M.D. 263
27. Immediate Conjunctival Hypersensitivity Reactions
    in the Guinea Pig after Systemic Sensitization
    E. Lee Stock, M.D. 269

Index 277

ANIMAL MODELS
OF OCULAR DISEASES

Chapter 1

THE SELECTION OF ANIMAL MODELS FOR SCIENTIFIC INVESTIGATIONS

JOSEPH S. SPINELLI, D.V.M.

Introduction

Although the term "laboratory animal" usually refers to the rat, mouse, guinea pig, rabbit, dog, or cat, any member of the animal kingdom may be used in the laboratory. Each of the thousands of animal species, including insects, have unique anatomical, physiological, and pathological characteristics. While few have been utilized for research purposes, many have great potential as laboratory animals. A thorough search of the literature would show that many animal species seem to have been uniquely designed to answer almost any biological problem that comes to mind. For example, marsupials' unique anatomy permits the direct observation of embryonic and fetal development, and there are miniature strains of various animals such as pigs and goats that are particularly adaptable for laboratory study.

THE PROCESS OF SELECTING AN ANIMAL SPECIES

There is a concern among many involved in the production, care, and use of laboratory animals that decisions about the selection of an individual species as a model for biomedical research are often made impulsively and are not based on a thorough analysis of which species best meets the needs of a particular investigation. Unless one is repeating someone else's work or complying with the terms of a preexisting protocol, the worst reason for selecting a particular type of animal as a biological model is that "other people use it." Before selecting an animal species for use in a particular line of investigation, experimenters should ask three major questions: Which animal species possesses the unique anatomical and physiological characteristics consistent with the needs of the experiment? Are there animal species that have naturally occurring disease states similar to those being studied? What will it cost to purchase and maintain the animals under consideration? Each of these will be discussed more completely.

Anatomical and Physiological Characteristics

By determining the unique anatomical and physiological characteristics of a given species, one can judge whether the species would be suitable for a given line of scientific investigation. For example, rabbits may have value because their eyes are large, allowing for accurate clinical observation of corneal lesions.

The average life span and generation interval of the animal type being considered, and the number of offspring produced at each birth and during the breeding life of the animal type, may also have an important bearing on the selection of a species.

Inbred Strains

The anatomy and physiology of a given animal species can be manipulated through the development of inbred strains. Almost every one of the 50,000 to 100,000 gene pairs becomes fixed in a homozygous state after 20–25 successive generations of a single pair brother/sister mating. After the 20–25 successive generations of a single pair brother/sister mating, the inbred strain will have become as genetically homozygous as possible. The residual heterozygosity is extremely small and in succeeding generations disappears at the same rate as the spontaneous mutation rate. In other words, after 20–25 generations, the strain is as inbred as it will get. A further increase in homozygosity by inbreeding is balanced by a decrease due to new mutations.

Inbred Mice

Over 200 strains of inbred mice have been developed. By mating a female of one inbred strain with a male of another, the same kind of heterozygous F-1 hybrid population can always be produced. Only the F-1 hybrid generation of such crosses is genetically homozygous. With approximately 200 inbred strains of mice from which to choose, 39,800 reciprocal hybrids are possible. Inbred strains offer the advantage of providing reproducible types of individuals whose genetic characteristics are predictable. Once an inbred strain has been developed, information as to its characteristics can be accumulated by studying many different individuals of the same genotype.

Monitoring Inbred Strains

Once a decision is made to use a given inbred strain, one must assure that the animals are truly members of that inbred strain. One cannot depend upon the appearance of an animal to determine its strain. Mix-ups, even among highly reliable vendors, have been reported.[1] Both breeders and users must incorporate monitoring techniques to assure purity in a given inbred strain. Various methods are now available to genetically monitor inbred strains of rodents. These are described below. Further discussion and detailed references for each of these techniques are available.[2]

Colony Management

Sound protocols and assurance that those protocols are being followed are the best insurance against potential problems in colony management. Spontaneous mutations can cause a drift in the traits of inbred strains. Therefore, in order to assure maximum genetic similarity, it is important to keep even inbred strains as closely related to each other as possible. For example, a large colony of inbred mice should be produced from a small central core. Each inbred strain should be produced from a small central foundation stock whose members are, in turn, ancestors of the production stocks used to supply investigators.

Whenever possible, animals with similar physical characteristics should be raised in separate rooms. All escaped animals should be humanely killed since there is a risk that they might be returned to an improper cage.

Biochemical Markers

For the most part, biochemical markers are enzymes. Electrophoresis is the most commonly used method to determine the variation in biochemical markers.

Skin Grafting

Skin grafting has been used for years to assure that a strain is inbred. This method involves the exchange of skin grafts between animals from within a given population or from different populations to see whether they are uniform with respect to the histocompatibility genes. If the grafts are accepted, this is an indication that there is a high degree of inbreeding and homogeneity between the animals. Although skin grafting requires little training and equipment, final results are usually not available until 60–100 days after grafting. An advantage of the technique is that it monitors several hundred histocompatability genes located on virtually every chromosome.

Serologic Techniques

Serologic techniques can be used to identify immunogenic markers. Generally, tests are conducted relative to a major histocompatibility complex found on the surface of cells. Similar to biochemical methods, serologic techniques generally test for the expression of a relatively few gene loci. However, the expression of the tested loci is well defined between strains.

Mandibular Analysis

Genetic monitoring can also be accomplished by analyzing mandibular shape. This shape is known to be genetically distinct and differs markedly between inbred strains of rodents. Rodents of approximately the same size and weight are used for comparative purposes. At least eleven anatomical reference points of the mandible are measured. Like skin grafting, this technique simultaneously assays a large number of gene loci.

Microbiologically Defined Animals

An important consideration in determining the selection of a potential laboratory animal is whether microbiologically defined animals of that species are available. Animals come to the laboratory with a variety of microbial life. Microbial "loads" vary: some animals are completely free of demonstrable microorganisms while others are infected with pathogenic organisms. Ideally, the only pathogenic organisms that should infect the laboratory animals are those under study. However, even when animals appear healthy, they may be infected with pathogenic microorganisms that could produce clinical disease. Therefore, it is best to use animals totally free of pathogenic organisms in order to limit the introduction of undesirable variables into one's work. Also, there are times when there is an advantage to using axenic or germ-free animals in research.

Gnotobiotic Animals

A gnotobiotic animal is one that is maintained in the absence of all other organisms or in the presence of specifically known biological companions.

Axenic Animals

Axenic animals are those raised and maintained in the absence of all other organisms. When axenic animals are purposely infected with known biological agents, they are referred to as gnotobiotic, or defined flora, animals.

Pathogen-Free Animals

Pathogen-free animals are those that are free of all microorganisms capable of causing disease.

The Maintenance of Microbiologically Defined Animals

Sophisticated facilities must be utilized in order to maintain animals in a gnotobiotic state. A variety of systems including corridor facilities and the maintenance of animals in a sterile laminar air flow cabinet are used for this purpose. A key component is management. If animals are to be maintained in a gnotobiotic state, all material contacting them must be adequately sterilized and protocols rigidly adhered to.

Naturally Occurring Disease States

The second major factor to consider when selecting a potential laboratory animal is whether the type of animal being considered has naturally occurring disease states similar to those being studied. One needs merely to review the titles of papers in this book to determine the importance of this consideration. As a subset of this criterion, the question can be asked, "Does a disease manifest itself in a more desirable manner in the animal type under consideration than in other animal types?" For example, scrapie has an incubation period of years in sheep, but of only weeks in mice. It is therefore, far more practical to study that condition in the latter species.

Costs

Regardless of the scientific considerations, one eventually has to deal with practical matters, such as cost and maintenance, in determining which animal will be best suited for research. The expense and difficulty of maintaining a statistically significant population of very large animals, such as whales or elephants, would preclude them from most types of ophthalmologic research.

There is an important issue relating to costs at the time that one applies for research grants that all of us know but too often forget: budgets for grant years should take inflation rates into consideration, and should not be based on purchase and per diem prices in effect at the time the grant is written. A failure to add the appropriate inflation figure may result in a reduction in the number of animals that can be used in experimental procedures.

Adequate Facilities

The cost of maintaining animals is largely determined by the relative ease or difficulty of their housing and care. These are considerations that account for the popularity of traditional laboratory animal species, because most animal facilities are equipped to take care of them and animal care personnel and investigators are familiar with their handling. This is not to say that both groups cannot learn to care for and handle nontraditional species. However, it is important that the investigator check with animal care staff to be sure that adequate facilities are available for housing and maintenance.

Numbers of Animals

Whether a particular species is practical to use depends in part on the number of animals available. Animals on the endangered list cannot be used, and others are virtually impossible to house.

Environments for the Study of Animals

Cypress and Hurvits[3] describe three major types of environments in which animals can be studied. These are the laboratory environment, the domestic environment, and the natural environment.

The Laboratory Environment

Animals are most frequently studied in the traditional animal facility, the investigator's laboratory. The advantages of this environment are that defined strains are available, the environment can be easily standardized, and records are easily maintained. The primary disadvantage is that the environment is highly artificial. Although a variety of animal facilities are available to researchers, studies are sometimes better carried out in specialized laboratory environments. Among these are special containment facilities for microorganisms and regional primate centers established throughout the country by the National Institutes of Health to facilitate research related to human health requiring the use of nonhuman primates. (The primate centers are listed in Table 1-I.)

TABLE 1-I
LIST OF REGIONAL PRIMATE CENTERS IN THE UNITED STATES

1. Oregon Regional Primate Research Center
   505 Northwest 185th Avenue
   Beaverton, Oregon 97005

2. Regional Primate Research Center
   University of Washington
   Seattle, Washington 98195

3. New England Regional Primate Research Center
   One Pine Hill Drive
   Southborough, Massachusetts 01772

4. Yerkes Regional Primate Research Center
   Emory University
   Atlanta, Georgia 30322

5. Wisconsin Regional Primate Research Center
   1223 Capital Courts
   Madison, Wisconsin 53706

6. Delta Regional Primate Research Center
   Tulane University
   Covington, Louisiana 70433

7. California Primate Research Center
   University of California, Davis
   Davis, California 95616

THE CALIFORNIA PRIMATE RESEARCH CENTER. In California, the regional primate center is located on the Davis campus of the University of California, as the California Primate Research Center (CPRC). The CPRC is operated as both a regional and a national resource for the biomedical research community. The facility is supported by a base operating grant from the Division of Research Resources at NIH. This grant is used to operate the physical facilities of the CPRC and to provide partial support for research programs by core scientists permanently assigned at the CPRC. Other scientists are invited to make use of the facilities at CPRC, either for their individual projects or as members of research teams participating in health-related research. Research projects are generally supported by funding sources other than the CPRC base operating grant; however, partial "seed" support is at times available for priority projects that have a high probability of success and that will lead to future extramural funding. Core units at the CPRC include Perinatal Biology and Reproduction, Respiratory Diseases, Experimental Biology, and Primate Medicine. The CPRC is located on a 300 acre tract of land adjacent to the UC Davis campus. Basic facilities include offices, fully equipped research laboratores, an electron microscopy facility (transmission and scanning), a computer facility, a library with bibliographic services, and conference and lecture rooms. The facility includes indoor and outdoor animal holding areas, as well as a hospital unit with support services for surgery, radiology, clinical pathology, pathology, therapeutics, and a nursery. Several small research and animal buildings bring the total operational indoor space to more than 60,000 square feet. Equipped research laboratories are available upon request for both permanent core investigators and visiting scientists.

The colony consists of approximately 2000 nonhuman primates of eleven species. Over 1200 of these animals are rhesus monkeys. Species available for research at the CPRC are *Callicebus moloch* (titi monkey), *Macaca fascicularius* (cynomolgus or crab eating monkey), *Macaca mulatta* (rhesus monkey), *Macaca radiata* (bonnet monkey), *Papio cynocephalus* (yellow baboon), *Papio papio* (guinea baboon), and *Saimiri sciureus* (squirrel monkey).

The colonies supported by the base grant include a research colony and a breeding colony. In addition, another colony of rhesus monkeys is under contract from the National Institute of Child Health and Human Development (NICHD). Neonates from this colony are used by investigators on projects approved by NICHD.

The CPRC provides safe and spacious housing for nonhuman primates that are used in research. Most animals on research trials and timed-mated breeding animals are housed indoors. Animals housed outdoors are either in half-acre field cages or in modified "corncrib" units. There is also a two-acre field cage for behavioral studies on squirrel and titi monkeys.

Over 100 local and visiting scientists use the CPRC each year. Graduate, professional, and postdoctoral students participate annually in a variety of research and training programs. There are residency programs in primate medicine and primate pathology, and a training course for animal technicians. Many foreign visitors are hosted each year for both brief and long-term studies in numerous biomedical disciplines and specialties.

The Domestic Environment

Domestic animals can be important for the study of various biomedical problems. Household pets, pet horses, farm animals, and zoo animals all present an opportunity to study naturally occurring diseases in populations that approximate human living conditions. The disadvantage of using domesticated animals is that they are not as convenient as laboratory animals nor is the environment completely under the investigator's control.

When thinking about using domestic animals one should also consider animals housed in zoos. Zoos are more frequently employing full or part-time veterinarians who have special residency training in zoo practice. The quality of care and the welfare of zoo animals has been dramatically improved during the last two decades, and the collection of zoo animals can offer opportunities to observe naturally occurring diseases that do not appear in other domestic animal populations. Medical and veterinary faculties working together can enrich the literature concerning the types of problems that occur in zoo animals and can develop new models for the study of human diseases.

Natural Environment

Animals can also be studied in their natural habitat. The advantage of this is that one has the opportunity to observe conditions that occur in the natural environment. The disadvantages include the difficulty of studying animals in this setting and that some species of wild animals can transmit serious diseases to humans.

A question may arise as to where one would go to find a natural environment these days, since most natural habitats have been severely compromised by humans. There are any number of tales told about investigators who have placed research equipment in the back country of national parks only to have it severely disturbed by hikers. One answer to this problem is the Natural Land Water Reserve System operated by the University of California, which is made available to academicians from anywhere in the world. This little-known resource, virtually unused by those of us in the health sciences, offers a unique opportunity for studying animals in their natural habitat.

THE U.C. NATURAL LAND AND WATER RESERVE SYSTEM (NLWRS). Established in 1965, the NLWRS was created to preserve a representative sample of California's rich ecological diversity before it became lost to urbanization and damaged by intensive extraction of natural resources. From an initial base of seven reserves, the NLWRS has grown to 26 (Fig. 1-1), representing 106 of the 178 major habitat types documented in California. Each reserve functions as an outdoor classroom or laboratory for teaching and research in the field-oriented natural sciences in much the same way that agricultural forestry field stations function in support of their disciplines. In a sense, the reserve system serves as an ecosystem library and an irreplaceable storehouse for biotic and genetic diversity of the state's natural habitats. In California, more than 500 species of birds can be observed, and well over 300 species breed here. There are 196 mammalian species native to the state of California, and a comparable diversity of reptiles, amphibians, and insects. This high biotic diversity affords innumerable biomedical research opportunities virtually at our doorstep. The 26 reserves of the NLWRS system support populations of a large percentage of California's mammalian biota. Of the state's 196 native species of mammals, 113 or 58 percent are found in NLWRS reserves. An additional 11 of 22 nonnative species, or 50 percent, are also present. A checklist of mammalian species for all 26 reserves is shown in Table 1-II. It should be noted that this list is incomplete, as several reserves have not had faunal surveys. Listing of a species is no indication that it is abundant on a reserve; in some cases only single sightings have been made. Indeed one of the values of the reserve system is that it offers a refuge for formally listed rare, threatened, or endangered species.

Aside from the question of abundance, the checklist is conservative concerning the simple presence of a species. Only those species with a confirmed sighting, its vocalization, or its sign are affirmatively entered in the checklist. Those species that are unconfirmed but highly probable on a reserve are indicated with a different symbol. In the absence of information needed to assess the probability of presence, certain species have been entirely deleted from a reserve listing. For example, the presence of 25 mammalian species has been confirmed at the Landis Hill Big Creek Reserve, yet museum records in previous studies indicate the past presence of 25 additional species for the surrounding area of southwestern Montery county. Populations of some of these species may be depressed due to habitat changes associated with the suppression of fires. As the Big Creek Reserve is more intensely studied and as fire is reintroduced, many of these 25 additional species may be trapped or sighted in the reserve. However, none of these 25 species have been tabulated in the checklist.

While further studies may tend to expand the list of species for each reserve, changing land use practices and associated habitat destruction adja-

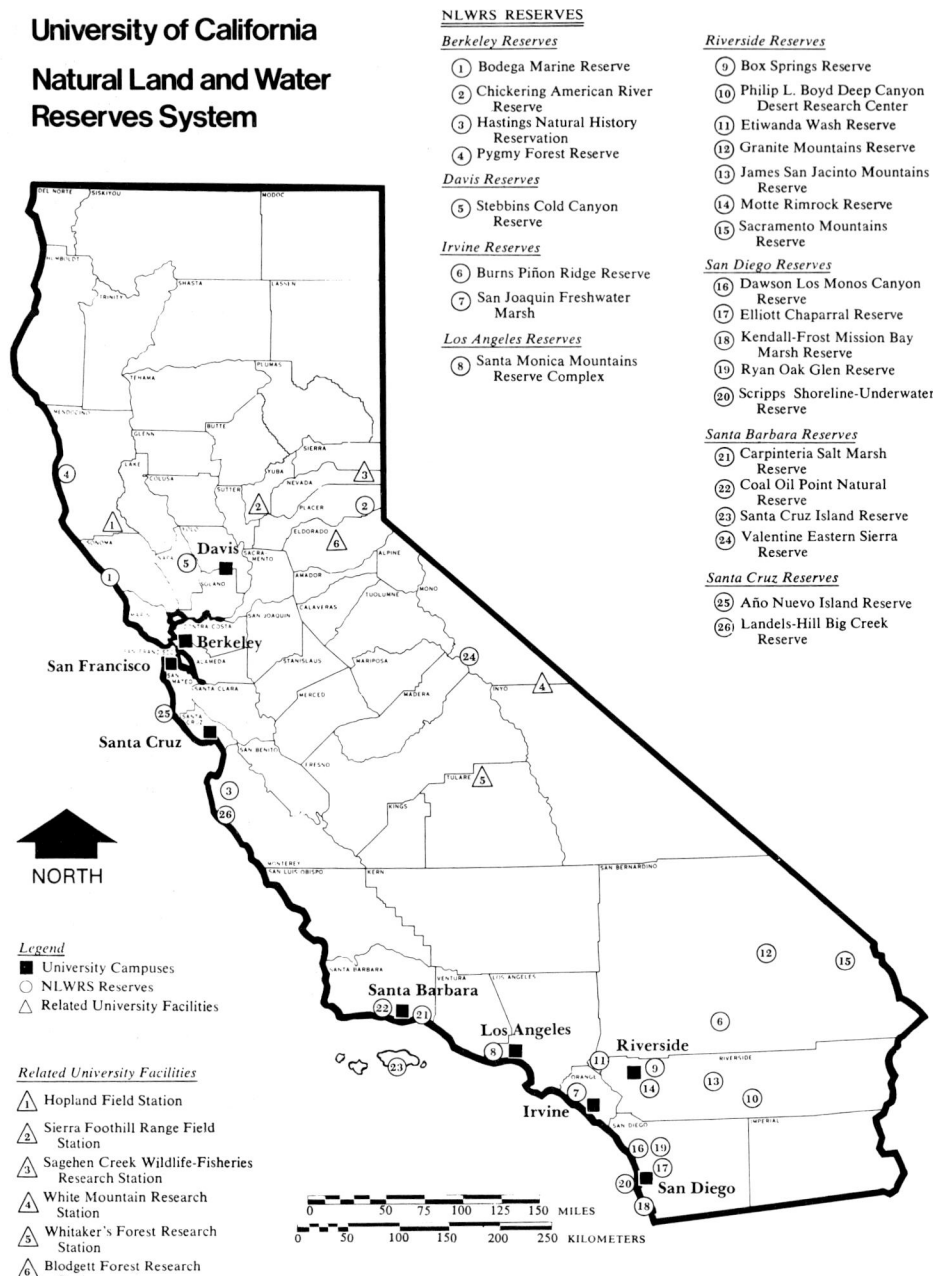

Figure 1-1. University of California Natural Land and Water Reserves System. (Copyright, Joseph S. Spinelli)

Selection of Animal Models

TABLE 1-II
A CHECKLIST OF MAMMALS FOR THE UNIVERSITY OF CALIFORNIA NATURAL LAND AND WATER RESERVE SYSTEM (MARCH 1982)

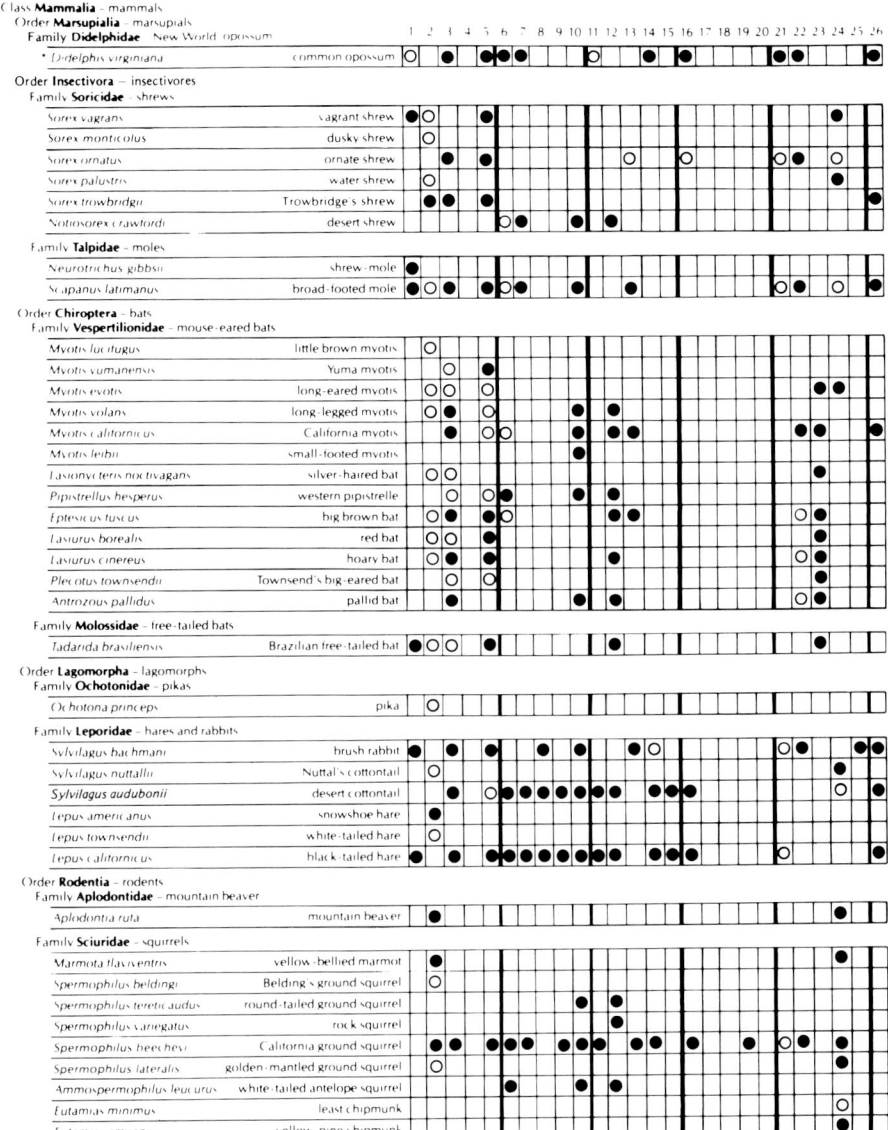

(Copyright, Joseph S. Spinelli)

TABLE 1-II (CONTINUED)

Species	Common name	1	2	3	4	5	6	7	8	9	10	11	12	13	14	15	16	17	18	19	20	21	22	23	24	25	26
Eutamias panamintinus	Panamint chipmunk											●															
Eutamias speciosus	lodgepole chipmunk	○																							●		
Eutamias senex	Allen's chipmunk	●																									
Eutamias quadrimaculatus	long-eared chipmunk	○																									
Eutamias sonomae	Sonoma chipmunk					●																					
Eutamias merriami	Merriam's chipmunk			●			●				●		●											●			●
Sciurus griseus	western gray squirrel	●	●		●						●	○	●											●			●
Tamiasciurus douglasii	Douglas' squirrel	●																						●			
Glaucomys sabrinus	northern flying squirrel	●											○														
Family Geomyidae – pocket gophers																											
Thomomys bottae	southwestern pocket gopher	●	●	●		●	●	●	●		●	●	●	●	●		○				○	○	●		○		●
Thomomys monticola	mountain pocket gopher	○																							●		
Family Heteromyidae – heteromyid rodents																											
Perognathus longimembris	little pocket mouse					●					●		●														
Perognathus inornatus	San Joaquin pocket mouse																								●		
Perognathus parvus	Great Basin pocket mouse					●																					
Perognathus formosus	long-tailed pocket mouse										●		●														
Perognathus penicillatus	desert pocket mouse										●																
Perognathus fallax	San Diego pocket mouse				●		●	○	●	●	●	●		●													
Perognathus californicus	California pocket mouse			●		●			●	●		○		○		○					●						●
Perognathus spinatus	spiny pocket mouse										●																
Dipodomys heermanni	Heermann's kangaroo rat			●																							
Dipodomys panamintinus	Panamint kangaroo rat											●													○		
Dipodomys stephensi	Stephen's kangaroo rat								○				●														
Dipodomys merriami	Merriam's kangaroo rat				●						●		●	●													
Dipodomys agilis	Pacific kangaroo rat									●	●	●		●	●	●											
Dipodomys venustus	narrow-faced kangaroo rat			●																							
Dipodomys microps	chisel-toothed kangaroo rat								○																		
Dipodomys deserti	desert kangaroo rat										●		●														
Family Cricetidae – New World mice and rats																											
Reithrodontomys megalotis	western harvest mouse	●		●			●	●			○		●								○	○	●	●	○		●
Peromyscus californicus	California mouse			●				●		●	●		●				○				○	●					●
Peromyscus crinitus	canyon mouse					●				●	●																
Peromyscus eremicus	cactus mouse					●		●		●	●		●														
Peromyscus maniculatus	deer mouse	●	●	●			●	●	●	●	●	●	●	●		●							●	●	●		
Peromyscus boylii	brush mouse	○	●		●					●	○	●	●	●								●		○			
Peromyscus truei	pinyon mouse			●		●	●			●		●	●														
Onychomys torridus	southern grasshopper mouse						●				●		●	○										○			
Neotoma lepida	desert wood rat						●	●		●	●	●	●		●	●								○			
Neotoma fuscipes	dusky-footed wood rat		●		●	●		●				●	●			●					●			●			●
Neotoma cinerea	bushy-tailed wood rat	●																						●			
Phenacomys intermedius	heather vole	○																						●			
Microtus montanus	montane vole	○																						●			
Microtus californicus	California vole	●		●		●			●	○	●	●			●	●		○				○	●				
Microtus longicaudis	Long-tailed vole	○																						●			
Lagurus curtatus	sage brush vole	●																						●			
Ondatra zibethicus	muskrat	●																									
Family Muridae – Old World mice and rats																											
Rattus norvegicus	Norway rat	●																				○	○				
Rattus rattus	black rat										○											○					
Mus musculus	house mouse	●		●		●		●	○		●	○		○		●						○	●				
Family Zapodidae – jumping mice																											
Zapus princeps	western jumping mouse	○																							●		
Family Erethizontidae – New World porcupines																											
Erethizon dorsatum	porcupine	●		●																					●		

Selection of Animal Models

TABLE 1-II (CONTINUED)

Order **Cetacea** – whales, porpoises, and dolphins
 Suborder **Odontoceti** – toothed whales
  Family **Delphinidae** – porpoises and dolphins

Species	Common name	1	2	3	4	5	6	7	8	9	10	11	12	13	14	15	16	17	18	19	20	21	22	23	24	25	26
Tursiops gilli	Pacific bottle-nosed dolphin																				●						

 Suborder **Mysticeti** – baleen whales
  Family **Eschrichtidae** – gray whales

Species	Common name	1	2	3	4	5	6	7	8	9	10	11	12	13	14	15	16	17	18	19	20	21	22	23	24	25	26
Eschrichtidus robustus	gray whale	●																						●			●

Order **Carnivora** – carnivores
 Family **Canidae** – canids

Species	Common name	1	2	3	4	5	6	7	8	9	10	11	12	13	14	15	16	17	18	19	20	21	22	23	24	25	26
Canis latrans	coyote	●	●	●		●	●	●	●	●	●	●	●	●	●	●			●		○			●		●	●
Canis familiaris	house dog			○		○		○	●			○		●		●	○	○	●		●	●	●		●		
Vulpes vulpes	red fox	●	●																								
Vulpes macrotis	kit fox								●		●																
Urocyon cinereoargenteus	gray fox	●	●	●		●	●	●	●	●	●	●	●	●			○					●					●
Urocyon littoralis	island fox																					●					

 Family **Ursidae** – bears

Species	Common name	1	2-26
Ursus americanus	black bear	●	

 Family **Procyonidae** – procyonids

Species	Common name	1	2	3	4	5	6	7	8	9	10	11	12	13	14	15	16	17	18	19	20	21	22	23	24	25	26
Bassariscus astutus	ringtail	●				●	○		○		●	○	●	○													●
Procyon lotor	raccoon	●	●	●			●	●		●	○		●				○		●		○	○					●

 Family **Mustelidae** – mustelids

Species	Common name	1	2	3	4	5	6	7	8	9	10	11	12	13	14	15	16	17	18	19	20	21	22	23	24	25	26
Martes americana	marten		○																				●				
Mustela ermina	ermine		○			○																	●				
Mustela frenata	long-tailed weasel	●	○	●			○	●	●		●	●		○	●						○	●	●				
Mustela vison	mink		○			●																					
Taxidea taxus	badger	●	○	●			●	●		○	●		●		○		○					○		●			
Spilogale gracilis	western spotted skunk			●		●	●	●	●		●	●	●	○	●		○				○		●				
Mephitis mephitis	striped skunk	●	○	●		●	○	●	●	●	●		●	●			●				○	●		●		●	●
Enhydra lutris	sea otter																							●			

 Family **Felidae** – cats

Species	Common name	1	2	3	4	5	6	7	8	9	10	11	12	13	14	15	16	17	18	19	20	21	22	23	24	25	26
Felis concolor	mountain lion	●	●	●			●			●	●	●		●	○												●
Felis domesticus	house cat					○		●		●		●		●		●	○	○	○		○	○	○		●		
Lynx rufus	bobcat		●	●		●	●	●	●	●		●	●	●		●								○		●	

 Family **Otariidae** – eared seals

Species	Common name	1	2-26
Callorhinus ursinus	northern fur seal	●	col 24: ●
Arctocephalus townsendi	Guadalupe fur seal		col 24: ●
Eumetopias jubata	northern sea lion	●	col 24: ●
Zalophus californianus	California sea lion	●	col 19: ●; col 22: ●

 Family **Phocidae** – hair seals

Species	Common name	1	others
Phoca vitulina	harbor seal	●	col 23: ●; col 24: ●
Mirounga angustirostris	northern elephant seal	●	col 23: ●; col 24: ●

Order **Perissodactyla** – odd-toed ungulates
 Family **Equidae** – horses and asses

Species	Common name	col 13
Equus asinus	wild burro	●

Order **Artiodactyla** – even-toed ungulates
 Family **Suidae** – pigs

Species	Common name	2	26
Sus scrofa	feral pig	●	●

 Family **Cervidae** – cervids

Species	Common name	1	2	3	4	5	6	7	8	9	10	11	12	13	14	15	16	17	18	19	20	21	22	23	24	25	26
Odocoileus hemionus	mule deer	●	●	●		●	●	●	●	●	●	○	●	●	●		●			●			●		●		●

 Family **Bovidae** – bovids

Species	Common name	1	2	3	4	5	6	7	8	9	10	11	12	13	14	15	16	17	18	19	20	21	22	23	24	25	26
Ovis canadensis	mountain sheep (or bighorn sheep)								●		●																
Ovis aries	domestic sheep										●											○					●
Bos taurus	domestic cattle		○										●												●		●

The numbers at the top of this table correspond to the reserve numbers shown in figure 1 on the inside of the front cover.

● – Presence confirmed by sightings, signs or vocalizations
○ – Presence unconfirmed, but highly probable
* – Species not native to California

cent to NLWRS reserves will have a tendency to reduce the numer of species present.[4-8] Rare, endangered, or threatened species are particularly susceptible to local extinction on a reserve due to land use changes that reduce available habitat. Thus for any reserve the species' composition is likely to be in a state of flux, a situation not apparent in the checklist.

A brochure describing the NLWRS, its component reserves, and information needed for permission to use a reserve is available.* Collection of animals on NLWRS reserves is by permit only, subject to reserve regulations and the approval of the reserve manager. Mammal collecting in the past has been limited primarily to live trapping for tag and release studies. Because the reserves function as a refuge for the benefit of animal species, the possibility of taking live specimens for breeding or direct laboratory use will vary depending on such factors as the size of a population on a given reserve, the status of the species, the number of specimens desired, the timing of collection, and the overall reserve policy. In other words, the welfare of the animal species will always be the first consideration in deciding whether animals can be made available from a reserve. When collecting for these purposes is not permitted on a reserve it may be possible to collect on adjacent public or private lands with the necessary permission.

Apart from NLWRS regulations, a scientific collecting permit is required "to take or possess in any part of the state, for scientific, educational, or propagation purposes, mammals, birds and the nests and eggs thereof, fish, amphibia or any other form of plant or animal life," pursuant to Section 1002 of the California Fish and Game Code and Section 650 and 652 of Title 14 of the California Administrative Code. The permits, available from the Wildlife Protection Branch of the State Department of Fish and Game, may regulate the time, number of species, number of specimens, and the collecting methods to be used. State-designated, fully protected species (pursuant to Section 4700 of the California Fish and Game Code) and all state and federal rare, threatened, and endangered species are subject to additional regulations including, in some instances, review and approval by the state Fish and Game Commission. Mammals in these two categories are shown in Tables 1-III and 1-IV. Marine mammals are also regulated by the Marine Resources Branch of the California Department of Fish and Game and the National Marine Fisheries Services.

Sources of Information on Animal Models

Various organizations can provide information on potential animal models. THE INSTITUTE OF LABORATORY ANIMAL RESOURCES. The Institute of

---

*Write to the Director, University of California Natural Land and Water Reserve System, 2111 Bancroft Way, Room 544, Berkeley, California 94618, or call (415) 642-2211.

TABLE 1-III
STATE RARE AND ENDANGERED MAMMALS

San Joaquin antelope squirrel	Rare
Mojave ground squirrel	Rare
Moro Bay kangaroo rat	Endangered
Giant kangaroo rat	Rare
Fresno kangaroo rat	Endangered
Salt marsh harvest mouse	Endangered
Amargosa vole	Endangered
Sierra Nevada red fox	Rare
San Joaquin kit fox	Rare
Wolverine	Rare
Guadalupe fur seal	Rare
California bighorn sheep	Rare
Peninsula bighorn sheep	Rare

TABLE 1-IV
STATE DESIGNATED FULLY PROTECTED MAMMALS
(PURSUANT TO SECTION 4700, CALIFORNIA FISH AND GAME CODE)

Morro Bay kangaroo rat
Salt marsh harvest mouse
Pacific right whale
Ringtail cat
Wolverine
Northern elephant seal
Guadalupe fur seal
Southern sea otter

Laboratory Animal Resources has developed an information exchange program on animal models and genetic stocks. The program goal is to establish a central agency to collect, maintain, and disseminate information on vertebrate models and genetic stocks useful for biomedical research. The objectives of the program are to inform biomedical scientists of the various animal models for research and to verify information that will assist them in identifying, selecting, and locating a particular strain of animal or model. The information accumulated within the program includes key references describing animal models, data on sources of supply, and characteristics of these animals. The data are made available without charge to interested individuals through periodic publications and in response to specific inquiries.*

THE JACKSON LABORATORY. The Jackson Laboratory maintains a subject-strain bibliography in order to make the literature on the biology of the

---

*Inquiries can be directed to: Animal Models and Genetic Stocks Information Exchange Program, Institute of Laboratory Animal Resources, National Academy of Sciences, 2101 Constitution Avenue N.W., Washington, D.C. 20418.

laboratory mouse more readily available to its scientific staff, as well as to investigators elsewhere. The bibliography includes more than 68,000 references to journals, papers, and books, mentioning specific inbred strains, named genes, or named transplanted tumors of mice. The services* are available to research workers at a fee that covers the actual cost of the search and the preparation of a list of selected references.

MEDLARS. The National Library of Medicine's computer-based Medical Literature Analysis and Retrieval System (MEDLARS) is available through a nationwide network of centers at more than 1,000 universities, medical schools, hospitals, government agencies, and commercial organizations. MEDLARS includes a variety of on-line data bases containing citations to specific articles in serials or presentations reported in congressional proceedings, references to books and serials catalogued at the National Library of Medicine, and actual chemical and toxicity data.

THE REGISTRY OF COMPARATIVE PATHOLOGY. The Registry of Comparative Pathology at the Armed Forces Institute of Pathology is intended to serve as a national center where scientists can obtain consultative assistance on questions concerning comparative pathology and information on animal models of human disease.

Basically, the principle purpose of the Registry of Comparative Pathology is to gather in one place information and material that can serve as a central resource to provide consultative assistance to scientists working in the broad field of comparative pathology. It also provides materials of interest on a wide variety of animals for research and education, and it collects and catagorizes information on animal models of human disease.†

REFERENCES

1. Kahan, B., et al: Histocompatibility and isoenzyme differences in commercially supplied "BALB/c" mice. *Science, 217*:379–381, 1982.
2. Anonymous: Genetic monitoring. *Charles River Digest, 21*(3): July 1982. (Charles River Breeding Laboratories, Inc., 251 Ballardvale Street, Wilmington, Massachusetts 01887.)
3. Cypress, R. H., and Hurvits, A. I.: In Melby, E. C., and Altman, N. H. (Eds.): *Animal Models in Handbood of Laboratory Animal Science*, Vol 2. Cleveland, CRC Press, 1974.
4. Diamond, J. M.: The island dilemma: Lesson of modern biogeographic studies for the design of natural reserves. *Biological Conservation, 7*:129–146, 1975.
5. Diamond, J. M.: In May, R. M. (Ed.): *Theoretical Ecology*, Oxford, Backwell, 1976.

---

*Requests for services should be directed to: Bibliographic Service Library, The Jackson Laboratory, Bar Harbor, Maine 04609.

†Information or assistance may be obtained from: Registrar, Registry of Comparative Pathology, American Registry of Pathology, Armed Forces Institute of Pathology, Washington, D.C. 20306.

6. Feeney-Burns, L., et al.: Ultrastructure and acid phosphatase activity in hereditary cataract of deer mice. *Invest Ophthalmol Vis Sci, 19*:777–788, 1980.
7. Schaffer, M. D.: Minimum population sizes for species conservation. *BioScience, 31*(2):121–134, 1981.
8. Terborgh, J.: Preservation of natural diversity: The problem of extinction prone species. *BioScience, 12*:715–722, 1974.

SECTION I
INFECTIOUS DISEASES

Chapter 2

THE RABBIT MODEL OF HERPETIC KERATITIS

JOHN C. MERRIAM, M.D.

Introduction

The word "herpes" is derived from a Greek verb meaning "to creep." According to Juel-Jensen and MacCallum,[1] the word has been used for at least 2,500 years to describe various "spreading lesions of the skin, such as cancer, infections like lupus vulgaris, erysipelas and ringworm, and various forms of eczema." Although the term formerly had a broader sense than today, it is possible that ulceration of the lips in intermittent fevers described in *Epidemics VI* of the Hippocratic *Corupus* was due to herpes simplex.[1] As Juel-Jensen and MacCallum point out, the imprecise use of the word continued through the middle ages and is found in the writing of Celsus and Galen.

The first accurate account in English of presumed herpes simplex of the face is credited to a Warwick physician, James Cooke, who discussed the disease *Mellificum Chirurgiae* in 1676.[1] Thereafter, authors attempted to subclassify the various manifestations of cutaneous herpes. In *Delineations of Cutaneous Diseases* (1817), Thomas Bateman recognized six different types of herpes: "H. phlyctaenodes" (zoster of the face or limbs), "H. zoster" (zoster of the trunk), "H. circinatus" (ringworm), "H. labialis," "H. praeputialis" (genital herpes), and "H. iris" (probably erythema multiforme or a fungal infection).[1] In *A Dictionary of Practical Medicine* (1890), Pringle[2] described two principal manifestations of herpes—catarrhalis and zoster. He further subdivided the former into herpes facialis and herpes genitalis; this nosology anticipated the contemporary distinction between type 1 and type 2 herpes simplex, based on a variety of biologic and chemical properties.[3]

Horner is credited with the first description of "herpes corneae febrilis" in 1871.[4] However, the clinical term "dendritic keratitis" was first defined and named by Grut and then by Emmert in 1885. Experimental work with the

---

This work was supported in part by Grants EY-07058 and EY-01597 from the National Institutes of Health, Bethesda, Maryland. Dr. Merriam is a Heed Foundation Fellow.

herpes virus began in the late nineteenth century when Vidal (1873) and Steiner (1875) showed by human inoculation that cutaneous herpes simplex was infectious.[5] In 1912 Grüter successfully inoculated the rabbit eye with material from human keratitis and vesicles of herpes labialis, thereby proving the transmissibility of herpes simplex from man to experimental animal.[6] When he published his work in 1920, Grüter also reported transmitting the agent from an infected rabbit cornea to the normal cornea of a blind man. Lowenstein[7] expanded on Grüter's work and showed that herpetic material from the genital tract as well as cutaneous infections could produce keratitis in the rabbit. Doerr and Vöchting, and others, subsequently showed that in some rabbits, keratitis was followed by encephalitis, convulsions, coma, and death.[8-10]

The Rabbit Model

These early studies demonstrated the utility of the rabbit model of herpetic keratitis, and this animal has become the standard experimental model for the disease. There is a voluminous literature on the rabbit model of herpetic keratitis, which includes investigations into natural history, pathology, immunology, medical therapy, and experimental surgery. All studies have employed one of three techniques for producing experimental herpetic keratitis.

In the early demonstrations of the transmissibility of the agent from man to rabbit, the subject cornea was lightly abraded or scarified before herpetic material was applied to the eye. Recently, investigators have attempted to use a more precisely reproducible model. A review of the literature reveals that trephines, fine needles, spatulas, and capillary tubing have been used to produce various numbers and patterns of epithelial abrasions including interlocking circles, grids, etc.[11-15] Kaufman et al.[11] used a 5 mm trephine set to a depth of 0.05 mm to produce three interlocking circles in the central cornea before applying a drop of virus suspension and rubbing the lids over the globe. Jawetz and co-workers[12] scarified the corneal epithelium with the edge of a sterile Lindner spatula to produce ten horizontal and ten vertical scratches across the diameter of the cornea before applying virus suspension. Corwin et al.[13] used a sterile 27 gauge needle to produce five horizontal and five vertical scratches in the epithelium, extending across only half the diameter of the cornea. Okumoto and associates[14] dipped a sterile platinum scraper into virus suspension prior to "crosshatching" the cornea. Jones and Al-Hussaini[14] used a sterile capillary tube containing the desired concentration of virus suspension to produce as many as two inoculation sites in each of eight meridia, and an additional one in the center of the cornea. Thus, with this technique, a single rabbit eye can be used to study the infectivity of a number of virus dilutions. Shiota, Inoue, and Yamane[15] described a modification of Jones and Al-Houssaini's technique, using a 1.0 mm capillary tube to make 25 inoculations in a single eye. A variety of modifications of the other techniques, using more, fewer, or different sizes of trephinations or scratches, are found throughout the literature. However, these techniques have two potential drawbacks: the depth of inoculation is poorly controlled, and it does not appear that inoculation of the human eye depends on abrasion of the cornea.

In 1943 Gallardo[16] showed that keratitis could be produced in the rabbit without first damaging the corneal epithelium. Inoculation of the eye with a drop of virus suspension in the lower conjunctival cul-de-sac and gentle massage of the closed eyelids routinely produced disease. Many of the preclinical studies of various antiviral agents have employed this technique.[17-24]

An accurate comparison of therapeutic and experimental studies is difficult because of the many variables in disease production. Inoculation techniques, virus strains, inoculum sizes, and the sex and type of outbred rabbit (albino, pigmented, chinchilla, etc.) may all be significant variables. The spectrum of the natural history of dendritic keratitis in the rabbit is best illustrated with specific examples. Jawetz et al.[12] inoculated white New Zealand rabbits with two strains of HSV (strains PH and W) after producing ten horizontal and vertical scratches in the cornea. The virus content of corneal epithelial cells peaked at approximately 48 hours and declined to zero by 10–12 days in both strains. Clinically, however, with strain PH, keratitis was noted by day 2, peak inflammation occurred at day 4–6 postinoculation, and the eyes healed by day 14 to 18. Fine, linear scars were seen in otherwise clear cornea at day 21. In contrast, strain W keratitis was established by day 2 and peaked at day 4–8 postinoculation. Although the acute inflammation later subsided, vascular invasion occurred in the majority of animals. A dense stromal opacity occupied the central cornea by day 16 and persisted indefinitely.

In 1973, Oh and Stevens[25] compared the clinical manifestations of infection of the nonscarified rabbit eye with eight strains of type 1 and seven strains of type 2 HSV (Fig. 2-1). In general, infection with type 1 HSV produced a slight to moderate conjunctivitis. Punctate erosions were seen by day 3 or 4, and these coalesced to a dendritic or geographic ulcer that reached peak severity by day 7 after inoculation. The lesions then began to regress and disappeared by day 14 without scarring. In some animals, a pannus was noted at day 9, although it never extended more than 3 mm from the limbus and disappeared by day 21 (Figs. 2-2, 2-3). Iritis was graded as slight to moderate in intensity and resolved completely by day 20.

The infections caused by the seven strains of HSV-2, like those caused by HSV-1, were somewhat variable (Figs. 2-1 and 2-4). In general, however, infections were not clinically apparent until day 5–12 postinoculation, notably later than the strains of HSV-1. Punctate erosions coalesced to den-

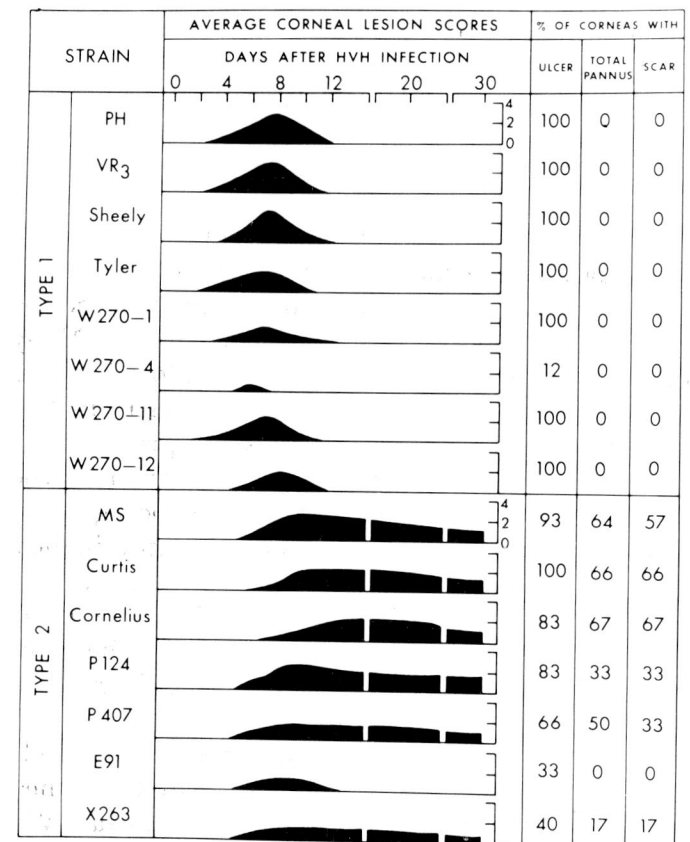

Figure 2-1. Clinical course of corneal lesions produced by 10^5 TCID$_{50}$ of types 1 and 2 HVH in rabbit eyes.

dritic or geographic ulcers, usually involving the stroma. By day 5–6 after appearance of the ulcer, more than two-thirds of the corneal surface was involved. With the exception of the infections produced by strain E91, all strains eventually produced total pannus, severe corneal opacification, and scarring. Conjunctivitis subsided by day 25, but the corneal pannus and scarring persisted for the two months of observation (Fig. 2-5).

Although inoculation with or without scarification of the corneal epithelium produces dendritic keratitis in the rabbit, neither technique reliably leads to stromal or disciform keratitis. In 1972, Sery, Nagy, and Nazario[26] described the direct inoculation of 200 herpes simpex virus particles (Strain H-4) into the central corneal stroma to produce stromal keratitis. Corneal edema began at day 6–37 (mean of 15 days), and disciform keratitis was found without a preceding dendritic keratitis in 11 of 25 cases.[27] In 1976 Metcalf et al.[28] described an alternative model of stromal keratitis. They injected into

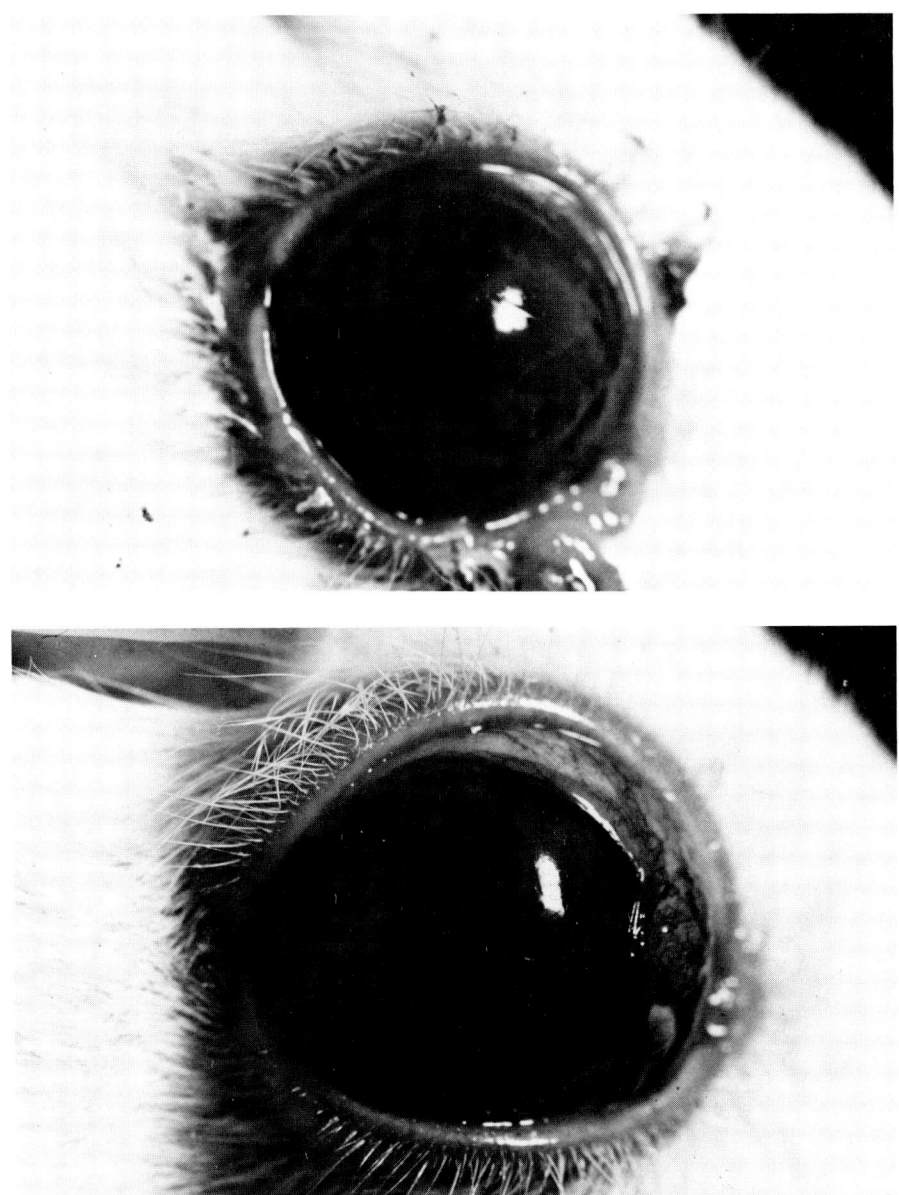

Figure 2-2. Corneal lesions produced by type 1 HVH (Sheely strain): Inoculum of 10^5 TCID$_{50}$ of virus was dropped on intact corneas of rabbit eyes. Top: Postinfection day 7; geographic corneal ulceration is evident. Bottom: Postinfection day 14; corneal ulcer disappeared completely without leaving scars. Iritis is present.

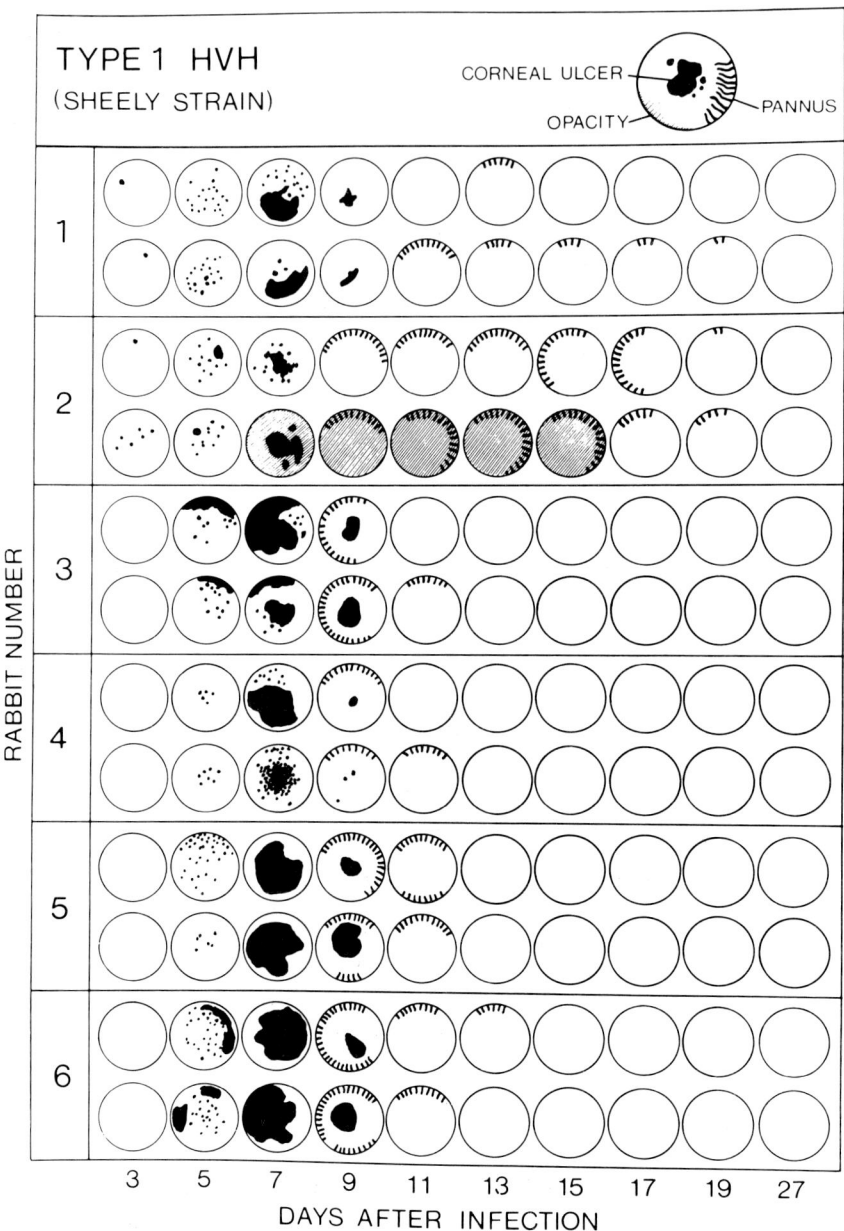

Figure 2-3. Topography of chronological changes observed in corneas infected with Sheely strain of type 1 HVH.

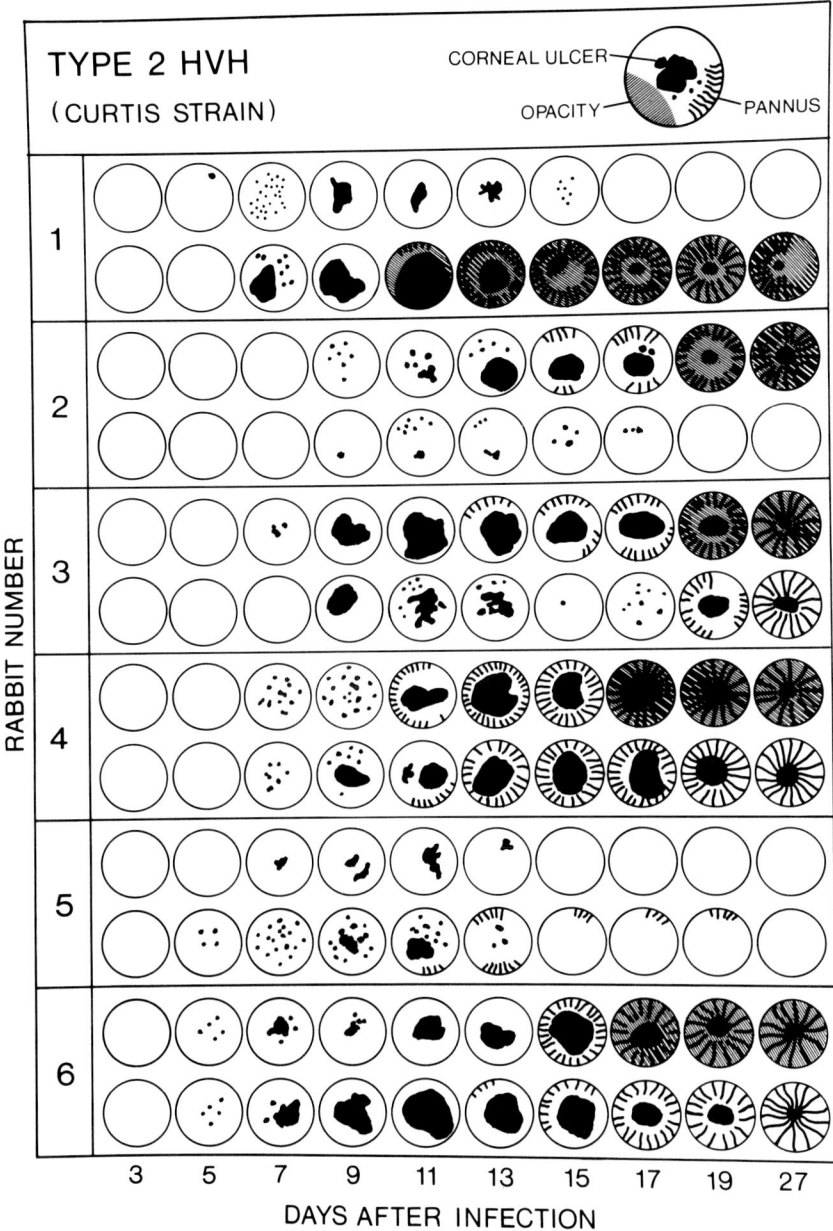

Figure 2-4. Topography of chronological changes observed in corneas infected with Curtis strain of type 2 HVH.

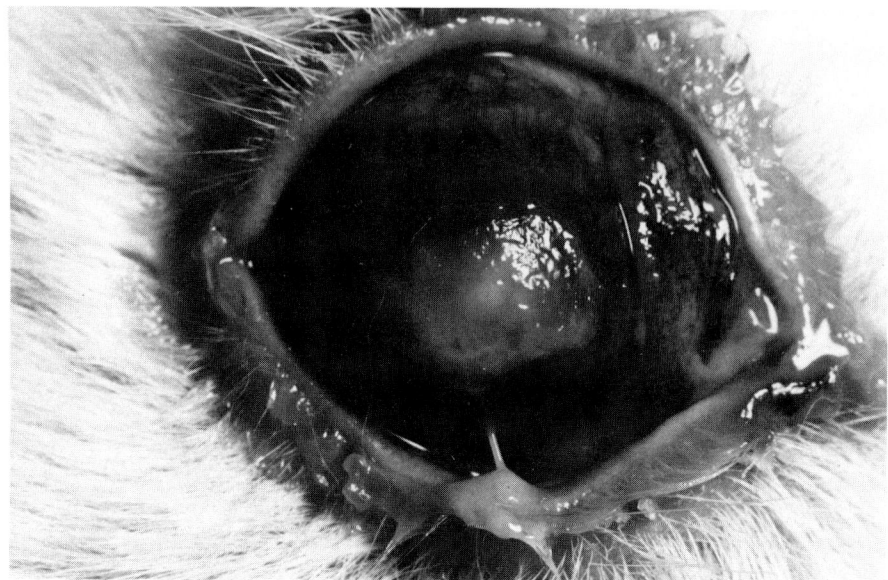

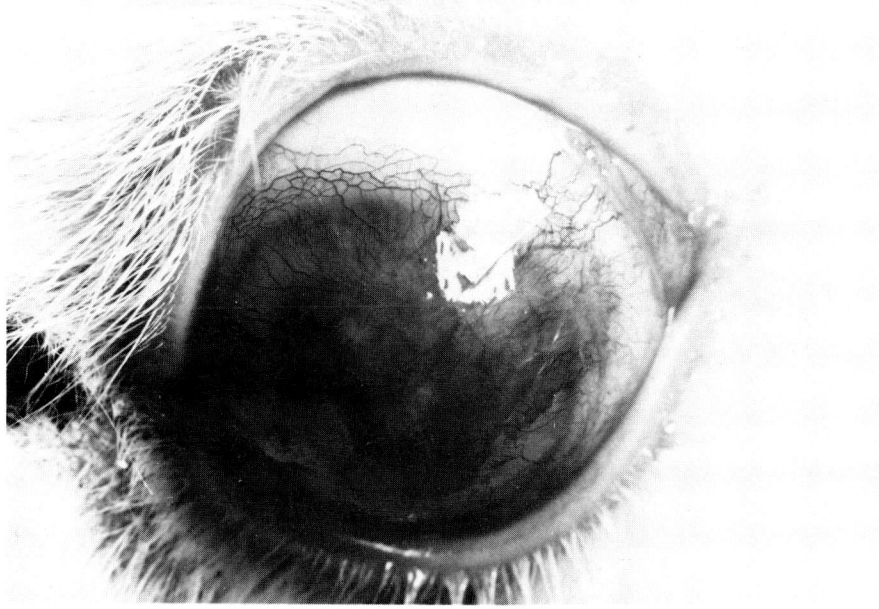

Figure 2-5. Corneal lesions produced by type 2 HVH (Curtis strain): Inoculum of 10^5 $TCID_{50}$ of virus was dropped on intact corneas of rabbit eyes. Top: Postinfection day 13; extensive corneal ulceration with pannus. Bottom: Postinfection day 60; opaque and scarred cornea with total pannus.

the central cornea 0.02 ml of a suspension of the RE strain of HSV, a strain that has a propensity to produce stromal keratitis without a fatal encephalitis.[29] The initial appearance of punctate and dendritic epithelial keratitis was followed by a "high incidence" of stromal edema, appearing 7–22 days after injection and lasting about two weeks. Approximately one-quarter of these eyes had a persistent necrotizing keratitis, resulting in permanent scarring and vascularization of the cornea.

Pathology and Immunopatholgy

Stevens and Oh[30] compared the histopathology of the keratitis produced by two strains of type 1 and type 2 *Herpesvirus hominis*. Outbred male New Zealand rabbits were inoculated in the intact cornea with virus suspensions of Sheely and VR_3 HSV-1 and Curtis and MS HSV-2. The cornea infected with type-1 HSV recovered rapidly from the initial loss of epithelium, and inflammation of the stroma was generally superficial. In contrast, infection with the two strains of HSV-2 produced persistent epithelial cell loss and deeper and more severe stromal inflammation. At the peak of the inflammatory response, the eyes infected with HSV-2 showed markedly more inflammation of the corneal endothelium, iris, and choroid than those infected with HSV-1. At other times, no strain differences were noted. The MS strain of HSV-2 was generally more virulent than the Curtis strain of HSV-2. Little difference in virulence was noted between the two strains of HSV-1. In none of the rabbit eyes was the retina or optic nerve involved.

Using female New Zealand rabbits, Hudson and colleagues[31] confirmed that HSV-2 infection (strain MS) develops more slowly than HSV-1 infection (strain P) of the cornea, and persists longer and with more inflammation.

Ultrastructural studies revealed equal synthesis of type 1 and 2 nucleocapsids in epithelial cell nuclei. However, type 2 virions appeared to degenerate within cytoplasmic vesicles or tubules. Extracellular type 2 particles were rarely seen, although abundant numbers of type 1 virions were found between cells and on the basement membrane. These observations may explain the relatively slow development of HSV-2 lesions. Light microscopy showed that HSV-2 lesions were raised, an observation that Oh and Stevens[25] made clinically. Hudson et al.[31] suggest that the appearance of HSV-2 lesions may be due to stromal swelling, but their detailed electron micrographs do not provide an explanation for the phenomenon nor the severe damage caused by HSV-2.

Immune mechanisms may be important in the pathogenesis of stromal damage. Meyers and Pettit[32,33] infected the abraded corneal epithelium of New Zealand rabbits with the W-strain of type-1 HSV. Virus proliferation in the epithelium produced no significant chemotaxis.[32] However, when the disease had progressed to stromal keratitis, significant chemotaxis was noted; HSV antigen, antiviral antibody, and complement were found in the stroma.[33]

The pathogenesis of disciform keratitis is poorly delineated. Irvine and Kimura[29] produced disciform keratitis in pigmented, outbred rabbits by applying a suspension of the RE strain of herpes virus to the abraded cornea. Total body x-radiation suppressed the host immune response without affecting the development of stromal keratitis. Endothelial cell damage appeared to correlate with the time course and severity of stromal edema, and the authors concluded that direct endothelial damage was more important than immune mechanisms.

Sery and Nagy[27] studied the cellular infiltrates induced by direct intrasomal injection of H-4 HSV. Most animals had a predominantly mononuclear cell reaction during the acute inflammation. In contrast, Meyers and Pettit[32] found a predominantly polymorphonuclear cell response after applying virus to the abraded cornea. Sery and Nagy[27] suggest that differences in protocol and experimental models may account for the discrepancy.

After the intrastromal injection of the RE strain of HSV, Metcalf et al.[28] found plasma cells and lymphocytes at the limbus, and polymorphonuclear leukocytes (PMN's), lymphocytes, and macrophages in the central cornea. Lymphocytes appeared with electron microscopy to be intimately associated with keratocytes, suggesting that cell-mediated immunity may be critical to the pathogenesis of stromal keratitis.[34] In another study, Metcalf and Helmsen[35] confirmed that HSV antigens were found in association with the surface of keratocytes at the time of necrotizing keratitis, when active viral replication could be demonstrated. When keratitis was limited to the epithelium, where active viral replication could be demonstrated, HSV antigen was found in the nuclei, on nuclear membranes, and on cell surface membranes of epithelial cell.[35]

In an elegant study of the time course of stromal keratitis after intracorneal injection of RE strain HSV, Metcalf and Reichert[36] found that cultures of the whole cornea were positive for HSV for two weeks after injections. Lymphocytes and plasma cells accumulated at the limbus, suggesting that in this model the limbus may behave as a lymphoid tissue for the development of immunocompetence. Neovascularization was associated temporally with the infiltration of inflammatory cells, predominantly PMN's with some lymphocytes and macrophages. Lymphocytes often were intimately associated with abnormal keratocytes. The authors contend that this observation, as well as other experimental work,[37] indicates that a T-cell attack on target keratocytes contributes to necrotizing keratitis and scarring.

Some studies suggest that other mechanisms also may affect the pathogenesis of stromal keratitis. Meyers-Elliott and Chitjian[38] showed that PMN depletion in male New Zealand rabbits drastically reduced the incidence of stromal infiltrates and injury after topical inoculation of the cornea with W-strain HSV-1. Similarly, depletion of the third component of complement, which is chemotactic for neutrophils, prevented stromal keratitis. The relative importance of humoral immunity and the modulating effect of antiviral antibodies on the cellular immune response are controversial.[39] The role of various lymphokines, migration inhibition factor, interferon, natural killer cells, and the mechanisms of latency and reactivation are other aspects of the pathogenesis of herpetic keratitis that are only beginning to be understood.[40]

In all the rabbit models described above, the persistence of stromal edema occurred in the apparent absence of actively replicating virus. This observation appears to support the concept that disciform keratitis is a hypersensitivity phenomenon rather than an active infection and to explain the fact that human disciform keratitis responds to topical steroids.[41] However, herpes virus has been found in the corneal stroma of rabbits experimentally infected with the PH strain of HSV;[42] herpes virus has been found in the corneal stroma of patients undergoing keratoplasty for chronic herpetic keratitis.[43] These discoveries bring into question the exact relation of the rabbit model of stromal keratitis to human disease.

Herpetic keratitis is easy to produce in the rabbit, and the rabbit eye is easy to examine. These characteristics have made the rabbit model the most popular system for the assessment of antiviral medications,[17-24,44-50] and other anti-inflammatory agents.[51] However, it has been long appreciated that the rabbit is far more sensitive to the herpes virus than man,[8-10] and investigators have generally used virus strains that were less likely to produce encephalitis to minimize loss of experimental animals. This difference between the disease in the animal and in man demonstrates that the rabbit model is an imperfect paradigm of human keratitis. As the immune response of the rabbit and man differ significantly,[52] the use of the rabbit to evaluate therapies that depend on stimulation of the host, such as interferon,[53-58] vitamin A,[59] and vaccination,[60] is particularly problematic.

Other animal models are available.[61-65] However, inbred strains of mice and rats that are immunologically well-defined may be most useful in studying the various components of the inflammatory response in the eye.[66-69]

The observation that different strains of herpes differ in virulence is not new[52] but has begun to attract renewed interest.[70] Using outbred New Zealand rabbits, Centifanto-Fitzgerald and associates demonstrated that the transfer of genetic information from a virus causing stromal disease to the genome of a virus causing epithelial disease resulted in recombinant viruses with one or more of the characteristics of the donor virus.[71] The authors suggest that the genetic properties of the infecting strain may be as important as, or perhaps more important than, host factors to the disease pattern. The elucidation of the roles of the virus genome and host defenses will require that genetically constant and immunologically defined animal models be used.

REFERENCES

1. Juel-Jensen, B. D., and MacCallum, F. O.: In *Herpes Simplex, Varicella, and Zoster.* J. B. Lippincott Co., Philadelphia, 1972.
2. Pringle, J. J.: Herpes. In J. K. Fowler (Ed.): *A Dictionary of Practical Medicine.* London, 1890, p. 344.
3. Lowrey, S. P., Melnick, J. L., and Rawls, W. E.: Biological markers for herpes viruses type 1 and 2. *J Gen Virol, 10*:1, 1971.
4. MacNab, A.: *Ulceration of the Cornea.* Baitliere, Tindall, and Cox, London, 1907, pp. 162–165.
5. Thygeson, P.: Historical observations on herpetic keratitis. *Surv Ophthalmol, 21*:82–90, 1976.
6. Grüter, W.: Experimentelle und Klinische Untersuchungen über den sogenannten Herpes Coreae. *Ber Dtsch Ophthalmol Ges, 42*:162–167, 1920.
7. Löwenstein, A.: Ätiologie Untersuchungen über den fieberhaften. *Munch Med Wochenschr, 66*:769, 1919.
8. Doerr, R., and Vöchting, K.: Études sur le virus de l'herpès fébrile. *Rev Gen Ophtal* (Paris), *34*:409–421, 1920.
9. Blanc, G., and Caminopteros, J.: Recherches expérimentales sur herpès. *Compt Rend de la Soc de Biol, 84*:629–630, 1921.
10. Levaditi, C., Harvier, P., and Nicolau, S.: Sur la présence dans la salive des *sujets* sains, d'un virus produisant la kérato-conjonctivite et l'encéphalite, chez le lapin. *Compt Rend de la Soc de Biol, 84*:817–818, 1921.
11. Kaufman, H. E., Nesburn, A. B., and Maloney, E. D.: IDU therapy of herpes simplex. *Arch Ophthalmol 67*:583–591, 1962.
12. Jawetz, E. et al: Studies on herpes simplex XI. The antiviral dynamics of 5-iodo-2-deoxyuridine *in vivo. J Immunol, 95*:635–642, 1965.
13. Corwin, M. E., et al: A double-blind study of the effect of 5-iodo-2-deoxyurdine on experimental herpes simplex keratitis. *Am J Ophthalmol, 55*:225–229, 1963.
14. Jones, B. R., and Al-Hussaini, M. K.: Therapeutic considerations in ocular vaccinia. *Trans Ophthal Soc UK, 83*:613–631, 1963.
15. Shiota, H., Inoue, S., and Yamane, S.: Efficacy of acycloguanosine against herpetic ulcers in rabbit cornea. *Br J Ophthalmol, 63*:425–428, 1979.
16. Gallardo, E.: Primary herpes simplex keratitis: clinical and experimental study. *Arch Ophthalmol, 30*:217–220, 1943.
17. Hettinger, M. E., et al: Ac_2IDU, BVDU, and thymine arabinoside therapy in experimental herpes keratitis. *Arch Ophthalmol, 99*:1618–1621.
18. Trousdale, M.D., et al: Evaluation of the antiherpetic activity of 21-fluoro-5-iodo-ara-C in rabbit eyes and cell cultures. *Invest Ophthalmol Vis Sci, 21*:826–832, 1981.
19. Trousdale, M. D., Nesburn, A. B., and Miller, C. A.: Assessment of acyclovir on acute ocular infection induced by drug-resistant strains of HSV-1. *Invest Ophthalmol Vis Sci, 20*:230–235, 1981.
20. Trousdale, M. D., Dunkel, E. C., and Nesburn, A. B.: Effect of acyclovir on acute and latent herpes simplex virus infections in the rabbit. *Invest Ophthalmol Vis Sci, 19*:1336–1341, 1980.

21. Pavan-Langston, D., Lass, J., and Campbell, R.: Antiviral drops: comparative therapy of experimental herpes simplex keratouveitis. *Arch Ophthalmol,* 97:1132–1135, 1979.
22. Pavan-Langston, D., Campbell, R., and Lass, J.: Acyclic antimetabolite therapy of experimental herpes simplex keratitis. *Am J Ophthalmol,* 86:618–623, 1978.
23. Pavan-Langston, D., North, R. D., and Geary, P. A.: ARA–AMP—Highly soluble new antiviral drug. *Ann Ophthalmol,* 8:571–579, 1976.
24. Lanier, J. D. et al: Proflavine and light in the treatment of experimental herpetic ocular infections. *Antimicrob Agents Chemother,* 6:613–619, 1974.
25. Oh, J. O., and Stevens, T. R.: Comparison of types 1 and 2 *Herpesvirus hominis* infection of rabbit eyes. I. Clinical manifestations. *Arch Ophthalmol,* 90:473–476, 1973.
26. Sery, T. W., Nagy, R. M., and Nazario, R.: Experimental disciform keratitis. 2. Local corneal hypersensitivity to a highly virulent strain of herpes simplex. *Ophthalmol Res,* 4:99, 1972.
27. Sery, T. W., and Nagy, R. M.: Cellular reaction in experimental herpetic disciform keratitis. *Am J Ophthalmol,* 84:675–680, 1977.
28. Metcalf, J. F., McNeill, J. I., and Kaufman, H. E.: Experimental disciform edema and necrotizing keratitis in the rabbit. *Invest Ophthalmol Vis Sci,* 15:979–985, 1976.
29. Irvine, A. R., and Kimura, S. J.: Experimental stromal herpes simplex keratitis in the rabbit. *Arch Ophthalmol,* 78:654–663, 1967.
30. Stevens, T. R., and Oh, J. O.: Comparison of types 1 and 2 *Herpesvirus hominis* infection of rabbit eyes. II. Histopathologic and virologic studies. *Arch Ophthalmol,* 90:477–480, 1973.
31. Hudson, J. B., Hollenberg, M. J., Wilkie, J. S., and Lewis, B. J.: Ultrastructural study of lesions induced in rabbit cornea by herpes simplex virus types 1 and 2. *J Infectious Dis,* 133:367–381.
32. Meyers, R. L., and Pettit, T. H.: Chemotaxis of polymorphonuclear leukocytes in corneal inflammation: Tissue injury in herpes simplex virus infection. *Invest Ophthalmol,* 13:187–197, 1974.
33. Meyers, R. L., and Pettit, T. H.: The pathogenesis of corneal inflammation due to herpes simplex virus. I. Corneal hypersensitivity in the rabbit. *J Immunol,* 111:1031–1042, 1973.
34. Metcalf, J. F., and Kaufman, H. E.: Herpetic stromal keratitis—evidence for cell-mediated immunopathogenesis. *Am J Ophthalmol,* 82:827–834, 1976.
35. Metcalf, J. F., and Helmsen, R.: Immunoelectron microscopic localization of herpes simplex virus antigens in rabbit cornea with antihuman IgG-antiferritin hybrid antibodies. *Invest Ophthalmol Vis Sci,* 16:779–786, 1977.
36. Metcalf, J. F., and Reichert, R. W.: Histological and electron microscopic studies of experimental herpetic keratitis in the rabbit. *Invest Ophthalmol Vis Sci,* 18:1123–1138, 1979.
37. Polack, F., Siverio, C., Bigar, F., and Centifanto, Y.: Immune host response to corneal grafts sensitized to herpes simplex virus. *Invest Ophthalmol,* 15:188–195, 1976.
38. Meyers-Elliott, R. H., and Chitjian, P. A.: Immunopathogenesis of corneal inflammation in herpes simplex virus stromal keratitis: role of the polymorphonuclear leukocyte. *Invest Ophthalmol Vis Sci,* 20:784–798, 1981.
39. Meyers-Elliott, R. H., and Chitjian, P. A.: Induction of cell-mediated immunity in herpes simplex virus keratitis: kinetics of lymphocyte transformation and the effect of antiviral antibody. *Invest Ophthalmol Vis Sci,* 19:920–929, 1980.
40. Nesburn, A. B.: Immunological aspects of ocular herpes simplex disease. In Suran, A., Gery, I., and Nussenblatt, R. B. (Eds.): Immunology of the Eye; Workshop III. *Immunology Abstracts,* sp. supp. pp. 21–42, 1981.
41. Pavan-Langston, D.: Diagnosis and management of herpes simplex ocular infection. *Int Ophthalmol Clin,* 15:19, 1975.

42. Tanaka, N., and Kimura, S.: Localization of herpes simplex antigen and virus. *Arch Ophthalmol*, 78:68–73, 1967.
43. Carter, C. A., Easty, D. L., and Walker, J. R.: Experimental ulcerative herpetic keratitis. II. Influence of topical corticosteroid in immunized rabbits. *Br J Ophthalmol*, 65:388–396, 1981.
44. Lass, J. H., et al.: Treatment of experimental herpetic interstitial keratitis with medroxyprogesterone. *Arch Ophthalmol*, 98:520–527, 1981.
45. Robbins, R. M., and Galin, M. A.: A model for steroid effects in herpetic keratitis. *Arch Ophthalmol*, 93:828–830, 1975.
46. Easterbrook, M., et al.: The effect of topical corticosteroids on the susceptibility of immune animals to reinoculations with herpes simplex. *Invest Ophthalmol*, 12:181–184, 1973.
47. Kimura, S. J., et al: The effect of corticosteroid hormones on experimental herpes simplex keratitis. *Am J Ophthalmol*, 51:945–948, 1961.
48. Kaufman, H. E., and Maloney, E. D.: Experimental herpes simplex keratitis: The effect of corticosteroids and epithelial curettage. *Arch Ophthalmol*, 66:125–128, 1961.
49. Jawetz, E., Okumoto, M., and Soune, M.: Studies on herpes simplex X. The effect of corticosteroids on herpetic keratitis in the rabbit. *J Immunol*, 83:486–490, 1959.
50. Trousdale, M. D., Dunkel, E. C., and Nesburn, A. B.: Effect of flurbiprofen on herpes simplex keratitis in rabbits. *Invest Ophthalmol Vis Sci*, 19:267–270, 1980.
51. Smolin, G., et al: Natural and cloned human leukocyte interferon in herpesvirus infections of rabbit eyes. *Arch Ophthalmol*, 100:481–483, 1982.
52. Jawetz, E., Coleman, V. R., and Merrill, E. R.: Studies on herpes simplex virus. VII. Immunological comparison of strains of herpes simplex. *J Immunol*, 75:28–34, 1955.
53. Kaufman, H. E., Ellison, E. D., and Centifanto, Y. M.: Difference in interferon response and protection from ocular virus infection in rabbits and monkeys. *Am J Ophthalmol*, 74:89–92, 1972.
54. Centifanto, Y. M., Goorha, R. M., and Kaufman, H. E.: Interferon induction in rabbit and human tears. *Am J Ophthalmol*, 70:1006–1009, 1970.
55. Kaufman, H. E., Ellison, E. D., and Waltman, S. R.: Double-stranded RNA, an interferon inducer, in herpes simplex keratitis. *Am J Ophthalmol*, 68:486–491, 1969.
56. Park, J. H., et al: Prophylaxis of herpetic keratoconjunctivitis with interferon inducers. *Arch Ophthalmol*, 81:840–842, 1969.
57. Tommila, V.: Treatment of dendritic keratitis with interferon. *Acta Ophthal*, 41:478–482, 1963.
58. Starr, M. B.: Vitamin A in experimental herpetic keratitis. *Arch Ophthalmol*, 99:322–326, 1981.
59. Carter, C. A., et al: Experimental ulcerative herpetic keratitis. IV. Preliminary observations on the efficacy of herpes simplex subunit vaccine. *Br J Ophthalmol*, 65:679–682, 1981.
60. Tabbara, K. F., Okumoto, M., and Smolin, G.: Experimental herpetic keratitis in the guinea pig. *Can J Ophthalmol*, 9:363–366, 1974.
61. Meyers, R. L., and Pettit, T. H.: Corneal immune response to herpes simplex virus antigens. *J Immunol*, 110:1575–1590, 1973.
62. Schardein, J. L., and Sidwell, R. W.: Antiviral activity of 9-B–D-arabinofuranosyladenine. III. Reduction in evidence of encephalitis in treated herpes simplex-infected hamsters. *Antimicrob Agents Chemother*, 155–160, 1968.
63. Sidwell, R.W., et al.: Antiviral activity of 9-B-D-arabinofuranosyladenine. II. Activity against herpes simplex keratitis in hamsters. *Antimicrob Agents Chemother*, 11:148–154, 1968.

64. Harper, I. A., and Sommerville, R. G.: Herpetic keratitis produced in the guinea pig by a new, standardized technique. *Arch Ophthalmol,* 73:552–554, 1965.
65. Allansmith, M., and Prendergast, R.: Task Group I recommendations. In Suran, A., Gery, I., and Nussenblatt, R. B. (Eds.): Immunology of the Eye; Workshop III. *Immunology Abstracts,* sp. supp. pp. 505–508, 1981.
66. O'Day, D., and Franklin, R.: Task Group III Recommendations. In Suran, A., Gery, I., and Nussenblatt, R. B. (Eds.): Immunology of the Eye. Workshop III, *Immunology Abstracts,* sp. supp. pp. 509–513, 1981.
67. Oakes, J. E., and Lausch, R. N.: Role of Fc fragments in antibody-mediated recovery from ocular and subcutaneous herpes simplex virus infections. *Infec Immun,* 33:109–113, 1981.
68. Metcalf, J. F., Hamilton, D. S., and Reichert, R. W.: Herpetic keratitis in athymic (nude) mice. *Infect Immun,* 26:1164–1171, 1979.
69. Thygeson, P.: Viruses and virus disease of the eye. II. Viruses of ocular importance. *Arch Ophthalmol,* 29:488–508, 1943.
70. Wander, A. H., Centifanto, Y. M., and Kaufman, H. E.: Strain specificity of clinical isolates of herpes simplex virus. *Arch Ophthalmol* 98:1458–1461, 1980.
71. Centifanto-Fitzgerald, Y. M., et al: Ocular disease pattern induced by herpes simplex virus is genetically determined by a specific region of viral DNA. *J Exp Med,* 155:475–489, 1982.

Chapter 3

HERPES SIMPLEX RETINOCHOROIDITIS IN NEWBORN RABBITS

JANG O. OH, M.D., PH.D.

Introduction

Ever since Batignani[1] reported the first case of neonatal infection with herpes simplex virus (HSV) in 1934, neonatal HSV infection has been recognized with increasing frequency. Over 90 percent of isolates recovered from infections of newborns are type 2-HSV.[2] Ocular manifestations of neonatal HSV infection (conjunctivitis, keratitis, chorioretinitis, optic neuritis, cataract, uveitis, and microphthalmia) occur in about 10 percent of neonates with disseminated infection and in 33 percent of those with localized infection.[3]

Herpetic chorioretinitis in newborn infants has been associated exclusively with type 2 HSV. As Table 3-I shows, 27 patients have been described with chorioretinitis as a manifestation of neonatal herpetic infections, and when HSV isolates from 17 cases were typed, all were found to be type 2 HSV.[4-20] The dermatotropic nature of type 2 HSV has been thought to be partly responsible for this unique association of type 2 HSV with chorioretinitis,[21,22] but the pathogenic mechanisms by which the internal ocular structure becomes affected remain unclear.

Experimental animal models are invaluable tools for the study of pathogenic mechanisms of any disease, yet almost no attempt to construct animal models of neonatal herpetic chorioretinitis have been made.[23] Recently we have successfully produced retinochoroiditis in the newborn rabbit eye by using type 2 HSV to infect the animal's skin, a natural portal of entry for the virus in the newborn.[24] In this paper we describe the model and the various lesions produced by type 2 HSV in the newborn rabbit.

Supported in part by NIH research grants EY-00964 and EY-01578. Drs. Dean Brick, Steven E. Sicher and Robert Friedlaender collaborated in this study. Mr. Petros Minasi and Mrs. Marcella Kopal provided excellent technical assistance.

TABLE 3-I
REPORTED CASES OF NEONATAL HERPETIC CHORIORETINITIS

Authors	Year	No. of cases	HSV type
Smith et al. (4)*	1941	1	NT
Florman et al. (5)	1952	2	NT
Mitchell et al. (6)	1963	1	NT
Cogan et al. (7)	1964	1	NT
Yen et al. (8)	1965	1	NT
Bahrani et al. (9)	1966	1	NT
Golden et al. (10)	1969	1	NT
Hagler et al. (11)	1969	2	HSV-2
Cibis et al. (12)	1971	1	HSV-2
Pettay et al. (13)	1972	1	NT
Cibis (14)	1975	1	HSV-2
Nahmias et al. (15)	1976	6	HSV-2
Yanoff et al. (16)	1977	1	HSV-2
Tarkkanen et al. (17)	1977	4	HSV-2
Chalhub et al. (18)	1977	1	HSV-2
Cibis et al. (19)	1978	1	NT
Mousel et al. (20)	1979	1	HSV-2
Total		27	17

NT: not typed *( ): Reference number

Reproduced by permission. From J. O. Oh and P. Minasi, In R. Sundmacher (Ed.), *Herpetic Eye Diseases*, 1981. Courtesy of J. F. Bergmann Verlag, Munchen.

MATERIALS AND METHODS

Newborn rabbits

New Zealand white rabbits were acquired at midterm pregnancy from a local commercial vendor. Each rabbit was placed in a separate cage with a breeding box. We used newborn rabbits between 17 and 34 hours old.

Virus

The Curtis strain of type 2 HSV was grown in primary cultures of rabbit kidney cells maintained in a medium consisting of 95% Medium 199, 5% rabbit serum, and antibiotics. The final titer of the virus preparation was 10^5 50% tissue culture infectious doses ($TCID_{50}$) per ml.

Virus Inoculation of the Skin

Using a 26-gauge hypodermic needle attached to a tuberculin syringe, we injected 0.05 ml of virus suspension (containing 10^3 $TCID_{50}$ of HSV) into each of two skin sites on the back of the newborn rabbits, one on each side of the midline, subcutaneously.

Collection of Blood and Tissue Specimens for Virus Assay and Histopathology

The rabbits were killed by intraperitoneal injection of sodium phenobarbital, and the visceral organs were exposed by an aseptic technique. For the virus isolation attempt, 2 ml of cardiac blood was collected immediately from each rabbit in a syringe containing 10 units of heparin. Various organs (heart, lungs, thymus, liver spleen, kidneys, adrenal glands, skin, brain, and eyes) were then removed aseptically, and a piece of each organ (except one whole eye and one whole adrenal gland of each rabbit) was fixed in Bouin's fixative for histopathologic study. The remaining tissues, including the second adrenal gland and the second eye of each rabbit, were frozen at $-60°C$ until used for virus isolation.

Virus Isolation from Cardiac Blood

We added an equal volume of sterile physiological saline to the heparinized blood and separated the leukocytes in Ficoll-Hypaque gradient as described by Boyum.[25] The separated leukocytes were washed three times in 3 ml of phosphate buffered saline (PBS) at pH 7.3 and inoculated into two tubes of Vero cells. We also collected plasma layer and inoculated 0.5 ml of it into each of two tubes of Vero cells for virus isolation. The tubes were incubated in a stationary position at 36°C, and the culture medium was completely changed one day later. We examined the cells for cytopathic effects (CPE) daily for seven days. The virus isolates were identified as HSV by a neutralization test using anti-HSV-2 rabbit serum.

Virus Isolation from Tissues

We ground a 1 cc piece of each tissue with a mortar and pestle, adding 1 ml of crystalline alumina (90 mesh to facilitate the grinding). Tissue homogenate, prepared by adding 2 ml of a medium consisting of 95% Eagle's minimum essential medium, 5% fetal calf serum, and antibiotics, was centrifuged at 800 G for ten minutes at 4°C. The supernatant fluid was considered to be a 10^{-1} dilution of the specimen, and serial tenfold dilutions were made with the medium. We then inoculated Vero cell tubes with 1 ml of each dilution, incubated the tubes in a stationary position at 36°C, and examined them for CPE daily for seven days. The reciprocal of the highest dilution showing CPE was considered to be the infectivity titer of the tissue homogenate per ml.

Histopathologic Studies

All tissues fixed in Bouin's fixative were processed and embedded in paraffin, and 5 micron sections, stained with hemotoxylin and eosin, were examined microscopically.

Measurement of Skin Lesions

The lesions produced by the subcutaneous injection of HSV were examined daily, and their diameters were measured in millimeters. To calculate the average size of the lesions produced on a given day, we divided the sum of the diameters of all the lesions on all of the rabbits on that day by the total number of skin sites injected.

RESULTS

Production of Skin Lesions

One day after subcutaneous injection of type 2 HSV (10^3 TCID$_{50}$), the skin showed slightly elevated erythematous lesions 2–3 mm in diameter at the injection sites. The lesions steadily increased in size and became vesicles by day 3 (Fig. 3-1a). On day 4, their size reached 11 mm, and crust was formed at the center of most of the lesions (Fig. 3-1b). On postinfection day 4, all the animals showed signs of systemic illness, including lethargy, irritability, restlessness, and hindleg paralysis; they had seizures and ate poorly, and all died by day 5.

When we examined the histopathology of the acute lesions on day 4, there were extensive, acute inflammatory reactions throughout the entire thickness of the skin and scattered foci of necrosis (Fig. 3-2). The infiltration of polymorphonuclear leukocytes was minimal, however. The epidermis was eroded over the area of necrosis, and the epithelium adjacent to the erosions contained multinucleated giant cells and typical Cowdry type A intranuclear inclusions.

Dissemination of HSV from Skin to Visceral Organs and Eyes

Gross autopsy showed signs of disseminated virus infection. Most of the lesions, which appeared as early as postinoculation day 3, occurred in livers (Fig. 3-3) and spleens. The adrenal glands showed microscopic foci of necrosis and hemorrhage in both cortex and medulla. Pneumonitis, myocarditis, and hemorrhagic nephritis also occurred in some animals. Perivascular cuffing and encephalitis were present in the brain. Typical Cowdry type A intranuclear inclusions were found in the liver, spleen, adrenal gland, and the skin.

In the eye, full-thickness retinal folds (Fig. 3-4a) with occasional focal necrosis (Fig. 3-4b) were observed in about 40 percent of the rabbits killed on postinoculation day 5. Strong fluorescence was observed at the retinal lesions at an entire layer of the retina when it was treated with fluorescein-labelled anti-HSV antiserum. In only a few cases did we see iritis (Fig. 3-5) or choroidal involvement, and only a minimal inflammatory reaction was associated with either of these changes.

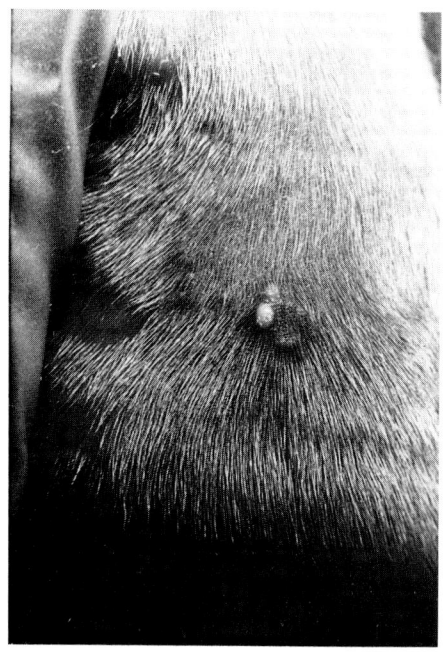 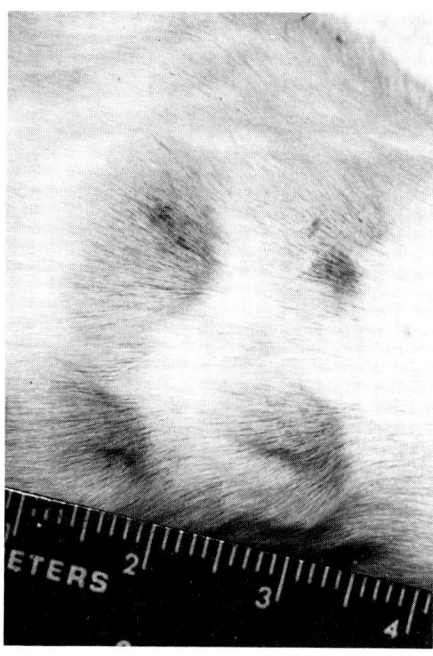

Figure 3-1. Skin lesions produced by type 2 HSV in newborn rabbits.
a. Vesicular lesions (Reproduced by permission. From D. C. Brick, J. O. Oh, and S. E. Sicher, *Invest Ophthalmol Vis Sci, 21*:681–688, 1981.)
b. Large indurated lesions with crust (Reproduced by permission. From J. O. Oh and P. Minasi, *Infect Immun, 27*:168–174, 1980. Courtesy American Society for Microbiology, Washington, D.C.)

Virologic Studies of Visceral Organs and Eyes

Infectious HSV could be recovered only from skin on postinoculation day 1; on day 2 it could be recovered from the skin in high titer (10^3 to 10^4 $TCID_{50}$) and from the lungs in low titers (Fig. 3-6); on or after day 3, the virus could be recovered in high titers from many organs. HSV could first be isolated from the eyes on day 4 and was present in one-third of the eyes cultured on either day 4 or day 5. Titers of the virus in the eyes ranged from 10^2 to 10^3 $TCID_{50}$.

Isolation of HSV from Blood

Infectious HSV could not be recovered from the blood before day 3 (Table 3-II). It could be found in the blood of 38 percent of the rabbits on day 3, 44 percent on day 4, and as many as 78 percent on day 5.

On day 3, HSV could be isolated from the mononuclear fraction of the blood of two rabbits and from the mononuclear and plasma fractions of one rabbit. On days 4 and 5, however, it could be recovered more often from both

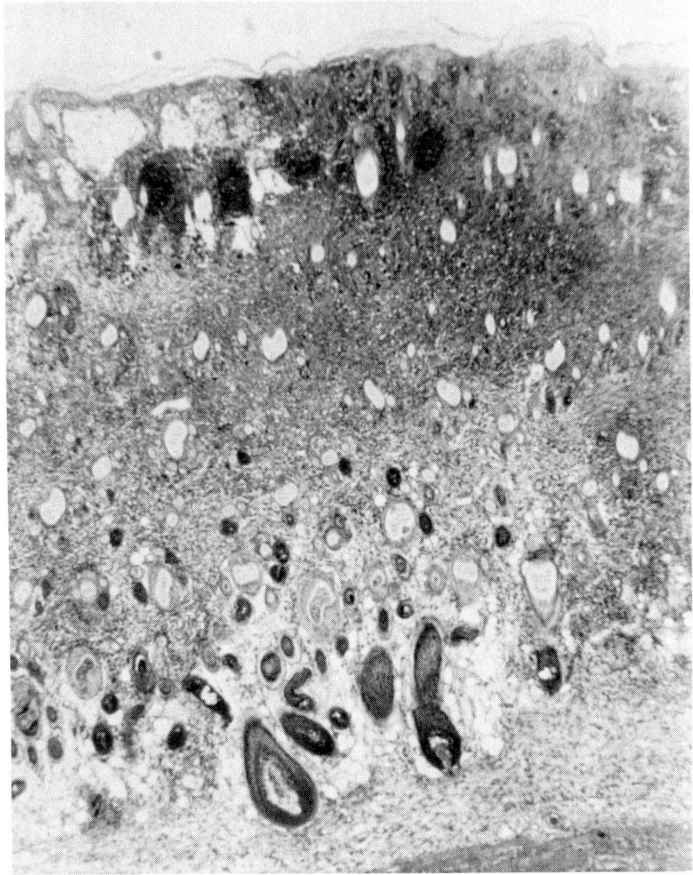

Figure 3-2. Histopathology of skin lesions produced by type 2 HSV. (Hematoxylin and eosin, ×300). Severe inflammation affects entire layer of skin, which is thickened and edematous. Note complete denudation of epithelium and foci of necrosis.

mononuclear cells and plasma. Overall, the virus was isolated from mononuclear cells in five rabbits, only plasma in one rabbit, and both mononuclear cells and plasma in eight rabbits.

Isolation of HSV from Sensory Ganglia

During its early stages, skin infection with type 2 HSV was accompanied by corresponding sensory ganglion infection. Table 3-III shows infectious HSV could be isolated from the homogenate of the cervicothoracic ganglia of seven of eight rabbits as early as day 2 after the skin inoculation and from the same ganglia of almost all the rabbits thereafter (days 3 and 4). The trigeminal ganglia were free of the infection during this period.

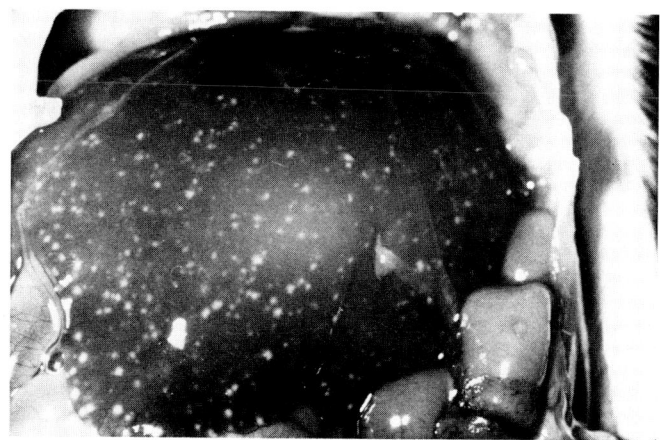

Figure 3-3. Hepatic lesions of a newborn rabbit with subcutaneous inoculation of type 2 HSV postinoculation day 4. Note numerous well-demarcated lesions are seen throughout the surface of the liver.

DISCUSSION

We have described and characterized a new experimental animal model for the study of neonatal herpetic chorioretinitis. The model's unique feature is that the eye lesions are produced in the newborn rabbit by infecting the skin with type 2 HSV, a natural route of infection for HSV in newborn infants. In contrast to a previously reported animal model,[23] in which a newborn rat was inoculated to produce eye lesions by an unnatural route (intracerebral), our model, infected through a natural portal of entry (skin), produced retinal lesions in 40 percent of newborn rabbits.

In a study of human infants, about 30 percent of patients with herpetic skin lesions developed chorioretinitis.[26] In our rabbit model, 2-HSV produced typical skin lesions; multiplied at the skin sites; disseminated to various organs, including the eye; and produced chorioretinal eye lesions. These manifestations are similar to those observed in human infants. The newborn rabbit model is thus quite ideal for the study of neonatal herpetic eye infection. Recently we have used it successfully to determine the protective effect of immunization and of antiviral agents on the neonatal herpetic eye infection.[27,28]

In the newborn rabbit model, typical retinal lesions were observed only in the eyes of the animals with 2-HSV skin infection. No such retinal lesions were seen in the eyes of normal rabbits or of animals whose eyes and skin were inoculated with heat-inactivated type 2 HSV. This would seem to

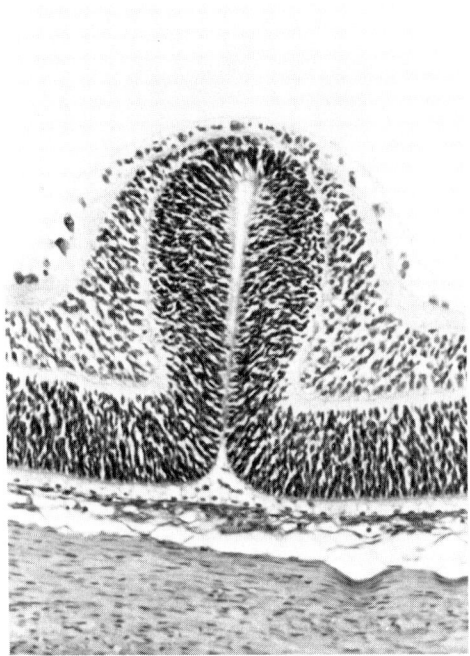 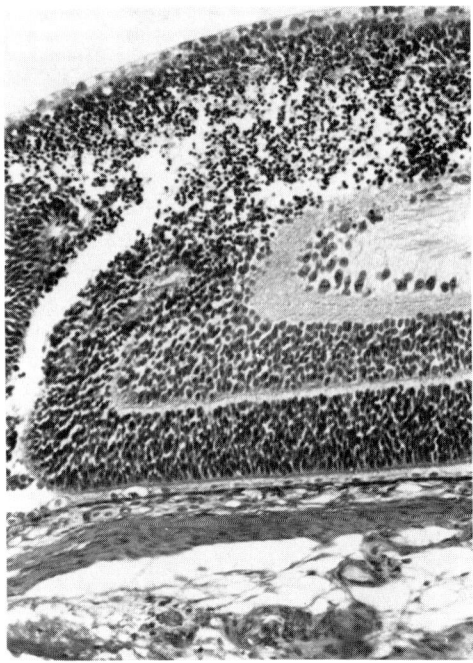

Figure 3-4. Retinal lesions in the eye of the newborn rabbit infected with type 2 HSV, post-inoculation day 4. (Hematoxylin and eosin, ×400).
a. A retinal fold.
b. A retinal fold with focal necrosis.
(Reproduced by permission. From J. O. Oh and P. Minasi, In R. Sundmacher (Ed.): *Herpetic Eye Diseases*, 1981. Courtesy of J. F. Bergmann Verlag, Munchen.)

indicate that the retinal lesions in the eyes of the HSV-infected newborn rabbits were virus-specific. No intranuclear inclusions typical of HSV could be found in these retinal lesions, however, although low titers of infectious HSV could be recovered from the whole eye and viral antigens by an immunofluorescence technique.

Other workers have found HSV-like particles in the retina of an infant with bilateral herpetic chorioretinitis[19] and in an experimental retinitis produced by HSV-2 in rats.[23]

Infectious HSV could be recovered from mononuclear cells of the peripheral blood and plasma of newborn rabbits as early as three days after the skin infection and was present in the eye one day later. It would seem, therefore, that in this model HSV reaches the eye from the skin lesions through the blood. In human infants, intranuclear inclusions were found in both vascular endothelial cells and the perivascular cuffing, and this also suggested hematogenous dissemination of the virus.[19] It is not clear, however, which of the mononuclear cell subsets in the newborn rabbit are associated with type

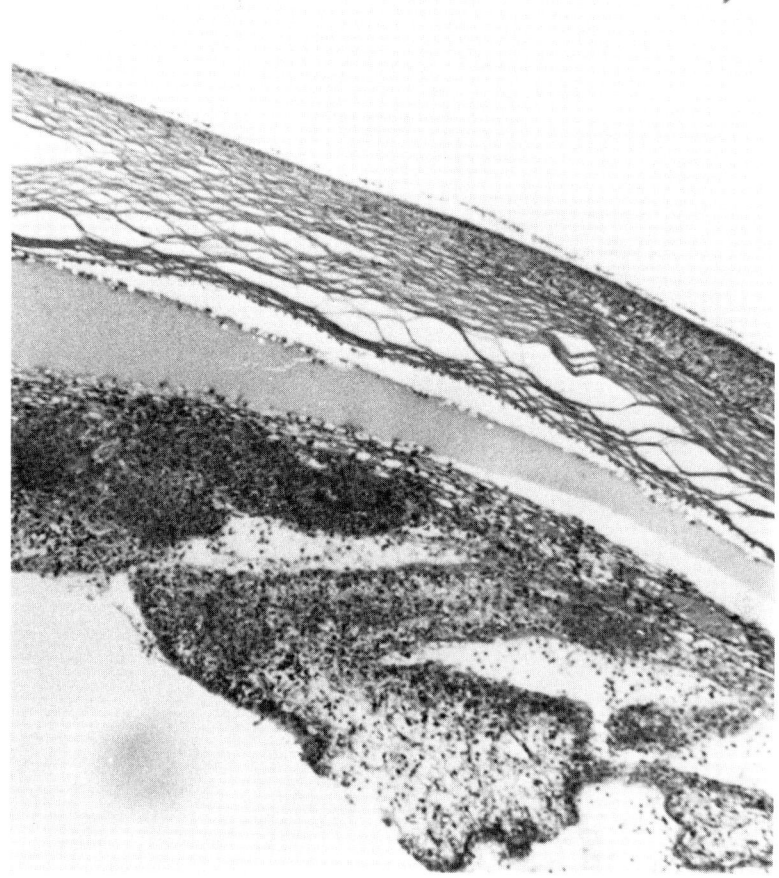

Figure 3-5. Iritis in the eye of the newborn rabbit infected with type 2 HSV, postinoculation day 4. (Hematoxylin and eosin ×400)

2 HSV, or if the virus multiplies in the mononuclear cells. In humans, HSV is known to multiply in both lymphocytes[29-32] and monocytes.[31-33]

Cervicothoracic ganglia of newborn rabbits were infected with type 2 HSV as early as two days after their skins were inoculated. Hematogenous dissemination of the virus to these ganglia was unlikely since the trigeminal ganglia of the same animals were not affected. It would seem, therefore, that the virus reached the ganglia by a neuronal route. Field and Hill[34] estimated that in the mouse, herpes virus travelled toward the ganglia at about 2 mm/hr. If this figure was applied to our newborn rabbits, only five hours would be needed by the virus to reach the cervicothoracic ganglia from the point of inoculation, a distance of about 10 mm. Therefore, it is not surprising to find type 2 HSV in cervicothoracic ganglia as early as two days after the inoculation to the skin.

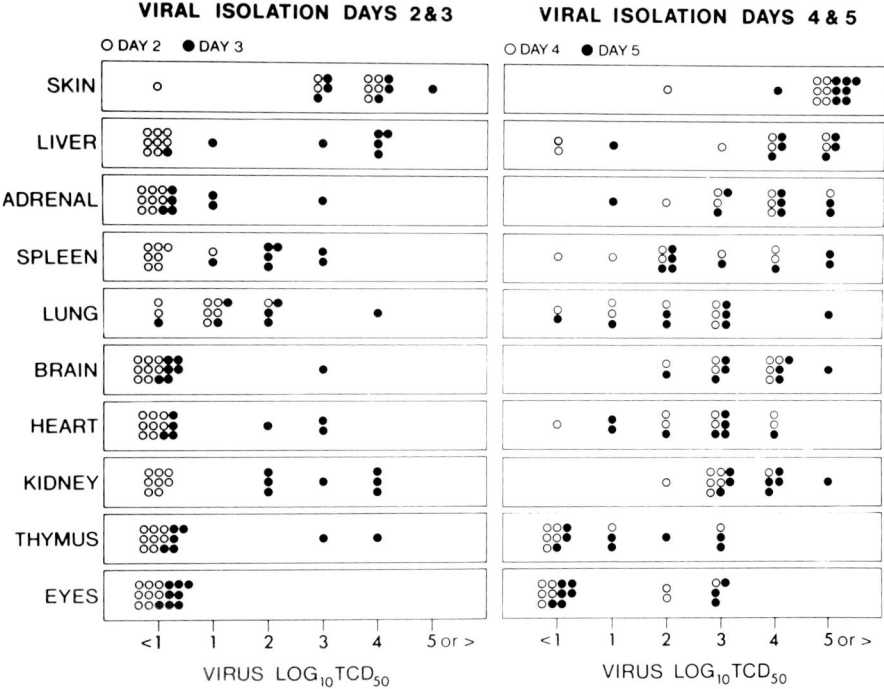

Figure 3-6. Virus titers of various organs of newborn rabbits inoculated subcutaneously with type 2 HSV. Each dot represents a virus titer in each organ of a rabbit. (Reproduced by permission. From D. C. Brick, J. O. Oh, and S. E. Sicher, *Invest Ophthalmol Urs Sci*, 21:681–688, 1981.)

TABLE 3-II
ISOLATION OF HSV-2 FROM CIRCULATING MONONUCLEAR CELLS
AND PLASMA OF NEWBORN RABBITS

Post Infection day	No. of specimens	HSV-2 isolated from			
		Mononuclear cells only	Plasma only	Mononuclear cells & plasma	Totals
1	5	0	0	0	0
2	11	0	0	0	0
3	8	2	0	1	3 (38%)
4	9	1	0	3	4 (44%)
5	9	2	1	4	7 (78%)
Totals		5	1	8	

Reproduced by permission. From D. C. Brick, J. O. Oh, and S. E. Sicher, *Invest Ophthalmol Vis Sci*, 21:681-688, 1981.

TABLE 3-III
ISOLATION OF HSV-2 FROM SENSORY GANGLIA OF NEWBORN RABBITS

Ganglia	Postinfection day			
	1	2	3	4
Cervicothoracic	0/5*	7/8	10/10	2/3
Trigeminal	0/5	0/3	0/3	0/3

*Number of animals yielding HSV-2/number of animals tested.
Reproduced by permission. From D. C. Brick, J. O. Oh, and S. E. Sicher, *Invest Ophthalmol Vis Sci, 21*:681-688, 1981.

Summary

The subcutaneous inoculation of the backs of 17–34 hour old New Zealand white rabbits with 10^3 $TCID_{50}$ of type 2 herpes simplex virus (HSV-2) induced cutaneous lesions within 24 hours, foci of disseminated infection in many organs (including the eye) on day 3 and thereafter, and the death of the animals on day 5 with infection of the central nervous system. Infectious HSV-2 could be isolated from the mononuclear cells and plasma of the peripheral blood, indicating the active role of both elements in the dissemination of the virus. Infectious HSV was also recovered from the corresponding sensory ganglia of the skin lesion (the cervicothoracic ganglia) as early as two days after the subcutaneous inoculation of the virus. About 40 percent of the animals developed ocular lesions consisting of retinal folds with or without necrotizing changes. Iritis and choroiditis also developed in some eyes. Infectious HSV-2 could be isolated from 33 percent of the eye on days 4 and 5. Thus, the newborn rabbit may serve as a suitable experimental animal for the study of HSV-2 induced chorioretinitis in the human newborn.

REFERENCES

1. Batignani, A.: Conjunctivite da virus erpetico in neonato. *Bull Ocul, 13*:1217–1220, 1934.
2. Nahmias, A. J.: Genital herpes simplex infection: Virologic and cytologic studies. *Obstet Gynecol, 29*:395–400, 1967.
3. Nahmias, A. J., and Hagler, W. S.: Ocular manifestations of herpes simplex in the newborn. *Int Ophthalmol Clin, 12*:191–213, 1972.
4. Smith, M. C., Lennette, E. H., and Reames, H. R.: Isolation of the virus of herpes simplex and the demonstration of intranuclear inclusions in a case of acute encephalitis. *Am J Pathol, 17*:55–68, 1941.
5. Florman, A. L., and Mindlin, R. L.: Generalized herpes simplex in an 11-day-old premature infant. *Am J Dis Child, 83*:481–486, 1952.

6. Mitchell, J. E., and McCall, F. C.: Transplacental infection by herpes simplex virus. *Am J Dis Child,* 106:207–209, 1963.
7. Cogan, D. G., Kuwabara, T., Young, G. F., and Knowx, D. L.: Herpes simplex retinopathy in an infant. *Arch Ophthalmol,* 72:641–645, 1964.
8. Yen, S. S. C., Reagan, J. W., and Rosenthal, M. S.: Herpes simplex infection in female genital tract. *Obst Gyn,* 25:479–492, 1965.
9. Bahrani, M., Bexerbaum, B., and Gilger, A.: Generalized herpes simplex and hypoadrenocorticism. A case associated with adrenocortical insufficiency in a prematurely born male, clinical, virological, ophthalmological and metabolic studies. *Am J Dis Child,* 111:437–445, 1966.
10. Golden, B., Ball, W. E., and McKee, A. P.: Disseminated herpes simplex with encephalitis in a neonate. *JAMA,* 209:1219–1221, 1969.
11. Hagler, W. S., Walters, P. V., and Nahmia, A. J.: Ocular involvement in neonatal herpes simplex virus infections. *Arch Ophthalmol,* 82:169–176, 1969.
12. Cibis, A., and Burde, R. M.: Herpes simplex virus-induced congenital cataracts. *Arch Ophthalmol,* 85:2202–223, 1971.
13. Pettay, O., Leinikki, P., Donner, M., and Laninleimu, K.: Herpes simplex virus infection in the newborn. *Arch Dis Child,* 47:97–103, 1972.
14. Cibis, G. W.: Neonatal herpes simplex retinitis. *Albrecht v Graefes Arch klin exp Ophthal,* 196:39–47, 1975.
15. Nahmias, A. J., Visintine, A. M., Caldwell, D. R., and Wilson, L. A.: Eye infections with herpes simplex viruses in neonates. *Surv Ophthalmol,* 21:100–105, 1976.
16. Yanoff, M., Allman, M. I., and Fine, B. S.: Congenital herpes simplex virus type 2, bilateral endophthalmitis. *Trans Am Ophthalmol Soc,* 75:327–337, 1977.
17. Tarkkanen, A., and Laatikainen, L.: Late ocular manifestations in neonatal herpes simplex infection. *Br J Ophthalmol,* 61:608–616, 1977.
18. Chalhub, E. G., Baenziger J., Feigen, R. D., Middlekamp, J. N., and Shackelford, G. D.: Congenital herpes simplex type II infection with extensive hepatic calcification, bone lesions and cataract: Complete postmortem examination. *Develop Med Child Neurol,* 19:527–534, 1977.
19. Cibis, G. S., Flynn, J. T., and David, E. B.: Herpes simplex retinitis. *Arch Ophthalmol,* 96:299–302, 1978.
20. Mousel, D. K., and Missall, S. R.: Pan uveitis and retinitis in neonatal herpes simplex infection. *J Ped Ophthalmol Strabismus,* 16:7–9, 1979.
21. Oh, J. O., and Minasi, P.: Herpetic chorioretinitis in newborn infants: An experimental study. In Sundmacher, R. (Ed.): *Herpetic Eye Diseases.* Munchen, J. F. Bergmann Verlag, 1981, pp. 191–199.
22. Oh, J. O. and Minasi, P.: Different susceptibility of skin to type 1 and type 2 herpes simplex viruses in newborn rabbits. *Infect Immun,* 27:168–174, 1980.
23. Percy, D. H., Galil, K. A., Hatch, L. A., Pancer, L. B., and Crawford, J. P.: Experimental type 2 herpes simplex ophthalmitis in the newborn rat. *Invest Ophthalmol Vis Sci,* 19:529–544, 1980.
24. Brick, D. C., Oh, J. O., and Sicher, S. E.: Ocular lesions associated with dissemination of type 2 herpes simplex virus from skin infection in newborn rabbits. *Invest Ophthalmol Vis Sci,* 21:681–688, 1981.
25. Boyum, A.: Separation of white blood cells. *Nature* (London), 204:793–794, 1964.
26. Nahmias, A. J., Visintine, A. M., Caldwell, D. R., and Wilson, L. A.: Eye infections with herpes simplex viruses in neonates. *Surv Ophthalmol,* 21:100–105, 1976.

27. Friedlaender, R. P., Oh, J. O., and Minasi, P.: Protective effect of immunization on herpetic eye lesions in newborn rabbits. *Invest Ophthalmol Vis Sci, 19*:(Suppl)156, 1980.
28. Sicher E., Oh, J. O., and Kopal, M.: Acyclovir therapy of neonatal herpes simplex virus type 2 infections in rabbits. *Antimicrob Ag Chemother, 20*:503–507, 1981.
29. Bahrani, M., Bexerbaum, B., and Gilger, A.: Generalized herpes simplex and hypoadrenocorticism. A case associated with adrenocortical insufficiency in a prematurely born male. Clinical, virological, ophthalmological and metabolic studies. *Am J Dis Child, 111*:435–445, 1966.
30. Kirchner, H., Kleinicke, C., and Northoff, H.: Replication of herpes simplex virus in human peripheral T lymphocytes. *J Fen Virol, 37*:647–649, 1977.
31. Plaeger-Marshall, S., and Smith, J. W.: Experimental infection of sub-populations of human peripheral blood leukocytes by herpes simplex virus. *Proc Soc Exp Biol Med, 158*:263–268, 1978.
32. Riando, C. R., Jr., Richter, B. S., Black, P. H., Callery, R., Chase, L., and Hirsch, M. S.: Replication of herpes simplex virus and cytomegalovirus in human leukocytes. *J Immunol, 120*:130–136, 1978.
33. Craig, C. P., and Nahmias, A. J.: Different patterns of neurologic involvement with herpes simplex virus types 1 and 2: Isolation of herpes simplex virus type 2 from the buffy coat of two adults with meningitis. *J Infect Dis, 127*:365–371, 1973.
34. Field, H. J., and Hill, T. J.: The pathogenesis of pseudorabies in mice: Virus replication at the inoculation site and axonal uptake. *J Gen Virol, 26*:145–148, 1975.

Chapter 4

HERPETIC KERATITIS IN NORMAL AND ATHYMIC MICE

JOSEPH P. METCALF, M.D.

Introduction

Previous studies of herpetic keratitis in rabbits suggest that the deep stromal disease producing permanent corneal scarring and opacity results from cell-mediated immunopathogenesis involving the direct destruction or injury of stromal keratocytes by cytotoxic lymphocytes.[1-3] That is, the host immune system recognizes stromal keratocytes with associated herpes virus antigens as "foreign" and initiates an immune response similar to a graft rejection.[4] In support of this hypothesis, herpes virus antigens have been identified on the surface membranes of stromal keratocytes in the rabbit cornea,[5] and lymphocytes in intimate contact with stromal keratocytes were frequently seen in diseased corneas from rabbits and humans.[1,2]

As a further test of this hypothesis, studies of herpetic keratitis were initiated in athymic (nude) mice.[6] The athymic mouse is deficient in thymus-dependent immune functions, and readily accepts xenografts from a variety of sources.[7] Thus, if our hypothesis is correct, they should not develop stromal keratitis whereas normal mice should. As shown in Figure 4-1, both athymic (nu/nu) and normal heterozygous (nu/+) mice developed a corneal infection after inoculation with herpes simplex virus (HSV). However, after day 8 postinfection, the corneas of the athymic mice became progressively clearer, even though the mice were dying of a systemic viral infection.

Although these observations are consistent with our working hypothesis, there are other differences in the immune response of athymic mice that could account for these results. For example, athymic mice do not produce anti-HSV antibodies in response to the virus infection.[8] Thus, chemotactic factors may not be released to attract inflammatory cells into the cornea.

Supported by Grant EY-03949 from the National Eye Institute, NIH, Bethesda, Maryland and a Grant-in-Aid from Fight for Sight, Inc., New York City, New York.
Presented in part at the Annual Meetings of the Association for Research in Vision and Ophthalmology, 1982, Sarasota, Florida.
I thank Mr. Richard Reichert, University of Florida, for assistance with these studies.

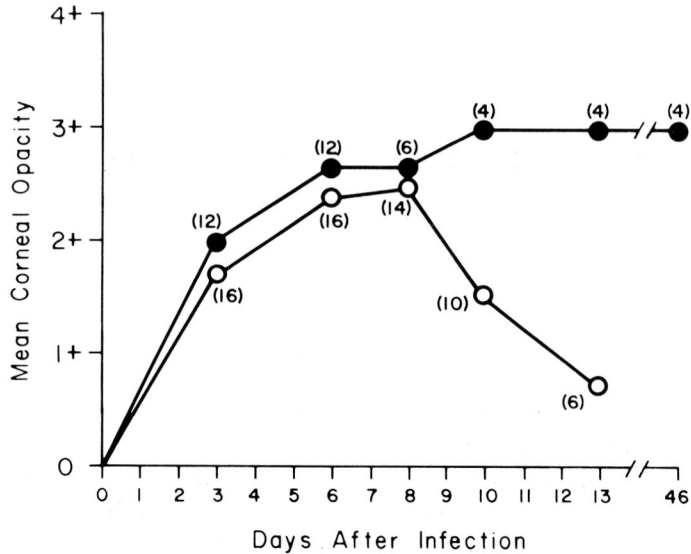

Figure 4-1. Comparison of herpetic keratitis in athymic nude (solid circles) and heterozymous littermates (solid circles). (From Metcalf et al.: *Infect Imm,* 26:1164, 1979. Courtesy ASM Publications, Washington, D.C.)

Furthermore, athymic mice are highly susceptible to HSV infection, and all of them die within 10–17 days following inoculation of the cornea.[6] Doses of the virus that have no effect on normal mice are lethal to athymic mice, and virus cultures of their eyes are positive for as long as the animals survive (Table 4-I).

TABLE 4-I

COMPARISON OF VIRUS CULTURES IN CORNEAS OF NORMAL AND ATHYMIC NUDE MICE AFTER CORNEAL INOCULATION WITH HSV

Days After Inoculation	Mice	
	Normal	Athymic
0 (1 hr.)	+	+
1	+	−
2	+	+
3	+	−
4	+	+
7	+	+
9	−	−
11	−	+
15	−	+
21	−	(dead)

If the failure of the athymic mice to develop stromal keratitis is due to the absence of thymic lymphocytes, then adoptive transfer of sensitized lymphocytes from normal mice to the athymic mice should restore their immune response capabilities. The reconstituted mice should then survive the viral infection, and also develop stromal keratitis as normal mice do. Therefore, studies of adoptive transfer of immune spleen cells from normal donors immunized to HSV, to athymic (nude) or normal recipients, with HSV-infected corneas, were carried out to define the role of cell-mediated immunity in herpetic stromal keratitis.

MATERIALS AND METHODS

Athymic (nu/nu) mice and their heterozygous (nu/+) BALB/c littermates were obtained from Grand Island Biological Company. These mice were maintained in a germ-free isolette and supplied with sterile food, water, and bedding throughout the study. Normal (+/+) BALB/c mice, obtained from Jackson Laboratories or Charles River, were maintained in a conventional manner.

The spleen cell donors were immunized by simultaneous or separate injections of live virus intraperitoneally (0.25 ml) and in the rear foot pads (0.05 ml in each). The RE strain of HSV, diluted to approximately $\times 10^4$ pfu/ml in Eagle's MEM without serum, was used to immunize the donor mice.[9]

RESULTS AND OBSERVATIONS

Effects of Adoptive Spleen Cell Transfer in Athymic Mice

The effects of adoptive spleen cell transfer in athymic mice are shown in Figures 4-2 through 4-4. The athymic controls died on day 10. They did not live long enough to display corneal clearing in this experiment. The normal controls developed necrotizing stromal keratitis and permanent corneal opacity, as observed previously in the rabbit.[10] However, the athymic mice that received the adoptive transfer of whole immune spleen cells survived the viral infection, but they failed to develop stromal keratitis as the normal mice did (Fig. 4-2). These results were unexpected and suggest that the whole spleen cell preparation contained cells that prevented dissemination of the virus without inducing stromal keratitis (Fig. 4-4a).

However, the athymic mice that received adoptive transfer of adherent-depleted spleen cells behaved like normal mice (Fig. 4-3), that is, about half of them survived the viral infection, and the survivors developed stromal

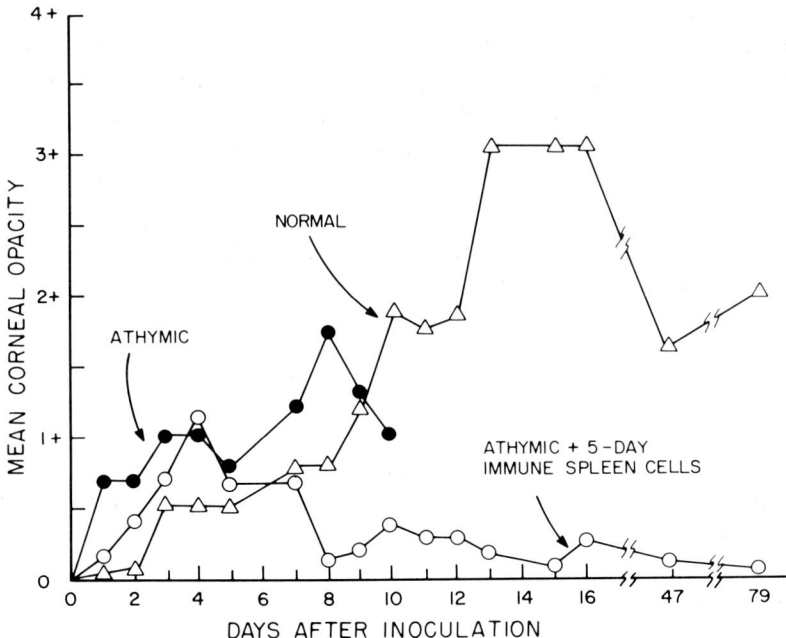

Figure 4-2. Effect of adoptive transfer of whole immune spleen cells on herpetic keratitis and survival of athymic (nu/nu) mice. Spleen cells were injected two hours after corneal inoculation.

keratitis (Fig. 4-4b), similar to changes observed in normal mice (Fig. 4-4c). Thus, it appears that the "adherent" cells prevented the expression of cell-mediated reactions and stromal keratitis by the nonadherent cells in the whole spleen cell preparation.

Effects of Adoptive Spleen Cell Transfer in Normal Mice

As shown in Figure 4-5, the protective effect of whole spleen cell transfer can also be demonstrated in normal mice. At two weeks postinoculation, however, some of the normal mice that received whole spleen cells developed stromal keratitis, as seen in the controls. It appears that the cytotoxic cells in the whole spleen cell preparation may have overcome the protective influence of the adherent cells in these mice.

Also, removal of the glass-adherent cells (Fig. 4-6) abrogated the protective effect of the whole spleen cells, as demonstrated in the athymic nude mice (Fig. 4-3). Thus, adoptive spleen cell transfer induces a course of herpetic keratitis in athymic (nu/nu) mice similar to that in normal mice.

Route of Immunization

In all of these experiments involving adoptive spleen cell transfer in both normal and athymic mice, the donor animals were immunized by both intra-

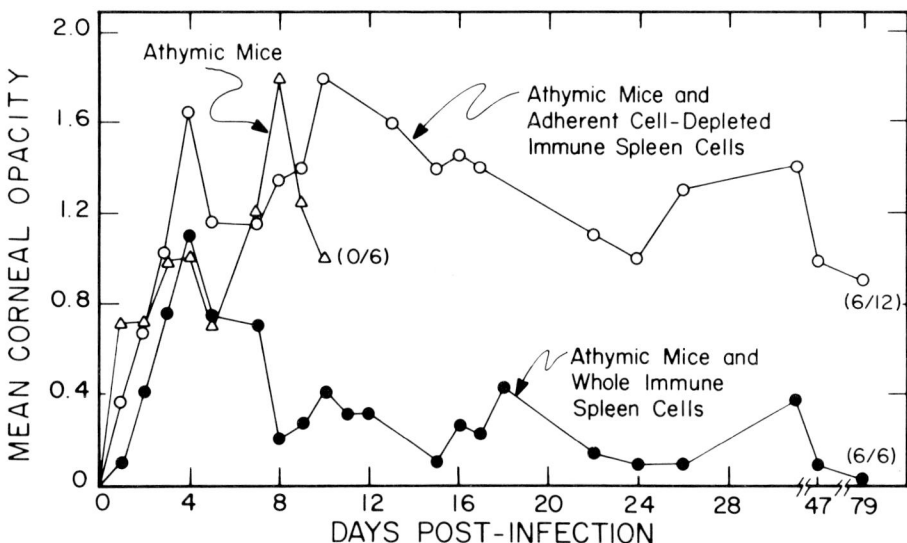

Figure 4-3. Effect of removing adherent cells from the spleen cell preparation on herpetic keratitis and survival of athymic (nu/nu) mice. Ratio of survivors to numbers of mice per group is shown in parentheses.

peritoneal and foot pad injections of live virus. Therefore, an experiment was carried out to determine whether immunization by both these routes is necessary to obtain immune spleen cells. As shown in Figure 4-7, a striking difference in herpetic corneal disease was seen when the recipients received spleen cells obtained from donors immunized by different routes. A clear-cut protective effect was not demonstrated in this experiment because the control animals developed little corneal disease. However, the mean corneal opacity of animals receiving whole spleen cells from donors immunized by both routes of injection was lower than the controls during the first two weeks post-infection.

In contrast, the group of mice receiving spleen cells from animals injected in the foot pads only developed corneal disease of much greater severity than the controls. After nine days, the most severely affected animals in this group died, and the mean corneal opacity approached control levels, increasing again after day 14.

The results of this experiment are also consistent with the notion that spleen cell preparations from mice immunized by both the intraperitoneal and foot pad routes of injection contain two cell types that affect the course of stromal herpes in the mouse. One of these cells, induced by the foot pad route of immunization, increases the severity of corneal disease in the eyes of mice infected with herpes. The other cell, induced by the intraperitoneal route of immunization, appears to be capable of preventing corneal disease

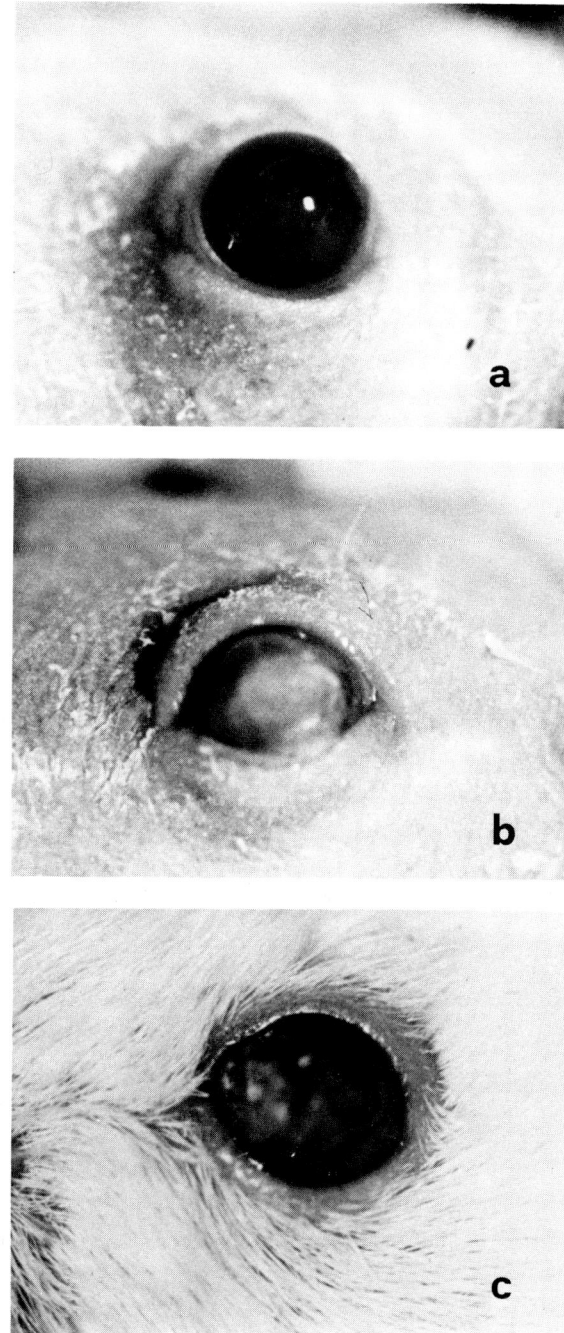

Figure 4-4. Eyes of mice three months after corneal inoculation with HSV. (a) Athymic (nu/nu) mouse that received adoptive transfer of whole immune spleen cells. (b) Athymic (nu/nu) mouse that received adoptive transfer of adherent-depleted spleen cells, showing stromal keratitis. (c) Herpetic keratitis in the cornea of a normal mouse.

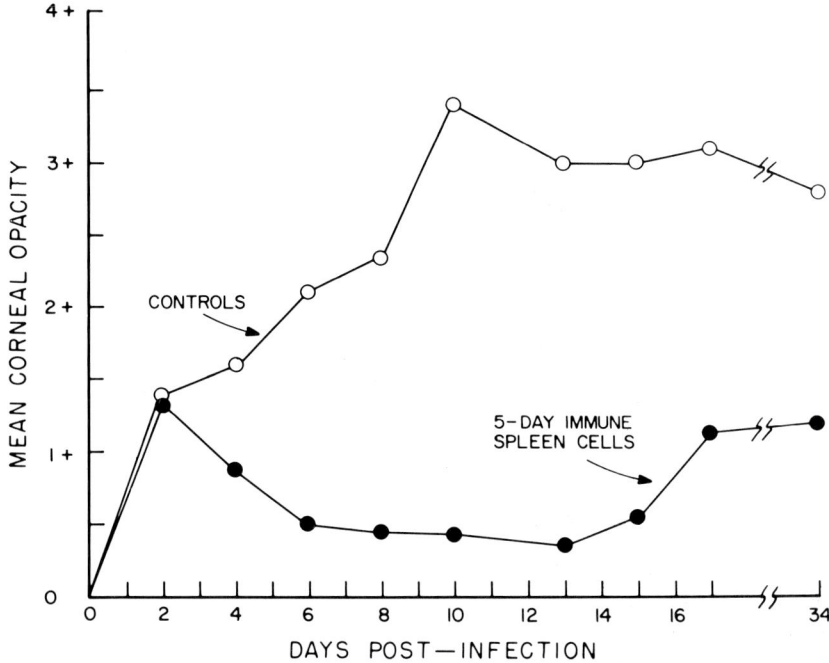

Figure 4-5. Protective effect of adoptive transfer of whole immune spleen cells against stromal keratitis in normal mice. Spleen cells were injected 24 hours after corneal inoculation.

in virus infected eyes, presumably by suppressing the cytotoxic activity of the foot-pad-induced cells. On the basis of the adherence studies (Figs. 4-3 and 4-6), the protective cell appears to be a macrophage.

DISCUSSION

The experiments described above involve adoptive transfer of immune spleen cells from appropriately immunized donor mice into recipient mice following corneal inoculation with HSV. Thus, one may ask whether these immune spleen cells influence the course of herpetic stromal keratitis in experimental animals following a primary corneal infection. If we examine the eyes of a group of mice with herpetic keratitis over a long period of time, spontaneous clearing of corneas with early necrotizing keratitis (neovascularization and cheesy white opacity) is frequently seen. For example, the group of normal mice (controls) shown in Figure 4-2 showed spontaneous corneal clearing between days 16 and 45 post-inoculation. Spontaneous clearing of stromal keratitis was also seen on days 26–42 postinoculation in a group of severely affected animals (Fig. 4-7), following adoptive transfer of immune spleen cells.

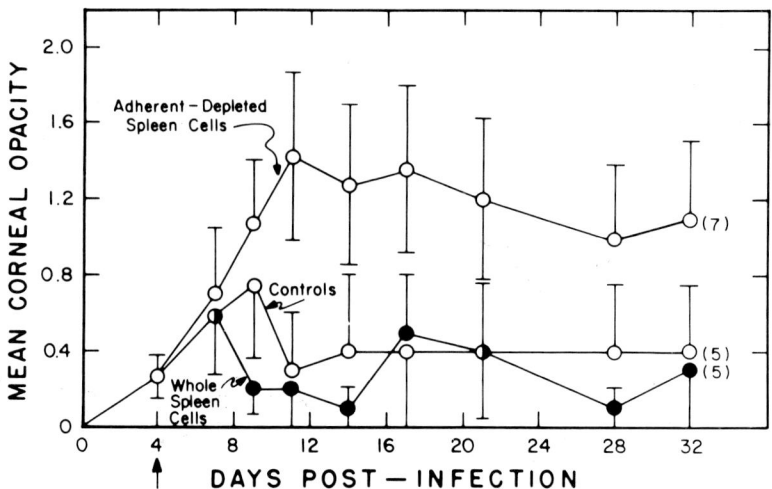

Figure 4-6. Effect of removing adherent cells from the immune spleen cell preparation on stromal keratitis in normal mice. The bars represent the standard error of the mean. Spleen cells were transferred four days after corneal inoculation of the recipients (arrow). Each group contained seven mice. Number of survivors is shown in parentheses.

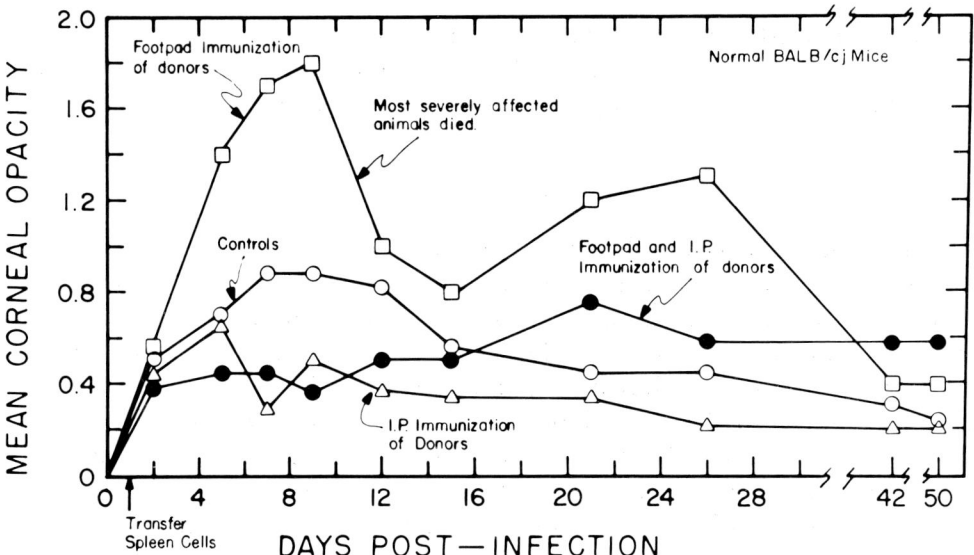

Figure 4-7. Comparison of route of immunization of the spleen cell donors on herpetic stromal keratitis in normal recipients. Spleen cells were transferred 24 hours after corneal inoculation (arrow).

Similarly, the development of necrotizing stromal keratitis in previously clear corneas is frequently seen. In the normal mice (controls) shown in Figure 4-2, stromal keratitis developed in the corneas of mice that had been clear until day 47. The net result of these changes in stromal disease was that half of the mice had clear corneas in both eyes and half had opaque corneas in both eyes. On day 79, there were no mice with a clear cornea in one eye and an opaque cornea in the other.

These observations strongly suggest that subtle differences in the immune system of these inbred mice determine the final outcome of the disease. That is, when corneal infection induces cytotoxic cells, a severe form of stromal disease will result. If the "protective cells" are stimulated, stromal disease will not develop, or spontaneous clearing of stromal disease will be observed if it has already appeared.

Additional evidence for the induction of cytotoxic immune cells that increase the severity of herpetic stromal keratitis is seen in the experiments reported by Williams, Nesburn, and Kaufman,[11] and more recently by Campbell, Pavan-Langston, et al.[12] These authors found that prior sensitization of rabbits by intradermal injections with live virus increased the severity of stromal disease when the immunized animals were later challenged by corneal inoculation. These observations are consistent with the results shown in Figure 4-7, showing that foot pad injections of live virus stimulated the induction of immune spleen cells, which increased stromal disease following adoptive transfer in mice.

Further studies are needed to identify and characterize the protective and cytotoxic spleen cells induced by immunization of mice with HSV, and to determine the mechanism by which they affect the course of herpetic stromal keratitis in experimental animals. However, it is clear from these observations that the mouse can be used as a "living test tube" in which the effects of specific immune cells on the course of herpetic stromal keratitis is studied.

SUMMARY

Immunization of mice by intraperitoneal and foot pad injections of live herpes simplex virus (HSV) stimulates the induction of two types of immune spleen cells that affect the course of herpetic keratitis following adoptive transfer into recipient animals. One cell type is a nonadherent, cytotoxic cell (T-lymphocyte?) induced by foot pad immunization of donor animals, which increases the severity of stromal disease following transfer to recipients with HSV-infected corneas. The other cell type is an adherent cell (macrophage?), induced by intraperitoneal immunization of donors. The adherent cell appears to suppress the expression of cytotoxic activity by the nonadherent cells, and thereby prevents the development of stromal keratitis in the recipient animals.

The identity and further characterization of these spleen cells remains to be determined. Adoptive transfer of immune cells in mice appears, however, to be an excellent model system in which to study the immunopathogenesis and immunotherapy of herpetic stromal keratitis.

REFERENCES

1. Metcalf, J. F., and Kaufman, H. E.: Herpetic stromal keratitis: Evidence for cell-mediated immunopathogenesis. *Am J Ophthalmol, 82*:827, 1976.
2. Metcalf, J. F., and Reichert, R. W.: Histological and electron microscopic studies of experimental herpetic keratitis in the rabbit. *Invest Ophthal Visual Sci, 18*:1123, 1979.
3. Sheppard, A. M., Adler-Storthz, K., and Smith, J. W.: Immune destruction of rabbit corneal cells infected with herpes simplex virus: Lymphocyte reactivity by antibody-dependent cellular cytotoxicity. *Invest Ophthalmol Vis Sci, 23*:227, 1982.
4. Henson, D., Helmsen, R., et al.: Ultrastructural localization of herpes simplex virus antigens on rabbit corneal cells using sheep antihuman IgG antihorse ferritin hybrid antibodies. *Invest Ophthal Visual Sci, 13*:819, 1974.
5. Metcalf, J. F., and Helmsen, R.: Immunoelectron microscopic localization of herpes simplex virus antigens in rabbit cornea with antihuman IgG antiferritin hybrid antibodies. *Invest Ophthal Visual Sci, 16*:779, 1977.
6. Metcalf, J. F., Hamilton, D. S., and Reichert, R. W.: Herpetic keratitis in athymic (nude) mice. *Infect Imm, 26*:1164, 1979.
7. Reed, N. D., and Manning, D. D.: Present status of xenotransplantation of nonmalignant tissue to the nude mouse. In Fogh, J., and Giovanella, B. C. (Eds.): *The Nude Mouse in Experimental and Clinical Research*. New York, Academic Press, 1978, pp. 167–185.
8. Burns, W. H., Billups, L. C., and Notkins, A. L.: Thymus dependence of viral antigens. *Nature, 256*:654, 1975.
9. Mishell, B. B., et al: Preparation of mouse cell suspensions. In Mishell, B. B., and Shiigi, S. M. (Eds.): *Selected Methods in Cellular Immunology*. San Francisco, W. H. Freeman, 1980, pp. 3–5.
10. Metcalf, J. F., McNeill, J. I., and Kaufman, H. E.: Experimental disciform edema and necrotizing keratitis in the rabbit. *Invest Ophthal Visual Sci, 15*:979, 1976.
11. Williams, L. E., Nesburn, A. B., and Kaufman, H. E.: Experimental induction of disciform keratitis. *Arch Ophthalmol, 73*:112, 1965.
12. Campbell, R., Pavan-Langston, D., et al.: Collagenase levels in a new model of experimental herpetic interstitial keratitis. *Arch Ophthalmol, 98*:919, 1980.

Chapter 5

MODELS OF CHLAMYDIAL CONJUNCTIVITIS IN NONHUMAN PRIMATES

PHILLIPS THYGESON, M.D.

Introduction

There seems to be no natural chlamydial conjunctivitis of monkeys or apes that is comparable to the chlamydial conjunctivitis of cats and guinea pigs. Nevertheless, monkeys and apes have been shown over the years to be susceptible to conjunctival inoculation with tissue or scrapings from human trachoma, inclusion conjunctivitis, and the cervices of mothers of inclusion blennorrhea babies. More recently, results have been obtained with cultured chlamydiae collected from trachoma, inclusion conjunctivitis, and nonspecific urethritis and cervicitis.

The induced disease is a spontaneously healing follicular conjunctivitis that often closely resembles human inclusion conjunctivitis in its appearance and clinical course. Without exception, however, so-called "experimental trachoma" has failed to develop the characteristic scars of trachoma, the characteristic limbal follicles and their cicatricial remains (Herbert's peripheral pits), or the typical trachoma pannus with its so-called "trachoma pustules" and "pannus ulcers." Claims have been made of pannus production and conjunctival scars as a result of repeated inoculations with cultured chlamydiae, but the scars and pannus described have borne little resemblance to those of human trachoma, and no one has ever reported the development of the most characteristic of all trachoma lesions, Herbert's limbal peripheral pits.[1]

So far as I know, no one has produced an experimental eye model with tissue material or cultures from lymphogranuloma venereum. My own inoculations with tissue scrapings, all of which were lethal for mice when inoculated into their brains, ended in failure.

A complication that reduces the value of subhuman primates as experimental models of human chlamydial conjunctivitis is their susceptibility to spontaneous folliculosis and spontaneous follicular conjunctivitis, both of which have caused serious confusion.[2,3] For example, it is now certain that Noguchi,[4] in his gold-medal-winning study of the etiology of trachoma (1928), confused spontaneous follicular conjunctivitis with experimental trachoma, and that this confusion led him to believe that *Bacterium granulosis*, a small gram-negative rod, was the etiologic agent of trachoma.

The Diagnostic Features of Trachoma

Trachoma is the most characteristic type of chlamydial conjunctivitis and was the first to be recognized. Unlike the other two types, inclusion conjunctivitis and lymphogranuloma venereum keratoconjunctivitis, trachoma shows clinical and pathologic signs that make its diagnosis, in the absence of cultural or serologic findings, absolutely certain. For example, Herbert's peripheral pits (the cicatricial remains of limbal follicles), and a group of other signs when they appear together, are both unequivocally pathognomonic.

The follicles of trachoma are soft and gelatinous, and their contents are easily expressible. In these respects, they are unlike the follicles of all other types of follicular disease. They also have a predilection for the upper tarsal conjunctiva, differing in this way from the follicles of inclusion conjunctivitis, which prefer the lower tarsus and fornices. The follicles of trachoma undergo necrosis and leave behind them highly characteristic stellate scars.

The pannus of trachoma also has a typical morphology and a predilection for the upper limbus. Severe forms are accompanied by round subepithelial infiltrates near the superior border of the pannus, the infiltrates often ulcerating and leaving shallow "pannus ulcers" that scar the cornea. The entropion-trichiasis of trachoma, unlike that of pemphigoid or erythema multiforme *major* (Stevens-Johnson type), is always much more prominent in the upper lid than in the lower.

Inclusion bodies (Halberstaedter-Prowazek inclusions) have been demonstrated in all cases of trachoma at onset[5] but may become difficult to find in the late stages. It should be borne in mind, however, that they are the first and most important pathologic finding in this unique disease.

Experimental Models and Their Problems

A satisfactory model of trachoma must show (1) demonstrable inclusions, at least at the onset of the disease, (2) conjunctival scars that are highly characteristic in type, (3) the typical pannus of trachoma, and most importantly, (4) the characteristic upper limbal follicles of trachoma and their cicatrizing remains, known as "Herbert's peripheral pits." Many attempts have been made to produce these lesions in the ape or monkey since the original inoculations that were made in orangutans in Java by Halberstaedter and Prowazek.[6] These first observers found inclusions in their inoculated animals but the animals failed to develop the lesions of trachoma other than conjunctival follicles.

Notable among the many reviews that have appeared in the literature dealing with experimental trachoma are those by Julianelle,[7] Morax,[8] Nataf et al.,[9] and Noguchi.[4] There can be no doubt that experimental trachoma, however unlike the human disease, has been produced. This must be the case, since classical trachoma has resulted from the inoculation of human volunteers with tissue from experimental animals after repeated passages of the experimental disease. Most important of these experiments are the inoculations made by Nicolle et al.[10] and Bland et al.[3] who produced experimental trachoma in the Algerian magot and grivet, respectively. The chlamydiae causing these experimental diseases were passed in series in the animals and then produced classical trachoma when inoculated into the conjunctivas of volunteers. It should be noted that the disease in these animals, although definitely trachomatous, lacked the cardinal diagnostic signs of trachoma in man. In the grivet, the experimental disease was so mild that it resembled spontaneous folliculosis.

In my long experience with experimental chlamydial conjunctivitis in nonhuman primates, all baboons and monkeys tested proved to be susceptible to tissue transfer and to cultures of material from both trachoma and inclusion conjunctivitis. On the other hand, tissue transfer from a single case of primary ocular lymphogranuloma venereum to the conjunctivas of two baboons led to systemic disease (meningoencephalitis) but failed to induce ocular lesions. As first observed by Morax[8] in 1928, experimental trachoma produced by tissue transfer was much milder than experimental inclusion conjunctivitis, the latter resembling in every respect (i.e., appearance, clinical course, and the presence of inclusions) the adult form of inclusion conjunctivitis in man. The much milder experimental trachoma was sometimes of considerably longer duration than the human disease but was always self-healing, and in its late stages was so mild as to resemble spontaneous folliculosis.

Both experimental inclusion conjunctivitis and experimental trachoma have been more severe when produced by cultured material. Again, experimental inclusion conjunctivitis has been by far the more severe disease. For example, the disease produced by Bour strain (serotype E) was so severe as to resemble purulent inclusion conjunctivitis of the newborn with its follicles obscured by papillary hypertrophy (see Fig. 5-1). While experimental trachoma was also a severe disease, chronicity could not be maintained and inclusions were found with the greatest difficulty.

Reactivation Attempts:

Attempts to reactivate these experimental infections with corticosteroid preparations were mildly successful in monkeys in which both experimental trachoma and experimental inclusion conjunctivitis had been induced by tissue transfer,[11] and strikingly successful in disease that had been induced by cultured material.[12] For example, Bour strain of inclusion conjunctivitis

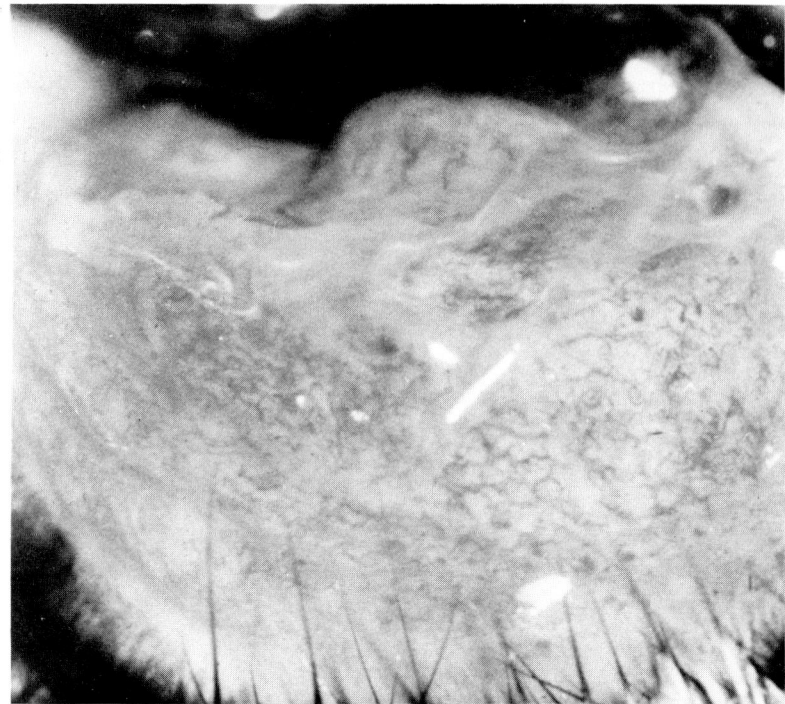

Figure 5-1. Animal model of human inclusion blennorrhea in cynomolgus monkey inoculated with Bour strain chlamydia, microimmunofluorescence (MIF) type E from adult inclusion conjunctivitis. Note characteristic acute mucopurulent papillary reaction.

agent produced typical experimental infection in four cynomolgus monkeys; however, after 66 days in two of four, and 113 days in the other two, the only remaining clinical signs were a few small follicles, and Giemsa-stained epithelial scrapings showed no inclusions. After treatment with a steroid preparation (subconjunctival prednisolone), all four animals had recurrences of their clinical signs, and the scrapings from one of each pair were inclusion-positive. The clinical course of the reactivated disease was short, and every animal healed without sequelae. Reactivation of the experimental trachoma produced by cultures of ASGH strain was accomplished in two of four animals but was less dramatic than it was with the Bour-strain-induced inclusion conjunctivitis and lasted longer.

In human trachoma, reactivation has occurred spontaneously in old age, presumably in response to the patient's reduced cellular immunity complicated by secondary bacterial infection, particularly with Koch-Weeks' bacillus (*Haemophilus aegyptius*) or by the topical use of corticosteroid preparations. In baboons and monkeys, reactivation of experimental trachoma has been accomplished only by the action of steroids or by repeated inoculation with cultures of trachoma agent. In my own experience, none of the animals inoculated with either trachoma or inclusion conjunctivitis have developed scars or pannus.

Models of Chlamydial Conjunctivitis Before and After Cultivation of the Agents

In a review of the literature published before the cultivation of the agents of trachoma and inclusion conjunctivitis, I found no claims of the development of a successful experimental trachoma model, but satisfactory inclusion conjunctivitis models were produced by Morax and a number of other workers. Since the cultivation of *Chlamydia trachomatis* the picture has changed, and there have now been several claims[13,14] that scars and pannus have been produced experimentally.

An opportunity was given me to examine the animals concerned in a claim by Wang and Grayston[13] (Seattle) that Bour agent (serotype E) had produced pannus, limbal follicles, and chronic disease typical of human trachoma. It was my opinion, however, that their experimental disease bore little resemblance to human trachoma, in spite of the fact that pannus and some chronicity had developed. No trachoma-type conjunctival scars were seen, and no Herbert's pits. It was reported later, however, that several animals inoculated with the same strain (Bour) did indeed develop conjunctival scars.

Another claim was made by Taylor et al.[14] (Baltimore) that models of chronic cicatrizing trachoma were produced by inoculating the eyes of cynomolgus monkeys at weekly intervals with an inclusion-conjunctivitis isolate (Bour strain, serotype E) or a trachoma isolate (serotype A). Efforts to produce similar models in rhesus monkeys were "less successful." The basis for the inoculations at weekly intervals seems to have been the mistaken idea that trachoma develops as the result of repeated infections with chlamydia of any serotype. This is certainly not the case, since there is abundant epidemiologic evidence that trachoma "breeds true" and is never caused by serotypes that produce inclusion conjunctivitis, genital infection, or lymphogranuloma.

It seems clear to me that both these claims (by the investigators in Seattle and Baltimore) are lacking in the essential requirements for a successful trachoma model. Like the well-established inclusion conjunctivitis model, a satisfactory trachoma model should duplicate the unique clinical and pathologic characteristics of trachoma, should contain demonstrable inclusions, should be produced by chlamydiae of serotypes A, B, or C, and should have soft, easily expressible follicles that cicatrize to form characteristic stellate scars on the upper tarsus and scars at the upper limbus (Herbert's peripheral pits). The trachoma scars that lead to trichiasis-entropion are important but not essential in a model. Only the three unique signs (expressible follicles, stellate scars of the upper tarsus, and Herbert's limbal pits) are indispensable.

Although no entirely satisfactory model of trachoma has been produced, apes and monkeys are still useful in trachoma research, provided spontaneous folliculosis and follicular conjunctivitis have been ruled out to avoid the mistake Noguchi made in 1928. If we exclude the experimental disease[15] that can be induced in the owl monkey (which may be acute but is of very short duration), any acute disease produced by a chlamydial strain indicates that the strain was an inclusion conjunctivitis strain and probably genital in origin.

This was the case with the Bour (serotype E) strain with which Wang and Grayston produced their experimental disease. This strain had been isolated originally from an adult male with unilateral follicular disease of subacute onset that I had mistakenly diagnosed as trachoma because of its micropannus. Further study showed that it was actually adult inclusion conjunctivitis, probably of genital origin. There was no trachoma in the patient's family or in the neighborhood, and endemic trachoma has not occurred in the San Francisco Bay area. On the other hand, follicular conjunctivitis of genital origin (caused by serotypes D, E, or F) has been quite common and was particularly common in the Bay area among the "hippies" of the 1960s.

Zoonotic Chlamydial Conjunctivitis in Man

Accidental transfer to man of the chlamydial conjunctivitis of cats (a feature of feline pneumonitis, caused by *Chlamydia psittaci*) has been reported twice,[16] and in both cases the disease resembled adult inclusion conjunctivitis. It is probable that the agent of ovine abortion has also infected the conjunctiva of man accidentally (Storz),[17] but the data are incomplete. There have been numerous undocumented reports of pneumonia and conjunctivitis in families with sick parakeets, and there is one documented example of chlamydial keratoconjunctivitis in a technician working with infected parakeets. The clinical disease in these cases bore no resemblance to either trachoma or inclusion conjunctivitis and was somewhat resistant to treatment with tetracycline. It showed no epithelial inclusions but yielded many positive cultures, some while the patient was taking tetracycline. There was no systemic involvement.

As to experimental models of these rare chlamydial conjunctivitides, all of them caused by *C. psittaci*, only the conjunctivitis of the cat, which seems to be a regular feature of feline pneumonitis, can be considered a model of the human infection.

REFERENCES

1. Thygeson, P.: Unpublished observations.
2. Wilson, R. P.: Folliculosis of the conjunctiva in animals. *4th Annual Report, Giza Memorial Ophthalmic Laboratory*. Giza-Cairo, Egypt, pp. 63–65, 1929.

3. Bland, J. O. W.: Spontaneous folliculosis of the conjunctiva in grivet and vervet monkeys and baboons. *14th Annual Report, Giza Memorial Ophthalmic Laboratory.* Giza-Cairo, Egypt, pp. 72–89, 1939–44.
4. Noguchi, H.: The etiology of trachoma. *J Exper Med,* 48 (No. 2, Supplement #2):63–65, 1929.
5. Wilson, R. P.: Trachoma. A selection of personal observations and experiences. *14th Annual Report, Giza Memorial Ophthalmic Laboratory.* Giza-Cairo, Egypt, pp. 13–37, 1939–44.
6. Halberstaedter, L., and von Prowazek, S.: Zur atiologie des Trachoms. *Deut med Woch,* 33:1285, 1907.
7. Julianelle, L. A.: *The Etiology of Trachoma.* New York, Oxford University Press, 1938.
8. Morax, V.: *Les conjonctivites Folliculaires.* Paris, Masson et Cie, 1933.
9. Nataf, R., Lepine, P., and Bonamour, G.: *Oeil et virus.* Paris, Masson et Cie, 1960.
10. Nicolle, C., Cuenod, A., and Blaizot, L.: Étude expérimentale du trachoma. *Arch Inst Pasteur Tunis,* 3:85, 1911.
11. Thygeson, P., and Crocker, T.: Observations on experimental trachoma and inclusion conjunctivitis. *Am J Ophthalmol,* 42:76, 1956.
12. Thygeson, P., Dawson, C., Hanna, L., Jawetz, E., and Okumoto, M.: Observations on experimental trachoma in monkeys produced by strains of virus propagated in yolk sac. *Am J Ophthalmol,* 50:907, 1960.
13. Wang, S. P., and Grayston, J. T.: Pannus with experimental trachoma and inclusion conjunctivitis agent infection of Taiwan monkeys. *Am J Ophthalmol,* 63:1133, 1967.
14. Taylor, H. R., Prendergast, R. A., Dawson, C. R., Schachter, J., and Silverstein, A. M.: An animal model for cicatrizing trachoma. *Invest Ophthalmol,* 21:422–433, 1981.
15. Murray, E. S., Fraser, C. E. O., Peters, J. H., McComb, D. E., and Nichols, R. L.: The owl monkey as an experimental primate model for conjunctival trachoma infection. *Trachoma and Related Disorders Caused by Chlamydia Agents.* Excerpta Medica, Amsterdam, pp. 386–396, 1971.
16. Schachter J., Ostler, H. B., and Meyer, K. F.: Human infection with the agent of feline pneumonitis. *Lancet,* 1:1063–1065, 1969.
17. Storz, J.: *Chlamydia and Chlamydia-Induced Diseases.* Springfield, Illinois, Charles C Thomas, p. 257, 1971.

Chapter 6

CHLAMYDIAL INFECTIONS IN CATS

KATHLEEN L. BOLDY, V.M.D.

Introduction

The infectious agents causing feline pneumonitis, psitticosis, trachoma, and various oculogenital and systemic syndromes have been identified. I will discuss the role of ocular chlamydial infections in cats as it applies to the continuing development of our knowledge concerning these important parasites and the effects on their hosts.

A Condensed Chlamydia Primer

Chlamydia species were formerly called *Bedsonia* or psitticosis-lymphogranuloma venereum-trachoma (PLT) organisms.[1,2] They are gram-negative, obligate intracellular parasites. Their complex developmental cycle involves the small, spheroidal, infectious chlamydial cell, the elementary body (EB). The EB is phagocytized by the host cell, then reorganizes to form larger, noninfectious initial or reticulate bodies (RB) that divide by binary fission. These multiplying chlamydial forms aggregate to microcolonies that are enveloped by a membrane forming the cytoplasmic inclusion. When large inclusions disband, the progeny of RBs that have differentiated back to EBs are ready to infect new host cells.[3,4]

The reproduction and subsequent infectivity of chlamydia are temperature-dependent. Surface antigens promote phagocytosis and inhibit phagolysosome formation. The heat lability of the organisms suggests that surface proteins are the principal virulence factors responsible for ensuring parasite uptake by host cells and circumventing destruction.[4,5]

The two recognized divisions of the genus *Chlamydia* are *C. trachomatis*, which includes the agents responsible for human trachoma, inclusion body conjunctivitis, lymphogranuloma venereum, and mouse pneumonitis; and *C. psittaci*, which contains the organisms producing psittacosis, bovine encephalomyelitis, guinea pig conjunctivitis, feline pneumonitis, and nonspecific conjunctivitis in sheep, goats, and cows.[1,3,6] There are biovariations of the two species, and recent studies show that amino acid requirements are different for a range of the more than 13 *C. trachomatis* serotypes and for four

C. psittaci strains. These requirements seem to reflect the host and/or syndrome differences.[7]

The Feline Syndrome

Current experimental and clinical observations indicate that the feline *Chlamydia psittaci* is primarily a conjunctival rather than a pulmonary or corneal pathogen, although there are a few exceptions.[8] Feline pneumonitis is characterized by a conjunctivitis with occasional mild rhinitis.[9,10,11]

Cats exposed to aerosols of feline *C. psittaci* exhibited a conjunctivitis that persisted for 22–45 days after a five to ten day incubation period. No signs of lower respiratory tract disease or significant pulmonary lesions were produced by the feline pneumonitis agent. Chlamydia were identified between postexposure days (PED) 7–14 in the cytoplasm of epithelial cells in Giemsa-stained conjunctival smears (Fig. 6-1). Conjunctivitis remained for at least 18 days after chlamydia were no longer detectable on cytology. Pyrexia appeared between PED 11–15 and remained for three to eight days. Low levels of chlamydial infectivity were present in conjunctiva and lung on PED 45.[12]

In the early stages of the clinical disease, the cat exhibits a unilaterally affected eye; the conjunctiva is chemotic, smooth, grayish pink, and shiny. The fellow eye may become involved in a few days. The initial ocular discharge is thin and watery, representing an increase in tears. Mucous exudate begins to form approximately two days after the disease is first noticeable. As the neutrophilic response intensifies, the secretion becomes mucopurulent. The conjunctiva loses most of the edema and becomes thicker and slightly more hyperemic. Follicular hyperplasia occurs rarely in chronic cases. If present, the rhinitis is serous at first and then becomes more mucoid. Sneezing accompanies the early stages, but it may persist throughout the chronic phase.[13]

Concomitant infection with other pathogens is a frequent natural event.[14,15] Ocular superinfections with bacteria, herpes virus, and mycoplasma often obscure the prototypical picture.[16] Hence, many of the papers describing feline pneumonitis as a cicatrizing conjunctival disease with corneal involvement, lasting longer than a year or progressing to cause the animal's death from pulmonary disease, are actually depicting a complex syndrome most probably involving herpes virus.[17,18]

In addition to multiple infections confusing the story of feline pneumonitis, other agents can mimic the chlamydial conjunctivitis and upper respiratory syndrome.[19] The gamut of feline upper respiratory disease includes a number of viruses, *Mycoplasma felis*, and *C. psittaci*. These can be differentiated clinically through the use of various laboratory tests such as cytology, microbiology, immunofluorescent antibodies, complement fixation, serum neutralizing antibodies, and tissue culture.[11,13]

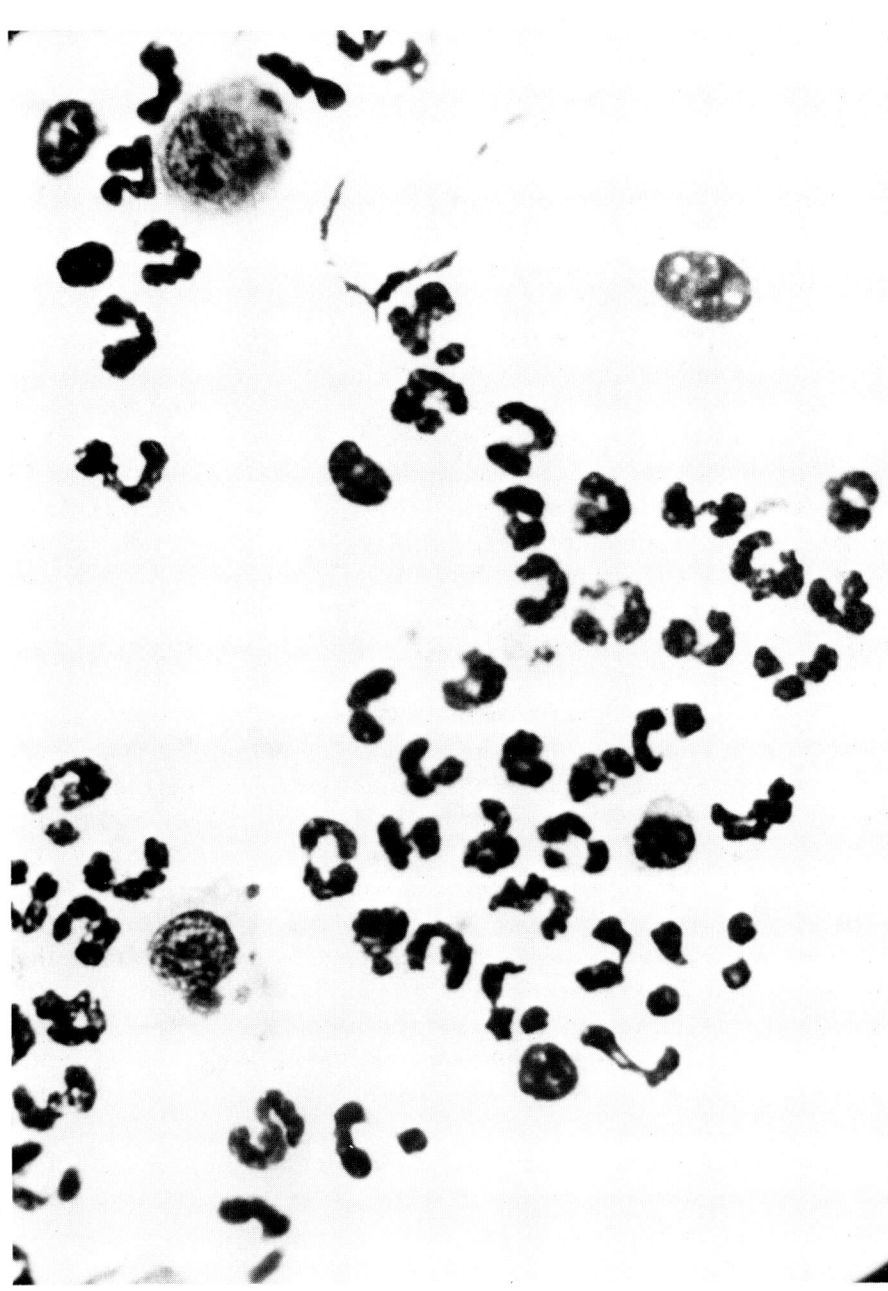

Figure 6-1. Polymorphonuclear cells are the main component of the inflammatory response seen in the conjuncti of cats affected with feline pneumonitis. Chlamydial inclusions can be seen in some of the epithelial cells.

Transmission of feline chlamydial disease can occur by inhalation of infective material, through direct contact, and with the "ocular promiscuity" suggested by Dr. Barrie Jones in his work with similar human disease.[20] *C. psittaci* has been cultured from asymptomatic queens' cervices after conjunctivitis developed in kittens postpartum.[17,21] Thus, an oculogenital relationship has been postulated, although no extensive studies have been published documenting the vertical transmission. In any case, transfer of the chlamydial agent through genital channels is not the major cause in the spread of the natural disease.

Presumptive diagnosis is made in most clinical circumstances by the presenting signs combined with cytological and immunofluorescent antibody examination. Isolation and identification of the chlamydial organism are needed for absolute verification, but the presence of a predominantly neutrophilic response correlates very well with recovery of the infectious agent.[6] The likelihood of finding cytological evidence of *C. psittaci* is greatest in the first two weeks of infection, although inclusions can persist much longer. Both feline and human chlamydial inclusions are best demonstrated with Giemsa stains.[13,22] (See Fig 6-2.) The outstanding appearance of the "cap" of purple granules near the nucleus helps to distinguish the inclusions of chlamydia from the smaller, lighter flecks of blue powder in mycoplasma infections or the variable spots of keratin granules, melanin, and stain precipitate on the epithelial cells.[23]

Serological studies of *C. psittaci* have been preliminary compared with the information known about *C. trachomatis*.[24] Complement-fixing antibodies are not reliable correlates of disease in either feline chlamydial conjunctivitis or trachoma. In man, immunofluorescence is the serological technique that offers the most acceptable combination of sensitivity, specificity, and convenience.[24,25] In cats, it has been applied mainly to the detection of chlamydial antigen in infected tissue. (Cross-reacting turkey strain *C. psittaci* is used at the University of California at Davis veterinary laboratory to diagnose infection using thick conjunctival smears in localized disease or sera in systemic syndromes.) Little work has been done on serotyping of isolates and titration of type-specific antibodies in feline pneumonitis.[26]

Immunization to prevent and treat the chlamydial disease of cats is seldom used clinically. In several studies,[27,28,29] cats receiving aerosol challenge following vaccination were infected easily; however, the duration and extent of disease were reduced in the vaccinated versus unvaccinated groups. Vaccination was not complete in any of the animals, but live vaccines afforded some protection, whereas inactivated vaccines provided no protection at all.

The zoonotic potential of feline pneumonitis is not great, yet it needs to be considered in cases of human conjunctivitis, fever, respiratory disease, and endocarditis where exposure to affected cats is historical.[2,30,31,32]

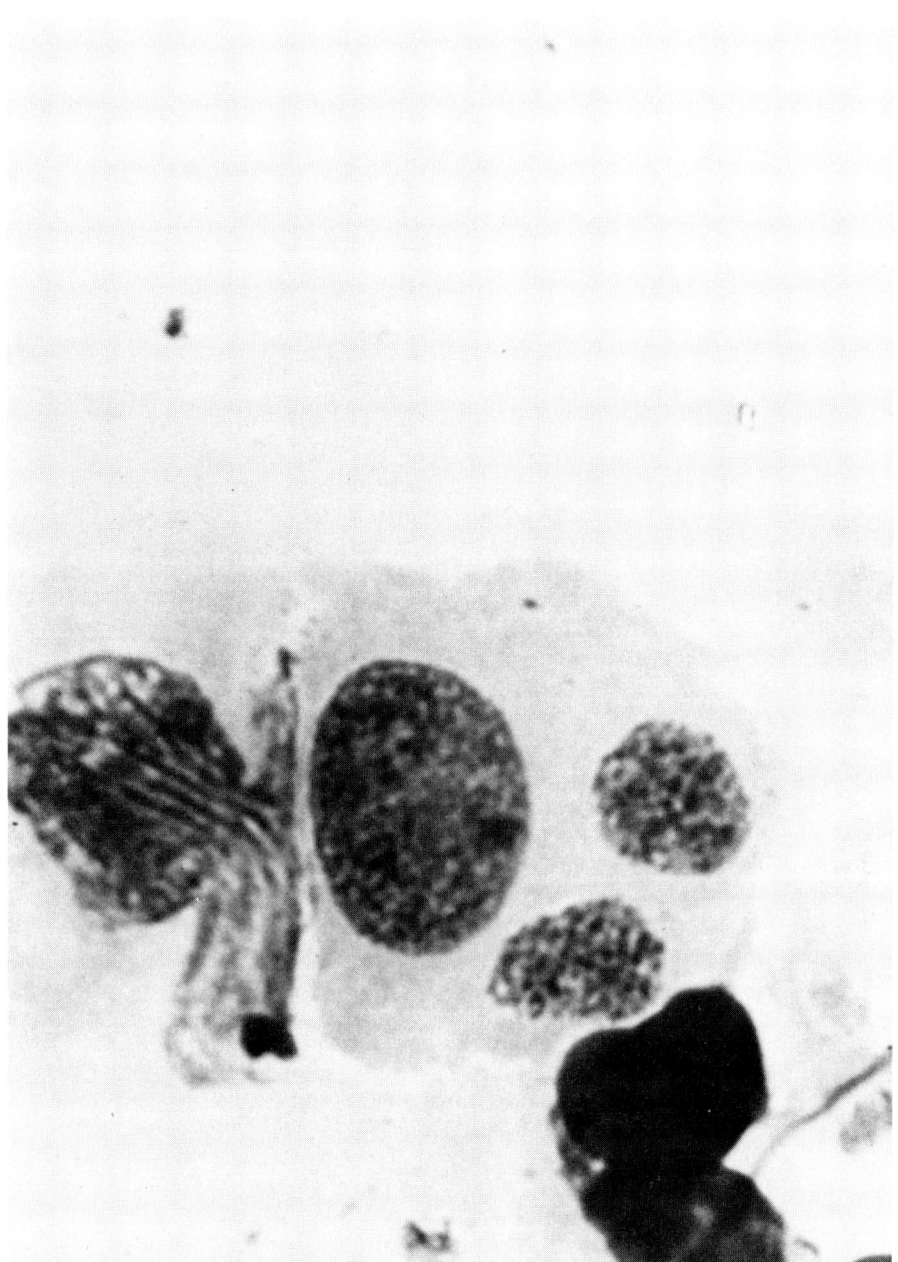

Figure 6-2. Conjunctival scraping showing typical chlamydial inclusions with Giemsa stain in a cat with conjunctivitis.

Conclusion

"Is the cat a valuable model for ocular disease?" The ocular chlamydial infections in cats do not truly mirror the diseases in humans. Uncomplicated, the feline syndrome does not extend to the cornea as either trachoma or inclusion conjunctivitis. Follicles rarely occur in the chronic state in the cat; cicatrizing conjunctivitis is not seen in this species with chlamydia alone.[33] The lymph node involvement in lymphogranuloma venereum is not present in feline pneumonitis. Even though the recent interest in neonatal pneumonia and conjunctivitis due to chlamydial infection is great, the cat is not the perfect analogue to examine. Lower respiratory involvement is seldom seen as part of the feline pneumonitis condition; experimental attempts to produce it by natural routes are not effective. The genital transmission from queen to kitten has promise,[34] but one must remember that the genital disease is asymptomatic and does not seem to play the major role in natural feline ocular disease.

Since the cytological response in the cat is different from that in humans,[2] a study of the feline immune mechanisms may be very satisfying. Why, indeed, is the feline syndrome nearly benign? Is it the difference in virulence factors of the chlamydial itself? Or is the parasite meeting with mechanisms that cripple its ability to produce extensive local damage? It may be interesting to investigate the cell-mediated response and the humoral antibody systems.

There are still many questions concerning the biology and pathology of chlamydia, some of which were posed by Dr. James Moulder in the recent international symposium of *Chlamydia*.[35] What regulates the developmental cycle? What is the nature of the surface receptors that bind chlamydia to host cells? Why are vaccines against chlamydial agents generally ineffective?[21,36,37] The questions easily continue.

REFERENCES

1. Thygeson, P.: Historical review of oculogenital disease. *Am J Ophthalmol*, 71:975–985, 1971.
2. Ostler, H. B., Schachter, J., and Dawson, C. R.: Accute follicular conjunctivitis of epizootic origin—feline pneumonitis. *Arch Ophthalmol*, 82:587–591, 1969.
3. Storz, J.: *Chlamydia and Chlamydial-induced Diseases.* Springfield, Charles C Thomas, 1971.
4. Friis, R. R.: Interaction of L cell and *C. psittaci*: entry of the parasite and host responses to its development. *J Bacteriol*, 110:706–721, 1972.
5. Caldwell, H. D., Kromhout, J., and Schachter, J.: Purification and partial characterization of the major outer membrane protein of *C. trachomatis*. *Infect Immun*, 31:1161–1176, 1981.
6. Shewen, P. E.: Chlamydial infections in animals: a review. *Can Vet J*, 21:2–11, 1980.
7. Pearce, J. H., and Allan, I.: Differential amino acid requirements of chlamydiae: regulation of growth and relationship with clinical syndrome. In Mardh, P. A. (Ed.): *Proceedings*

of the V International Symposium on Human Chlamydial Infections. Amsterdam, Elsevier Biomedical Press, 1982, pp. 29–32.
8. Dickie, C. W., and Sniff, E. S.: Chlamydia infection associated with peritonitis in a cat. *J Am Vet Med Assoc, 176*:1256–1259, 1980.
9. Hoover, E. A.: Feline pneumonitis. In Kirk, R. W. (Ed.): *Current Veterinary Therapy VII.* Philadelphia, Saunders, 1980.
10. Peiffer, R. L.: Feline ophthalmology. In Gellatt, K. N. (Ed.): *Veterinary Ophthalmology.* Philadelphia, Lea and Febiger, 1981, pp. 520–568.
11. Martin, C. L.: Feline ophthalmologic diseases: conjunctival diseases. *Mod Vet Pract, 62*:929–933, 1981.
12. Hoover, E. A., Kahn, D. E., and Langlass, J. M.: Experimentally induced feline chlamydial infection (feline pneumonitis). *Am J Vet Res, 39*:541–547, 1978.
13. Cello, R. M.: Clues to differential diagnosis for feline respiratory infections. *J Am Vet Med Assoc, 158*:968–973, 1971.
14. Gaskin, J. M.: Microbiology of the canine and feline eye. *Vet Clin North Am Small Anim Pract, 10*:303–316, 1980.
15. Wilkes, R. D.: Infectious diseases of neonatal cats. *Fla Vet J, 10*:11–14, 1981.
16. Shewen, P. E., Povery, R. C., and Wilson, M. R.: A survey of the conjunctival flora of clinically normal cats and cats with conjunctivitis. *Can Vet J, 21*:231–233, 1980.
17. Darougar, S., Monnickendam, J. A., El-Sheikh, H., Treharne, J. D., Woodland, R. M., and Jones, B. R.: Animal models for the study of chlamydial infections of the eye and genital tract. In Hobson, D, and Holmes, K. K. (Eds.): *Nongonococcal Urethritis and Related Infections.* Washington, D.C., Am Soc for Microbiol, 1980, pp. 186–198.
18. Darouger, S., Woodland, R. M., and Monnickendam, J. A.: Chlamydial infections in cats and guinea pigs as models for human chlamydial infections. *J Med Microbiol, 13*:xi, 1980.
19. Theobald, J.: Felidae. In Fowler, M. E. (Ed.): *Zoo and Wild Animal Medicine.* Philadelphia, Saunders, 1978, pp. 650–667.
20. Jones, B. R.: The prevention of blindness from trachoma. *Trans Ophthalmol Soc UK, 95*:210–213, 1975.
21. Cello, R. M.: Microbiological and immunologic aspects of feline pneumonitis. *J Am Vet Med Assoc, 158*:932–938, 1971.
22. Yoneda, C., Dawson, C. R., Daghfous, T., Hoshiwara, I., Jones, P., Messadi, M., and Schachter, J.: Cytology as a guide to the presence of chlamydial inclusions in Giemsa-stained conjunctival smears in severe endemic trachoma. *Br J Ophthalmol, 59*:116–124, 1975.
23. Lavach, J. D., Thrall, M. A., Benjamin, M. M., and Severin, G. A.: Cytology of normal and inflamed conjunctivas in dogs and cats. *J Am Vet Med Assoc, 170*:722–727, 1977.
24. Stephens, R. S., Kuo, C. C., and Tam, M. R.: Sensitivity of immunofluorescence with monoclonal antibodies for detection of *C. trachomatis* inclusions in cell culture. *J Clin Microbiol, 16*:4–7, 1982.
25. Woodland, R. M., Sheikh, H., Darougar, S., and Squires, S.: Sensitivity of immunoperoxidase and immunofluorescence staining for detecting chlamydia in conjunctival scrapings and in cell culture. *J Clin Pathol, 31*:1073–1077, 1978.
26. Lamont, H. C., and Nichols, R. L.: Immunology of chlamydial infections. In Nahmias, A. J., and O'Reilly, R. J. (Eds.): *Immunology of Human Infection.* New York, Plenum Publishing Corporation, 1981, pp 441–474.
27. Mitzel, J. R., and Strating, A.: Vaccination against feline pneumonitis. *Am J Vet Res, 38*:1361–1363, 1977.

28. Kolar, J. R., and Rude, T. A.: Duration of immunity in cats inoculated with a commercial feline pneumonitis vaccine. *VM/SAC, 76*:1171–1173, 1981.
29. Shewen, P. E., Povey, R. C., and Wilson, M. R.: A comparison of a live and four inactivated vaccine preparations for the protection of cats against experimental challenge with *C. psittaci*. *Can J Comp Med, 44*:244–251, 1980.
30. Ostler, H. B., Schachter, J., and Dawson, C. R.: Acute follicular conjunctivitis of epizootic origin—feline pneumonitis. *Arch Ophthalmol, 82*:587–591, 1969.
31. Regan, R. J., Dathan, J. R., and Treharne, J. D.: Infective endocarditis with glomerulonephritis associated with cat Chlamydia (*C. psittaci*) infection. *Br Heart J, 42*:349–352, 1979.
32. Schachter, J., Ostler, H. B., and Meyer, K. F.: Human infection with the agent of feline pneumonitis. *Lancet, 7605*:1063–1065, 1969.
33. Taylor, H. R., Prendergast, R. A., Dawson, C. R., Schachter, J., and Silverstein, A. M.: An animal model for cicatrizing trachoma. *Invest Ophthalmol Vis Sci, 21*:422–433, 1981.
34. Barron, A. L.: In March, P. A. et al. (Eds.): *Proceedings of the V International Symposium on Human Chlamydial Infections*. Amsterdam, Elsevier Biomedical Press, 1982, pp. 357–366.
35. Moulder, J. W.: In March, P. A. et al. (Eds.): *Proceedings of the V International Sympsium on Human Chlamydial Infections*. Amsterdam, Elsevier Biomedical Press, 1982, pp. 3–14.
36. Dawson, C. R.: Trachoma—antibiotics or vaccine? *Invest Ophthalmol, 13*:85–86, 1974.
37. Grayston, J. T., Woolridge, R. L., and Wang, S.: Trachoma vaccine studies in Taiwan. *Ann NY Acad Sci, 98*:352–367, 1962.

Chapter 7

CHLAMYDIAL CONJUNCTIVITIS IN THE GUINEA PIG

RAGA MALATY, M.D., PH.D.

Introduction

Guinea pig inclusion conjunctivitis (GPIC) was first described by Murray,[1] who recovered a chlamydial agent from a naturally occurring ocular infection. Since the inclusions recovered were loose and irregular and failed to show a glycogen matrix, and since the agent was not susceptible to sulfonamides or cycloserine, it was classified as a member of the *Chlamydia psittaci* group.[1,2] The disease can also involve the genital tract of male and female guinea pigs, and newborns of infected mothers were found to develop conjunctival GPIC soon after birth.[3,4]

Naturally Occurring GPIC

The naturally occurring ocular infection results in a mild, self-limited conjunctivitis.[1,5] The conjunctival changes consist of moderate hyperemia and edema, follicular hypertrophy, and a slight yellowish white discharge. These signs subside within a few weeks with no residual effect. Cytological examination of conjunctival scrapings show intracytoplasmic inclusions that appear loose and irregular. This is associated with a polymorphonuclear cellular response.

Experimental Ocular Infection With GPIC

Conjunctival inoculation of normal guinea pigs with GPIC organisms results in conjunctivitis one to five days postchallenge, depending on the size of the infecting dose.[1] An intense conjunctivitis with moderate hyperemia and diffuse infiltration accompanied by a watery-to-purulent discharge develops. Corneal involvement may be in the form of a superficial epithelial keratitis, and corneal vessels that are normally present become congested.[5,6] Kazdan et al.[5] observed dilatation of iris vessels and small fibrin clots in the anterior chamber in some of their animals during the first week after inoculation. This experimental infection is generally self-limited, lasting from three to four weeks, and shows no clinical evidence of conjunctival scarring. Cytological examination shows changes similar to those seen in the naturally occurring infection.

GPIC as a Model for Chronic Conjunctivitis

When a group of animals was rechallenged with increasing doses of GPIC one month after primary infection, only those receiving the higher doses of inoculum showed clinical and cytological signs of infection.[7] In addition, the disease resulting from rechallenge lasted only eight days. Cytological examination showed that chlamydial inclusions were limited to animals receiving the higher inocula, and the number of conjunctival epithelial cells showing inclusions was much lower than in the animals with primary infections. Histological examination of the cornea revealed a mononuclear cellular infiltration at the limbus in normal animals. Animals receiving the highest rechallenge inoculum were the only ones showing a different histological picture in the form of polymorphonuclear cells at the limbus and in the overlying epithelium. The central corneal stroma showed some round cells.

Guinea pigs inoculated with GPIC in the conjunctiva developed a chronic conjunctival inflammation that persisted for many months. Following these repeated inoculations, the animals developed a pannus in the superior region of the cornea, follicles on the palpebral conjunctivae, scarring of the lower palpebral conjunctiva, and deformities of the lower lid.[8] The number of chlamydial inclusions decreased with time after the repeated infections. Giemsa-stained scrapings of the conjunctiva show evidence of a decrease in polymorphonuclear response while the number of mononuclear cells becomes much higher. These responses and lesions are similar to those seen in trachoma, and studies on ocular infection with GPIC indicate that guinea pigs become partially immune following primary ocular infection.[1,5,6,7]

GPIC as a Model for Extraocular Chlamydial Infections

Experimental sexual transmission of GPIC has established the guinea pig as a model for human genital chlamydial infections and inclusion conjunctivitis. Intravaginal infection of pregnant female guinea pigs resulted in vaginal infection. This was demonstrated by detection of GPIC inclusions in the epithelial cells of genital tract smears, in histological sections, and by isolation of the agent.[3] Newborn guinea pigs of infected mothers developed conjunctival infections three to five days after birth. Male guinea pigs were also infected intraurethrally with GPIC and could transmit GPIC infections to females during mating.[4]

Complications of genital chlamydial infections have also been studied. Human infections have been complicated by salpingitis, endometritis, pelvic inflammatory disease, peritonitis, and perihepatitis. Direct inoculation of GPIC in the guinea pig uterine horn resulted in a self-limiting salpingitis.[9] However, some of these animals may develop a hydrosalpinx as a late complication of the acute infection.[10] Experimental vaginal infection of immunosuppressed guinea pigs resulted in a prolonged infection that spread to the fallopian tubes. Endometritis was also observed on histopathologic examination. GPIC was found in cells of the epithelial lining of the endometrium and in peritoneal mesothelial cells.[11] Administration of estradiol to female guinea pigs with genital chlamydial infection resulted in prolongation of the infection, which was complicated by an ascending infection with endometritis and cystic salpingitis.[12]

Proctitis is another problem that has been demonstrated by studies of the guinea pig. Intrarectal inoculation of GPIC resulted in infection in both males and females.[13] This animal infection is similar to human rectal infections reported in infants perinatally exposed to *Chlamydia* and in children in trachoma endemic areas.[14,15]

GPIC as a Model for the Study of Immunity in Chlamydial Infections

The earlier studies of GPIC infections have shown that primary infection renders the animals resistant to reinfection. This resistance wanes with time and can be overcome by high titer inoculum.[7] Immunity differs according to the site of primary infection. Mount et al.[4] demonstrated that ocular infection resulted in systemic immunity and showed resistance to both ocular and genital challenge with GPIC agent. Genital infection, on the other hand, did not afford resistance to infection via the ocular route. Male guinea pigs infected in the urethra with GPIC agent developed resistance to challenge of the urethra, but these animals remained susceptible to infection of the eye. Inoculation of the eye, however, resulted in immunity to both ocular and urethral infection.[16]

The GPIC model has been used extensively to study the role of humoral and cellular immune mechanisms in chlamydial infections. Serum and tear secretory antibodies can be demonstrated following experimental GPIC infection. Skin tests and migration inhibition tests indicate cell-mediated immunity.[17,18] Local antibody and cellular immunity appear simultaneously with the disappearance of the infectious agent. Cyclophosphamide treated guinea pigs inoculated with GPIC show persistence of agent and an accompanying delay in serum and tear secretory antibody response, although skin tests are positive ten days after infection.[19] Similar treatment of genitally infected animals showed that the infection was prolonged in the absence of a humoral immune response.[20]

The role of serum and tear antibodies in the host response to repeated GPIC infection has been studied in the guinea pig.[21] Resistance to challenge with a high dose inoculum was found to be associated with serum and tear antibodies. Immune tears or immune serum were applied to the external eye of guinea pigs two days before and five days after a high inoculum of GPIC. Treatment with immune serum resulted in delay in the growth of the agent, but only during the period of application. This was demonstrated by significant reduction in the number of intracytoplasmic inclusion bodies. The effect afforded a similar delay in the onset of infection but the infection was less severe (Fig. 7-1).

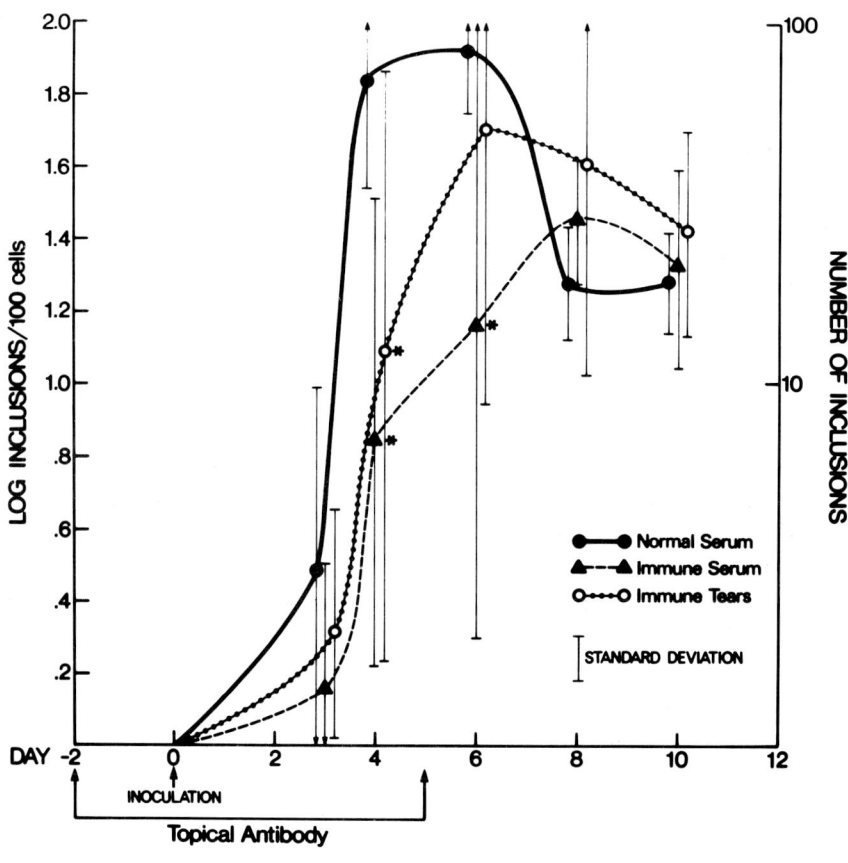

Figure 7-1. Effect of topical treatment with immune serum and immune tears on the growth of GPIC agent following conjunctival inoculation with 250 ELD_{50} GPIC. Topical antibody was applied 2 days before and 5 days after inoculation with GPIC. Conjunctival smears were taken before inoculation and 3, 4, 5, 6, 12, 16, 21, and 28 days after inoculation. Application of immune serum resulted in a significant reduction in the number of inclusions on days 4 and 5. With immune tears, retardation of the growth of the agent was significant only on day 4.

Serum antibodies are clearly associated with resistance to challenge infection with GPIC. However, the mechanism of immunity in the natural host has not been clearly defined. Attachment of antibody to the infective particles appears to allow lysosomal enzymes to enter the inclusion vacuole.[22] It is unclear why high titers of antibody are necessary for this mechanism to occur *in vivo*. The level of antibody may simply be an indication of the other immune mechanisms at work.

Vaccination Studies with GPIC

ENTERIC VACCINES: Oral administration of living GPIC suspensions to guinea pigs results in partial protection from mucosal infection whereby subsequent challenge to the conjunctiva or the vagina resulted in a less severe disease and a lower number of inclusions in mucosal cells.[23]

TOPICAL VACCINES: Heat-killed GPIC applied topically to the conjunctiva prior to challenge afforded no protection. No antibodies were detected at the time of challenge, but animals developed a secondary type of antibody response when challenged so that the local exposure appears to have "primed" them.[21]

Studies of Host-Parasite Relationships in GPIC

Peroxidase enzyme activity has been demonstrated in normal rat conjunctival epithelium.[24] Cytochemical studies of guinea pig conjunctival epithelium showed that peroxidase enzyme was not produced by normal cells. When guinea pigs were infected with GPIC, however, peroxidase was activated. The reaction appeared two days after inoculation and persisted for six to seven weeks. The enzyme was localized in the rough endoplasmic reticulum and perinuclear cisterna in all layers of the epithelium. Cells with and without chlamydial inclusions showed a positive reaction. The reaction remained outside the chlamydial vacuoles, however, and was not apparent in the lysosomes (Figure 7-2). It appears that the enzyme stimulated by infection is not directly responsible for the waning of the disease but is itself a result of an alteration in the host's metabolism produced by the infection.[25]

Summary

Several animal models have been used for the study of human chlamydial infections. Nonhuman primates have been used in the study of human ocular and genital chlamydial infections.[26-28] However, an animal model with a naturally occurring chlamydial infection may throw light on many aspects of the disease. Although the GPIC agent belongs to the *C. psittaci* group, the natural and experimental infections in its host show a close similarity to human *Chlamydia trachomatis* infections. The susceptible cells seem to be the same: columnar epithelial cells of the conjunctiva, vagina, fallopian tube, rectum, and urethra. Primary conjunctival infection results in a self-limited disease, while repeated infections result in conjunctival scarring and lid deformities resembling the sequelae of human trachoma. As in human chlamydial infections, venereal transmission and eye-to-eye trans-

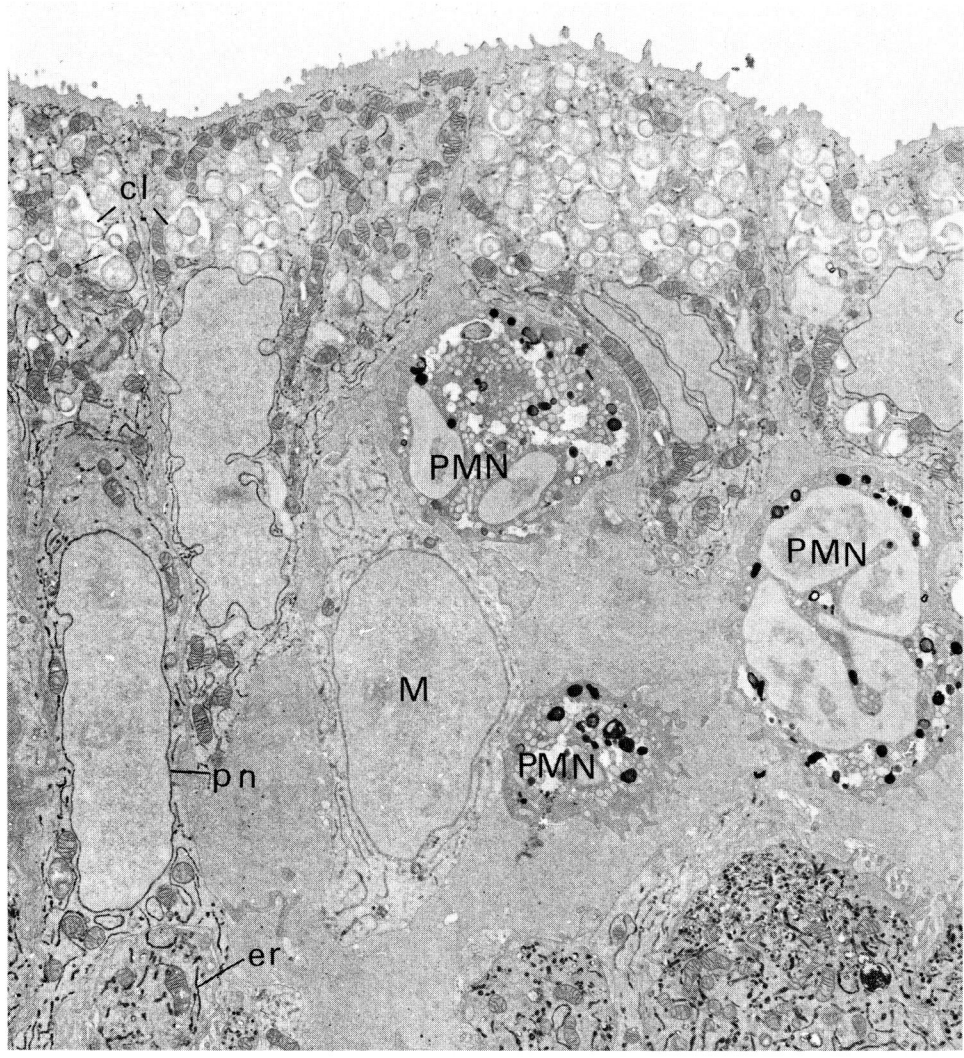

Figure 7-2. Tarsal conjunctiva from a guinea pig infected for 48 hours with *Chlamydia*, then tested for peroxidase. In this specimen, all the cells at the surface contain a large number of chlamydial inclusions (ci). Note that the irregular nuclei of the epithelial cells are outlined by the dense deposits of reaction product for peroxidase in the perinuclear cisternae (pn). Although reactive cisternae of RER (er) are liberally distributed throughout the cells, there is no reaction in the chlamydial inclusion. Three polymorphonuclear leukocytes (PMN) and a macrophage (M) have invaded the infected tissue. Some of the neutrophil granules are reactive for peroxidase, whereas others are not. The RER of the macrophage contains noticeably less peroxidase activity than that of the epithelial cells. The RER of the uninfected cells of the basal layers of the conjunctiva is reactive, as are the infected cells at the surface. ×5000.

mission may occur, and newborns passing through an infected birth canal may develop conjunctivitis. These similarities emphasize the value of the GPIC model in the study of human *C. trachomatis* infections.

REFERENCES

1. Murray, E. S.: Guinea pig inclusion conjunctivitis virus. I. Isolation and identification as a member of the psittacosis lymphogranuloma-trachoma group. *J Infect Dis, 114*:1–12, 1964.
2. Gordon, F. B., Weiss, E., Quan, A. L., and Dressler, H. R.: Observations on guinea pig inclusion conjunctivitis agent. *J Infect Dis, 116*:203–207, 1966.
3. Mount, D. T., Bigazzi, P. E., and Barron, A. L.: Infection of genital tract and transmission of ocular infection to newborns by the agent of guinea pig inclusion conjunctivitis. *Infect Immun, 5*:921–926, 1972.
4. Mount, D. T., Bigazzi, P. E., and Barron, A. L.: Experimental genital infection of male guinea pigs with the agent of guinea pig inclusion conjunctivitis and transmission to females. *Infect Immun, 8*:926–930, 1973.
5. Kazdan, J. J., Schachter, J., and Okumoto, M. A.: Inclusion conjunctivitis in the guinea pig. *Am J Ophthalmol, 64*:116–124, 1967.
6. Monnickendam, M. A., Darougar, S., Treharne, J. D., and Tilbury, A. M.: Guinea pig inclusion conjunctivitis as a model for the study of trachoma: Clinical, microbiological, serological and cytological studies of primary infection. *Br J Ophthalmol, 64*:279–283, 1980.
7. Ahmad, A., Dawson, C. R., Yoneda, C., Togni, B., and Schachter, J.: Resistance to reinfection with a chlamydial agent (guinea pig inclusion conjunctivitis agent). *Invest Ophthalmol Vis Sci, 16*:549–553, 1977.
8. Monnickendam, M. A., Darougar, S., Treharne, J. D., and Tilbury, A. M.: Development of chronic conjunctivitis with scarring and pannus, resembling trachoma, in guinea pigs. *Br J Ophthalmol, 64*:284–290, 1980.
9. Sweet, R. J., Banks, J., Sung, M., Donegan, E., and Schachter J.: Experimental chlamydial salpingitis in the guinea pig. *Am J Obstet Gynecol, 138*:952–956, 1980.
10. Schachter, J., Banks, J., Sung, M., and Sweet, R.: Hydrosalpinx as a consequence of chlamydial salpingitis in the guinea pig. In Mardh, P.-A., Holmes, K. K., Oriel, J. D., Piot, P., and Schachter, J. (Eds): *Chlamydial Infections*. Amsterdam, Elsevier Biomedical Press, 1982, pp. 371–374.
11. White, H. J., Rank, R. G., Soloff, B. L., and Barron, A. L.: Experimental chlamydial salpingitis in immunosuppressed guinea pigs infected in the genital tract with the agent of guinea pig inclusion conjunctivitis. *Infect Immun, 26*:728–735, 1979.
12. Rank, R. G., White, H. J., Matthews, H. M., and Barron, A. L.: Abstracts of 81st Annual Meeting, American Society for Microbiology, Washington, D.C., 1981.
13. Mount, D. R., and Barron, A. L.: Intrarectal infection of guinea pigs with the agents of guinea pig inclusion conjunctivitis. *Proc Soc Exp Biol Med, 153*:388–391, 1976.
14. Schachter, J., Grossman, M., Holt, J., Sweet, R., and Spector, S.: Infection with *Chlamydia trachomatis*: Involvement of multiple anatomic sites in neonates. *J Infect Dis, 139*:232–234, 1979.
15. Malaty, R., Zaki, S., Said, M. E., Vastine, D. W., Dawson, C. R., and Schachter, J.: Extraocular infections in children in endemic trachoma. *J Inf Dis, 146*:853, 1981.

16. Howard, L. V., O'Leary, M. P., and Nichols, R. L.: Animal model studies of genital chlamydial infections. Immunity to reinfection with guinea pig inclusion conjunctivitis in the urethra and eyes of male guinea pigs. *Br J Vener Dis, 52*:261–265, 1976.
17. Murray, E. S., Charbonnet, L. T., and MacDonald, A. B.: Immunity to chlamydial infections of the eye. I. The role of circulatory and secretory antibodies in resistance to reinfection with guinea-pig inclusion conjunctivitis. *J Immunol, 110*:1518–1525, 1973.
18. Watson, R. R., MacDonald, A. B., Murray, E. S., and Modabber, F. Z.: Immunity to chlamydial infections of the eye. III. Presence and duration of delayed hypersensitivity to guinea pig inclusion conjunctivitis. *J Immunol, 111*:618–623, 1973.
19. Modabber, F., Bear, S. E., and Cerny, J.: The effect of cyclophosphamide on the recovery from a local chlamydial infection. *Immunology, 30*:929–933, 1976.
20. Rank, R. G., White, H. J., and Barron, A. L.: Humoral immunity in the resolution of genital infection in female guinea pigs infected with the agent of guinea pig inclusion conjunctivitis. *Infect Immun, 26*:573–579, 1979.
21. Malaty, R., Dawson, C. R., Wong, I., Lyon, C., and Schachter, J.: Serum and tear antibodies to *Chlamydia* after reinfection with guinea pig inclusion conjunctivitis agent. *Invest Ophthalmol Vis Sci, 21*:833–841, 1981.
22. Friis, R. R.: Interaction of L cells and *Chlamydia psittaci*: entry of the parasite and host responses to its development. *J Bacteriol, 110*:706–721, 1972.
23. Nichols, R. L., Murray, E. S., and Nisson, P. E.: Use of enteric vaccines in protection against chlamydial infections of the genital tract and eye of guinea pigs. *J Inf Dis, 138*:742–746, 1978.
24. Iwata, T.: Cytochemical studies on endogenous peroxidase in conjunctival and corneal epithelial cells. *J Inf Dis, 138*:742–756, 1978.
25. Malaty, R., Nichols, B., Schachter, J., Togni, B., and Dawson, C.: Stimulation of peroxidase by chlamydial infection: Cytochemistry of guinea pig conjunctival epithelium. *Infect Immun, 25*:417–426, 1979.
26. Wang, S. P., and Grayston, J. T.: Pannus with experimental trachoma and inclusion conjunctivitis agent infections of Taiwan monkey. *Am J Ophthalmol, 63*:1133–1145, 1967.
27. Murray, E. S., Frazer, C. E. O., and Peters, J. H.: The owl monkey as an experimental primate model for conjunctival trachoma infection. In Nichols, R. L. (Ed.): *Trachoma and Related Disorders caused by Chlamydial Agents*, Amsterdam, Excerpta Medica, 1971, pp. 386–395.
28. Alexander, E. R., and Chiang, W. T.: Infection of pregnant monkeys and their offspring with TRIC agents. *Am J Ophthalmol, 63*:1145–1153, 1967.

Chapter 8

OCULAR TOXOPLASMOSIS

EDUARDO P. PENNA, M.D.

Introduction

Toxoplasma gondii, an obligate intracellular organism, was first recognized in the beginning of this century (1908) in acute infections of a North African rodent, *Stenodactilus gondi,*[1] and in rabbits in Brazil.[2] The name was derived from the Greek word *toxon* ("bow" or "arc") alluding to the lunate shape of the free *Toxoplasma,* plus the rodent name, "gondi."

Until recently, the parasites were recognized only as free and encysted intracellular organisms. Because spores, oocysts, and the life cycle were unknown, *Toxoplasma* was excluded from the *Sporozoa* and was considered a "parasitological curiosity."[3] The recent discovery of the coccidian stages of *Toxoplasma* in the cat intestine[4-7] has considerably broadened our understanding of toxoplasmosis and its transmission.

Toxoplasma gondii has been shown serologically and histopathologically in human beings, sheep, cattle, pigs, chickens, and many other species of warm-blooded animals and is now considered to infect at least one-third of animal and human populations in most areas of the world.[8]

Life Cycle and Epidemiology

Life cycle

Felines are the definitive hosts of *Toxoplasma gondii,* and numerous species of animals serve as intermediate hosts (Fig. 8-1). In the cat, *Toxoplasma* has two cycles and five stages. The enteroepithelial multiplicative stage is generally similar to that in other coccidia and leads to schizogony, gametogony, and oocyst production with sporogony occurring in two to five days in the external environment. Two additional stages representing the asexual cycle occur in extraintestinal tissues of cats. This cycle is similar to that in other mammalian and avian hosts: tachyzoites form groups during the acute infection and bradyzoites develop within cysts during chronic infections.[9]

During acute infections *T. gondii* is a slender, arc-shaped organism, approximately 2 to 4 microns wide and 4 to 7 microns long, with one tapered end that is used to penetrate the host cell.[10] When stained with Giemsa, it resembles the merozoite of a malaria parasite, with a reddish or purplish nucleus and a light blue cytoplasm. It was once believed that this proliferative

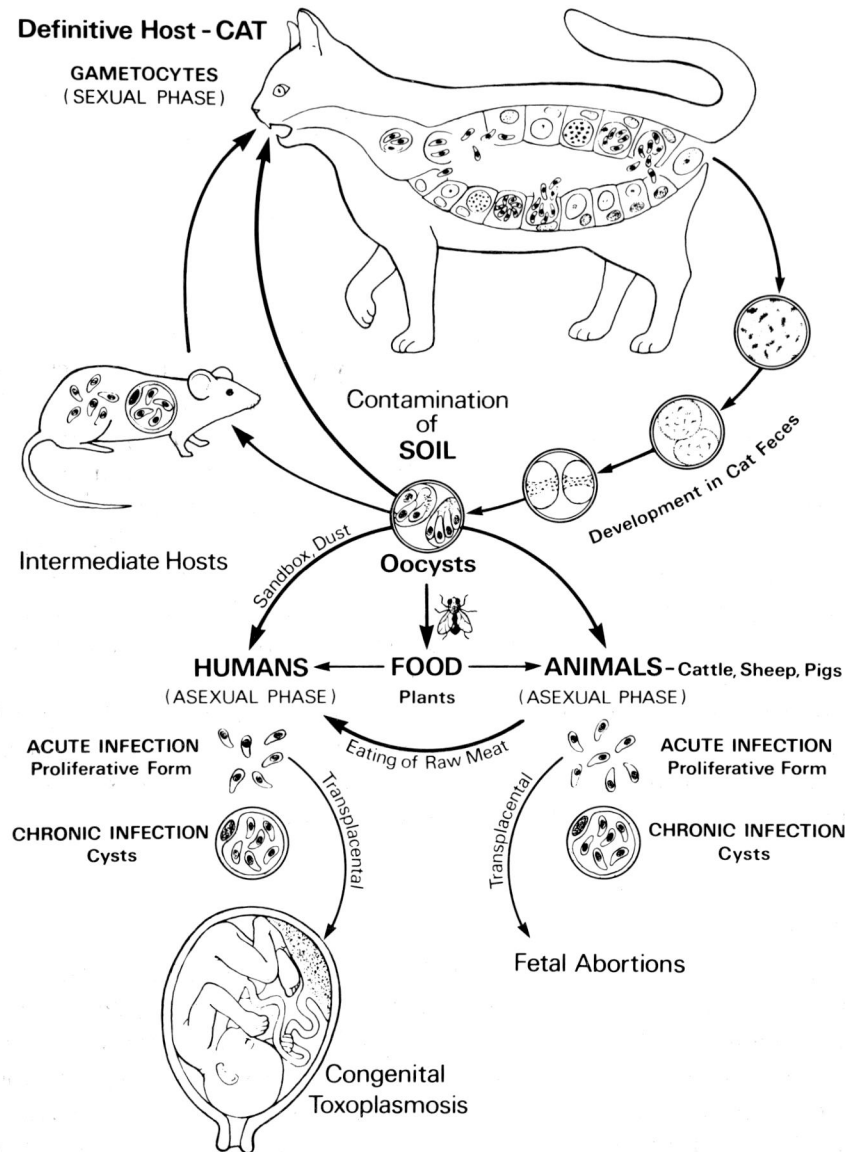

Figure 8-1. Life cycle of *Toxoplasma gondii*. (From Tabbara, K. F. "Ocular Toxoplasmosis." In Koch, DD, Parke, DW II, & Paton, D: *Current Management in Ophthalmology*. Copyright © 1983 by Churchill Livingstone Inc. Reprinted by permission of Churchill Livingstone, Inc., New York.)

form of *T. gondii* tachyzoite reproduced by a simple process of longitudinal division. However, it was discovered by Goldman and associates in 1958[11] that reproduction was by internal budding, or endodyogeny. This was one of the first clues relating *T. gondii* to the *Sporozoa*. The experimental work of Dubey and Frenkel[10] has shown that the proliferative form of *T. gondii* is found in the lamina propia of cat's intestine in from one to nine days after infection and longer in extraintestinal tissues after dissemination through the bloodstream. It can be detected, for instance, in the mesenteric lymph nodes and in lungs up to 19 days and in the brain up to 23 days before becoming encysted. In chronic infections, the proliferative form (tachyzoite) is not present but *T. gondii* persists for years in the tissues of its hosts, commonly in the brain and muscles, as encysted parasites (bradyzoite).[12] Originally, these structures were considered "pseudocysts" (aglomerations of parasites within the host cell wall), from which the host cell nucleus has been extruded. However, Frenkel[8] has shown that the wall of the cyst is a dense matrix of PAS-positive material deposited originally on the inner membrane of the host cell and thus is a true parasite cyst. The formation of cysts can be observed early in acute infections of animals (7 to 8 days) even without demonstrable humoral immunity;[10] thus, the cyst seems to be a stage in the cycle of the parasite and does not always require the influence of immune reactions in the host for its information. The organism reproduces slowly within the cysts and it also reproduces by endodyogeny.

Epidemiology

Felines are essential in the epidemiology of the *T. gondii* because they are the only host species known to excrete resistant isosporan oocysts in feces.[13] Cats probably acquire infection by ingesting cysts in the tissues of intermediate hosts. This explains why young kittens that are not very successful in capturing small rodents or birds until reaching five or six months of age have lower titers of antibody to *Toxoplasma* than mature cats.[14] Experimental studies[15,16] have demonstrated that most felines excrete oocysts after infection with *Toxoplasma*. The ingestion of each stage is followed by a characteristic prepatent period before oocysts appear in the feces: three to five days after ingestion of cysts, five to ten days after ingestion of trophozoites (feeding form), and 21–24 days after ingestion of cysts. Excretion lasts for one to three weeks and oocysts are rarely reexcreted after new infections. It has also been shown that the oocysts are the most infective form of *Toxoplasma* to cats.

Humans and animals acquire *Toxoplasma* infections mainly by ingesting cysts in undercooked meat and oocysts from sand boxes and soil contaminated with cat feces.[9] Experimental infections have shown that all mammals and birds can become infected and that *Toxoplasma* can be reisolated from tissues, especially from the brain and muscles, during the chronic phase of infection. Even the chicken, considered to be remarkably resistant to toxoplasmosis,[17] has been proven to develop parasitemia and cyst formation in the brain, muscle, ovary oviduct, kidney, and intestine.[18,19]

Various serological and parasitological surveys have revealed the widespread occurrence of *T. gondii* in animals raised for human consumption. Al-Khalidi and Dubey[20] observed that 10 percent of 500 horses slaughtered for pet food had antibody titers to *T. gondii* (dye test) and that 5 of 16 cats (31.2%) fed with the pooled equine tissues shed *Toxoplasma* oocysts in their feces. Makinde and Ezeh[21] found that 260 of 891 swine (29%) from 20 California counties were seropositive to *Toxoplasma* (indirect hemaglutination method). Riemann and associates[22] observed that four of ten goats studied were seropositive to *Toxoplasma* (dye test). Jacobs and Melton[18] observed the parasite in 12 of 62 pools (20%) of tissues from the ovaries and oviducts of apparently healthy hens. Catar and co-workers[23] isolated *Toxoplasma* from brains and diaphragmatic muscles of 43.3 percent of 30 pigs and from 9.4 percent of 85 cattle, studied with complement fixation test positive to 1:4. Jacobs et al.,[24] by using a positive *Toxoplasma* dye test, found the organism in 67 percent of sheep. The diaphragm was the most consistently parasitized, the psoas muscle next, and the brain the least.

The most common source of toxoplasmosis among animals is through congenital infection. All mammals may transmit infection congenitally when the acute phase of infection and pregnancy occur simultaneously. Experimental infections in pregnant sows,[25,26] bitches,[27] cows,[26] chickens,[18] sheep,[28] and cats[29] have shown that in all those animals congenital toxoplasmosis can cause abortion as well as stillborn and premature offspring. Naturally occurring congenital infections are prominent among sheep, and *T. gondii* is considered the major cause of abortions in sheep in New Zealand and England,[30,31] causing great economic loss. Plant and associates[28] diagnosed congenital infections in 37 of 38 flocks of lambs (10.1%). Hartley and Moyle[32] isolated *T. gondii* from 14 of 15 congenitally infected sheep and found the brain to be positive in 87 percent and muscle in 55 percent. Munday and co-workers,[31] studying material from ovine abortion/stillbirth outbreaks with undiagnosed causes, found that vibriosis and toxoplasmosis (27% each) were the main disease conditions. Acquired congenital toxoplasmosis has also been observed, although much less frequently, among goats,[33] cattle,[31] and cats.[34]

Other modes of uncommon toxoplasmosis transmission described in humans and animals are through blood transfusion,[35] by laboratory accident,[36] by ingestion of raw eggs,[18] and by drinking unpasteurized goat milk.[22]

Disease and Diagnosis

Disease

Considering the high prevalence of *Toxoplasma* antibody in nature, the common finding of *Toxoplasma* cysts in several slaughterhouse examinations of animal meat, and the rarity of clinical disease, it is clear that the majority of infections are asymptomatic in animals.[6] It seems that most animals after becoming infected with *Toxoplasma* present one mild acute phase, not clinically detected, with silent, systemic dissemination of the trophozoites to several organs, especially the muscles, brain, and eyes.

The symptomatic infections are manifested in either acute or chronic phases. The acute symptomatic infection terminates either with the death of the host, rarely seen, or with the development of immunity and chronic infection. Through experimental work, it has been shown that during the acute infection, after ingestion of *Toxoplasma* cysts or oocysts, the enteric infection spreads to the regional lymph nodes and via the portal circulation to the liver. From the lymph nodes, *Toxoplasma* reaches the thoracic duct and the lungs; from the liver, the organisms spread via the venous circulation to the lungs also. From there, the parasites are disseminated through arterial circulation. The multiplication of the parasite tachyzoites and the production of lesions depends upon several factors such as the amount of inoculum, the immunity of the host, and the virulence of the *Toxoplasma*. During the acute disease, *Toxoplasma* is frequently isolated from the blood and antibody titers are high. After some time, usually around two weeks,[9] cysts develop intracellularly, especially in neurons, retinal cells, and skeletal muscles.

During the chronic phase, cysts remain almost dormant in tissues and multiplication of the cystic bradyzoites is slow or negligible. Intact cysts may remain for months or years without invoking an inflammatory reaction.[6] An ever-increasing body of evidence indicates that cellular immunity is responsible for keeping the infection at bay in chronically infected human subjects or animals.[37] When immunity is impaired or abolished by other diseases, by administration of corticosteroids, or by cytotoxic agents, there may be a relapse of the disease caused by cyst rupture, after which the liberated bradyzoites enter new cells and multiply as tachyzoites. This condition is commonly seen in the ocular lesions of human toxoplasmosis, the most common form of the clinical disease during the chronic phase.[38]

Because most *Toxoplasma* infections are asymptomatic, whether acquired congenitally or not, signs and symptoms of the disease are rarely reported. In humans, the acute phase of toxoplasmosis appears as a mononucleosis syndrome characterized by fever, headache, mylagia, lymphadenopathy, splenomegaly, and high and rising titers of antibody to *Toxoplasma* in the serum.[39] Among the animals, only cats have a defined clinical entity. The acute feline toxoplasmosis is clinically characterized by anorexia, lethargy, high temperature, pneumonialike symptoms, and dyspnea a few days prior to death.[40] It is interesting that in cats, as in humans, the chronic infection is usually restricted to ocular involvement (without other systemic signs and symptoms). It is also thought that most cases of ocular toxoplasmosis are congenital, so that the cysts, after becoming localized in the eye structures during pregnancy, break down late in life. The ocular involvement is characterized by a necrotizing chorioretinitis that can be accompanied by anterior uveitis (iridocyclitis) with redness, flare, and keratic precipitates in the anterior chamber. Vanisi and Campbell[41] described ten cases of chorioretinitis in cats that were confirmed by histopathologic examinations. They found anterior uveitis in only three cats (30%) and noted that many cases of ocular toxoplasmosis in animals are probably overlooked because fundic examination is not routine among veterinarians.

The studies of Piper and associates,[16] however, yield a different opinion. In their studies of experimental toxoplasmosis they found that iridocyclitis was more frequent than chorioretinitis and that they could isolate the *Toxoplasma* from the iris and ciliary body in five dogs, three cats, and two pigs. These findings are important because *Toxoplasma* has never been found in the anterior segment of the eye in humans and ocular toxoplasmosis is considered to be a disease of the retina. Inflammation of the anterior uvea is a later manifestation of hypersensitivity to *Toxoplasma* antigens and is not associated with invasion of the anterior ocular structures by the parasite.

Diagnosis

A diagnosis of toxoplasmosis often depends upon a combination of signs, symptoms, serology, histopathology, and the isolation of *Toxoplasma*.[9] Histopathology and isolation are possible only in experimental studies and are not done routinely. Therefore, diagnosis is usually based upon the signs and symptoms associated with the serologic tests. As mentioned before, *Toxoplasma* antibody is commonly found in the normal population, so that a positive serologic test merely indicates past or present asymptomatic infection and does not necessarily indicate a disease. In fact, it is important to point out that antibody titers need not be high, since *Toxoplasma* can cause clinical disease even with low antibody titers.[9,42] Thus, a diagnosis of toxoplasmosis can be made in the presence of any sign or symptom of the disease associated with any level of *Toxoplasma* antibody. If possible, the best procedure is to do a second serologic test, and it can be assumed that the infection is an active disease if there is an increase in the titer of antibody to *T. gondii*.

The Sabin-Feldman dye test is considered the standard serologic test for *Toxoplasma* antibodies.[40] It is based on the phenomenon that *Toxoplasma* organisms normally stain with methylene blue but not with serum containing *Toxoplasma* antibodies. The highest dilution of serum in which 50 percent or more of the parasites remain unstained by the dye is considered to be the end point of the titer of the serum. The dye test is the most reliable because antibodies appear during the early stages of infection,[6] because they are measurable in from three to five days depending on the host, and because the titers persist longer than in any other tests. Because the Sabin-Feldman dye test requires a supply of normal human serum as an accessory factor and the maintenance of live parasites, which are dangerous to handle, it has lost popularity and is now used mostly in research work.

Of the other serologic tests, the indirect fluorescent method (IFA) has become the most widely used for clinical purposes because of its simplicity and because it yields results comparable to the dye test. Another advantage of the IFA is that it can detect IgG *Toxoplasma* antibody as well as IgM. This is important in the diagnosis of congenital toxoplasmosis because IgM, unlike IgG, does not cross the placenta. The test, therefore, reveals active infection in the newborn.

The other two most common tests, the complement fixation antibody test and the hemaglutination antibody test, are not very useful in the diagnosis of toxoplasmosis. With the complement fixation test, although it is simple and gives titers that are usually parallel to the dye test and the IFA, detectable levels of antibody appear two to three weeks after infection and persist only for a few months. The hemaglutination test is often difficult to interpret.[40]

Prevention and Treatment

Prevention

There are two major ways in which toxoplasmosis is acquired: through consumption of raw meat, and through contact with the feces of cats infected with *T. gondii*. With regard to the former, animals should be fed only cooked meat because the tissue cyst can be rendered noninfective by heating meat to 60°C (150°F). Since cats are the only animals known to produce the oocyst form, efforts should be made to prevent cats from becoming infected with posterior shedding oocysts.[43] Feeding cats dry or canned food, rather than allowing them to depend on hunting as their source of food, will reduce the likelihood of infection. If diet cannot be controlled, the litter pan should be cleaned daily, feces flushed down the toilet, and the pan disinfected with boiling water. Since soil contaminated by oocysts of *T. gondii* in feline feces is difficult to disinfect, gloves should be worn when working with soil that may contain cat feces.[9]

Treatment

The drugs most commonly used are the sulfonamides and pyrimethamines, which are effective individually and synergistically. Their pharmacological basis for the therapy of toxoplasmosis is the competitive inhibition of two sequential steps in the biosynthetic pathway leading to folinic acid, a substance essential to *T. gondii*.[9] This chemotherapy suppresses proliferating *Toxoplasma* but does little to affect the cysts. Treatment is usually directed at the symptoms of toxoplasmosis until the active immunity becomes effective and, as stated above, the mere presence of antibodies to *Toxoplasma* does not indicate disease or the need for treatment. Side effects, mainly thrombocytopenia and leukepenia, can be counteracted with foline acid, which the host can utilize but which *Toxoplasma* cannot. Certain other drugs, not based on the same mechanism, such as spiramycin, clindamycin, and tetracycline derivatives, have shown some effectiveness in experimental infections,[44,45] but are not now in common clinical use.

REFERENCES

1. Nicolle, C., and Manceaux, L.: Sur une infection à corps de Leishman (ou organismes voisins du gondi). *Compt Rend Acad Sci, 147*:763, 1908.
2. Splendore, A.: Un nuovo protozoa parasita dei conigli: incontrato nelle lesioni anatomiche d'una malattia che ricorda in moti punti il Kalazar dell'uomo. *Rev Soc Sci São Paulo, 3*:109, 1908.
3. Jacobs, L.: Toxoplasmosis in man and animals. *New Zealand Vet J 9*:85, 1961.
4. Hutchinson, W. M., Dunachie, J. P., and Work, K.: The fecal transmission of Toxoplasma gondii. *Acta Pathol Microbiol Scand, 74*:462, 1968.
5. Sheffield, H. G., and Melton, M. L.: Toxoplasma gondii: The oocyst sporozoite and infection of cultured cells. *Science, 167*:892, 1970.
6. Dubey, J. P., and Miller, N. L.: Toxoplasma gondii in cats: Fecal stages identified as coccidian oocysts. *Science, 167*:893, 1970.
7. Dubey, J. P., and Johnstone, I.: Fatal neonatal toxoplasmosis in cats. *J Am Anim Hosp Assoc, 18*:461, 1982.
8. Frenkel, J. K.: Toxoplasmosis: Mechanisms of infection, laboratory diagnosis and management. *Current Topics in Pathol, 54*:28, 1971.
9. Frenkel, J. K.: Toxoplasmosis: Parasite, life cycle, pathology and immunology. In D.M. Hammond and P.L. Long: *The Coccidia*. Baltimore, Park Press, 1973, p. 343.
10. Dubey, J. P., and Frenkel, J.K.: Cyst-induced toxoplasmosis in cats. *J. Protoxool, 24*:184, 1972.
11. Goldman, M., Carver, R. K., and Sulzer, A. J.: Reproduction of Toxoplasma gondii by internal budding. *J Parasit, 44*:161, 1958.
12. Miller, N. L., Frenkel, J. K., and Dubey, J. P.: Oral infections with toxoplasma cysts and oocysts in feline, other mammals and in birds. *J Parasit, 58*:928, 1972.
13. Munday, B. L.: Serological evidence of toxoplasma infection in isolated groups of sheep. *Res Vet Sci, 13*:100, 1972.
14. Wallace, G. D.: Isolation of Toxoplasma gondii from the feces of naturally infected cats. *J Infec Dis, 124*:227, 1971.
15. Dubey, J. P., Hoover, E. A., and Walls, K. W.: Effect of age and sex on the acquisition of immunity to toxoplasmosis in cats. *J Protozool, 24*:184, 1977.
16. Piper, J. W., Beh, K. J., and Helen, M. A.: Laboratory findings from ovine abortion and perinatal mortality. *Aust Vet J, 48*:558, 1972.
17. Jones, F. E., Melton, M. L., Lunde, M. N., Eyles, D. E., and Jacobs, L.: Experimental toxoplasmosis in chickens. *J Parasit, 43*:31, 1959.
18. Jacobs, L., and Melton, M. L.: Toxoplasmosis in chickens. *J Parasit, 52*:1158, 1966.

19. Kulasiri, C. S.: Infection of chicken with avirulent Toxoplasma gondii. *Exp Parasit, 17*:65, 1965.
20. Al-Khalidi, N. W., and Dubey, J. P.: Prevalence of Toxoplasma gondii infections in horses. *J Parasit, 65*:331, 1965.
21. Makinde, A. A., and Ezeh, A. O.: Serological survey of Toxoplasma gondii in Nigerian cattle: a preliminary report. *Br Vet J, 137*:485, 1981.
22. Riemann, H. P., Meyer, M. E., Theis, J. H., Kelso, G., and Behymer, D. E.: Toxoplasmosis in an infant fed unpasteurized goat milk. *J Pediat, 87*:573, 1975.
23. Catar, G., Bergendi, L., and Halkova, R.: Isolation of Toxoplasma gondii from swine and cattle. *J Parasit, 55*:952, 1969.
24. Jacobs, L., Moyle, G. G., and Ris, R. R.: The prevalence of toxoplasma in New Zealand sheep and cattle. *Am J Vet Res, 24*:673, 1963.
25. Moller, T., Fennestad, K. L., Erickson, L., and Work, K.: Experimental toxoplasmosis in pregnant sow. *Acta Pathol Microbiol Scand, 78*:241, 1970.
26. Stalheim, O. H. V., Hubbert, W. T., Boothe, A. D., Zimmerman, W. J., Hughes, D. E., Batnett, D., Riley, J. L., and Foley, J.: Experimental toxoplasmosis in calves and pregnant sows. *Am J Vet Res, 41*:10, 1980.
27. Chamberlain, D. M., Docton, F. C., and Cole, C. R.: Toxoplasmosis. II. Intrauterine infection in dogs, premature birth and presence of organisms in milk. *Proc Soc Exp Biol Med, 82*:198, 1953.
28. Plant, J. W., Beh, K. J., and Helen, M. A.: Laboratory findings from ovine abortion and perinatal mortality. *Aust Vet J, 48*:558, 1972.
29. Dubey, J. P., Hoover, E. A., and Walls, K. W.: Effect of age and sex on the acquisition of immunity to toxoplasmosis in cats. *J Protozool, 24*:184, 1977.
30. Beverley, J. K., and Watson, W. A.: Ovine abortions and toxoplasmosis in Yorkshire. *Vet Rec, 73*:6, 1961.
31. Munday, B. L., Ryan, F. B., King, S. J., and Corbould, A.: Preparturent infections and other causes of fetal loss in sheep and cattle in Tasmania. *Aust Vet J 42*:189, 1966.
32. Hartley, W. J., and Moyle, G. G.: Further observations on the epidemiology of ovine toxoplasma infection. *Aust J Exp Biol Med Sci, 52*:647, 1974.
33. Munday, B. L., and Mason, R. W.: Toxoplasmosis as a cause of perinatal death in goats. *Aust Vet J, 55*:485, 1979.
34. Jacobs, L.: Toxoplasma gondii: Parasitology and transmission. *Bull NY Acad Med, 50*:128, 1974.
35. Siegel, S. E., Lunde, M. N., Gelderman, A. H., Halterman, R. H., Brown, J. A., Levine, A. S., and Graw, R. G.: Transmission of toxoplasmosis by leukocyte transfusion. *Blood, 37*:388, 1971.
36. Dubey, J. P., Sharma, S. P., Jaranaek, D. D., Sulzer, A. J., and Teutsche, S. W.: Characterization of Toxoplasma gondii isolates from an outbreak of toxoplasmosis in Atlanta, Georgia. *Am J Vet Res, 42*:1007, 1981.
37. O'Connor, G. R.: The influence of hypersensitivity on the pathogenesis of ocular toxoplasmosis. *Trans Am Ophthal Soc, 68*:501, 1970.
38. Hogan, M. J., Kimura, S. J., and O'Connor, G. R.: Ocular toxoplasmosis. *Arch Ophthalmol, 72*:592, 1964.
39. Kean, B. W., Kimball, A. C., and Christenson, W. N.: An epidemic of acute toxoplasmosis. *JAMA, 208*:1002, 1969.
40. Petrak, M., and Carpenter, J.: Feline toxoplasmosis. *JAVMA, 146*:728, 1965.
41. Vanisi, S. J., and Campbell, L. H.: Ocular toxoplasmosis in cats. *JAVMA, 154*:141, 1969.

42. Henry, I., and Beverley, J. K.: Toxoplasmosis in rats and guinea pigs. *J Comp Pathol*, *87*:97, 1977.
43. Swartzber, J. E., and Remington, J. S.: Transmission of toxoplasma. *Am J Dis Child*, *129*:777, 1975.
44. Rolline, D. F., Tabbara, K. F., Ghosheh, R., and Nozik, R. A.: Minocycline in experimental ocular toxoplasmosis in the rabbit. *Am J Ophthalmol*, *93*:361, 1982.
45. Tabbara, K. D., Dy-Liacco, J., Nozik, R. A., O'Connor, G. R., and Blackman, H. J.: Clindamycin in chronic ocular toxoplasmosis. *Arch Ophthalmol*, *95*:542, 1975.

Chapter 9

EXPERIMENTAL MODELS OF TOXOPLASMOSIS

G. Richard O'Connor, M.D.

Introduction

Ocular toxoplasmosis is currently the most frequent cause of retinochoroiditis in man. The quest for a reliable animal model of ocular toxoplasmosis continues because our knowledge of this disease is far from perfect. Currently available treatment of this disorder is also unsatisfactory. Some lesions seem to progress despite the administration of antimicrobial agents that effectively kill the causative agent, *Toxoplasma gondii*, in tissue cultures or in acutely infected rodents. Some patients are plagued by multiple recurrences of inflammation, leading to the relentless destruction of the retina and causing loss of useful vision, while others are subjected to only one or two attacks in a lifetime. It appears that differences in strain virulence might account for the highly variable course of the disease that may be observed among different patients, but one cannot rule out differences in host susceptibility, differences in hypersensitivity to the organism, or differences in immunocompetence as the causes of this variability.

The ideal animal model of ocular toxoplasmosis should provide for the formation of lesions that closely resemble those of man in their morphology, in their clinical course, and in their histopathologic manifestations. The lesions should be readily reproducible in an eye that is anatomically and physiologically similar to that of man. They should be producible in an animal whose immunologic defense system is very similar to that found in man. The lesions should not be violently destructive, nor should they produce retinal detachments or severe opacities of the lens, for these changes would preclude serial observation of the lesions. For the same reason, experimentally induced infections of the eye should not cause such severe systemic reaction (e.g., encephalitis) as to bring about the premature death of the experimental animal. The retinochoroiditic lesions should be located in the posterior pole to allow photographic documentation. Serial observation is generally necessary over a period of several months.

This work was supported in part by Grants EY-01204 and EY-01597 from the National Institutes of Health, Bethesda, Maryland and in part by an unrestricted grant from Research to Prevent Blindness, Inc., New York City.

Historical Background

As early as 1951, Hogan[1] recognized the need for a reliable animal model of ocular toxoplasmosis. Reasoning that *Toxoplasma* probably gained access to the eye through the bloodstream, he injected living RH *Toxoplasma* parasites into the carotid artery of the rabbit and produced focal chorioretinal lesions in those animals. The lesions became clinically apparent within three or four days after inoculation, but their natural course could not be observed because the animals died of toxoplasmic encephalitis a few days later. Nevertheless, these early experiments provided specimens for the histopathologic analysis of blood-borne ocular infections with *Toxoplasma gondii*. Even here, however, the model was not optimally useful, for the retinal vasculature of the rabbit retina does not extend very far beyond the edges of the optic nerve head. Thus, it is not surprising that the lesions Hogan produced were primarily choroidal rather than retinal, and in this sense the model was not a good one.

Frenkel[2] in 1953 produced ocular lesions in pigeons by the intramuscular or intraperitoneal inoculation of living *Toxoplasma* organisms. While the majority of the birds succumbed to the infection within two to nine days, some survived for several months. Histologic examination of the tissues of these pigeons showed evidence of focal toxoplasmosis in the choroid, in the sclera, and in the extraocular muscles, but their retinas were left undisturbed.

Beverley, Beattie, and Fry[3] in 1954 produced severe anterior uveitis and cataract in eyes of rabbits by the intracameral inoculation of RH strain *Toxoplasma* organisms. The major purpose of their experiments was to determine whether the course of the ocular inflammation could be modified by the use of sulfonamides (4:4'-diaminodiphenyl sulphone) and/or systemic corticosteroids; in fact, they found that both agents were beneficial in the treatment of the disease they produced. One might reasonably ask whether this model has any relevance to human ocular toxoplasmosis. So far as is known, *Toxoplasma gondii* does not infect the anterior segment of the human eye. Furthermore, the rabbit's immunological defenses against the organism appear to be very different from those of man. Corticosteroids will quell inflammation in almost any lesion of the anterior segment, whether or not it is induced by a microorganism. Therefore, the value of the model described by Beverley et al.[3] is certainly open to question.

In 1954, Frenkel[4] published the results of his attempts to induce experimental ocular toxoplasmosis in the hamster. The hamster, like the guinea pig, is relatively well defended against *Toxoplasma*, but it was still necessary for Frenkel to give his animals supplements of sodium sulfadiazine in their drinking water in order to keep them alive. Hamsters were inoculated subcutaneously or intraperitoneally and observed for signs of ocular disease.

Parallel experiments were performed with *Besnoitia jellisoni*, a protozoan parasite that produces cysts much larger than those of *Toxoplasma*. Frenkel found that it was possible to see such cysts with the ophthalmoscope, and he observed them in hamster retinas three or four months after the initial inoculation of organisms by the subcutaneous route. One cyst, observed 107 days after the initial infection, was noted to burst. A cellular haze was apparent in the overlying vitreous four days later, and following the sacrifice of the animal, Frenkel was able to isolate this lesion and study it histologically. It showed large numbers of lymphocytes, polymorphonuclear leukocytes, and macrophages. Frenkel observed very little invasion of new cells by the liberated parasites and postulated that the inflammatory reaction represented a form of hypersensitivity to *Besnoitia* antigens. Frenkel also assumed that the same thing happened in *Toxoplasma* infections, but because of their small size, he was never able to observe *Toxoplasma* cysts in the act of rupturing. Nevertheless, Frenkel's work marked the birth of the hypersensitivity theory as an explanation for recurrent ocular toxoplasmosis. *Toxoplasma* cysts were assumed to rupture in the retina at various times after the initial infection, and the ensuing reaction was assumed to be due to hypersensitivity rather than to the multiplication of living organisms at the site of rupture. These studies were continued and extended in a subsequent paper published by the same author in 1961.[5] They have become the basis for the recommended treatment of ocular toxoplasmosis with systemic corticosteroids, but Frenkel[5] has repeatedly stated that there might be limited proliferation of the parasite at the time of cyst rupture, and for that reason, he has always recommended the use of antimicrobial agents with the corticosteroids.

In 1968, Nozik and O'Connor[6] published a description of experimentally induced toxoplasmic retinochoroiditis in the rabbit. The animals were infected by the injection of a small inoculum of Beverley strain *Toxoplasma* organisms into the suprachoroidal space. This was relatively easy to accomplish when the rabbits were placed under general anesthesia and the eyes were proptosed by gentle external mechanical pressure over the inferior orbital rim. Focal retinochoroiditis appeared near the posterior pole of the fundus four to six days after the inoculation. This produced moderate clouding of the vitreous, but the retinal lesion was visible at all times. Secondary reactions in the anterior uvea were generally mild and were treated with atropine drops alone. Activity in the experimentally induced fundus lesions lasted four to six weeks, at the end of which pigmented, atrophic scars developed. Histologic studies of the healing lesions showed cysts of *Toxoplasma* in the superficial retinal layers along with enormous numbers of lymphocytes and plasma cells.

Numerous attempts were subsequently made to bring about recurrences of inflammation in the retinal scars. The eyes were subjected to blunt trauma.[7] The animals were given intraocular and systemic injections of

Toxoplasma antigens.[8] In separate experiments they were given injections of epinephrine or of cortisone.[9] The only manipulations that succeeded in provoking a recurrence of retinochoroiditis were those that followed the intravenous inoculation of antilymphocyte serum or of normal horse serum.[10] Total body irradiation also succeeded in some instances in producing recurrences of toxoplasmic retinochoroiditis, presumably by weakening the cell-mediated defense system of the rabbit.

The rabbit model of ocular toxoplasmosis served a number of additional purposes. Because the normal period of inflammatory activity in the retinal lesion lasted four to six weeks, experiments were performed to determine whether this period could be shortened by the use of new antimicrobial agents. In this way, clindamycin[11] and minocycline[12] were evaluated for their effects on experimental ocular toxoplasmosis, and immunomodulatory agents such as BCG (Bacillus of Calmette and Guerin)[13] were also investigated.

In 1982, Culbertson, Tabbara, and O'Connor[14] described an animal model of ocular toxoplasmosis in the *Cynomolgus* monkey. Infection of the retina was accomplished by the intraretinal inoculation of *Toxoplasma* organisms of the RH strain. A specially modified hypodermic needle, attached to a flexible plastic tube, was passed across the vitreous cavity after a small incision had been made in the sclera in the pars plana region. The needle was advanced until its tip could be observed directly over the retina in the desired region of the fundus. Then a small inoculation of living *Toxoplasmas* was made under carefully controlled conditions. Focal necrotizing retinitis, closely resembling that of the acute lesion in man, was produced by this technique (Fig. 9-1). The lesion was well established about four days after inoculation. Considerable reaction was produced in the overlying vitreous, and a moderately severe iridocyclitis was observed in every case. The lesions showed some signs of persistent inflammatory activity, as judged by fuzziness of the edges or overlying vitreous cells, for three to four weeks. At that time, healing took place with the formation of atrophic, variably pigmented scars.

The *Cynomolgus* monkey appeared to be relatively resistant to the highly virulent RH strain of *Toxoplasma*. No signs of systemic or cerebral disease were produced by the infection, but all of the animals showed extensive antibody responses to the organism. Although several hundred thousand living organisms were injected, no death resulted from the primary infection. It is almost certain that 100 percent of a similarly inoculated group of rabbits would have died from such an infection, meningoencephalitis being the usual cause of death.

Treatment of infected monkeys with minocycline, a new long-acting derivative of tetracycline, produced a remarkable shortening of the course of the experimental lesions, bringing about resolution of the inflammatory process in about one week (unpublished data). The advantage of this drug is that it

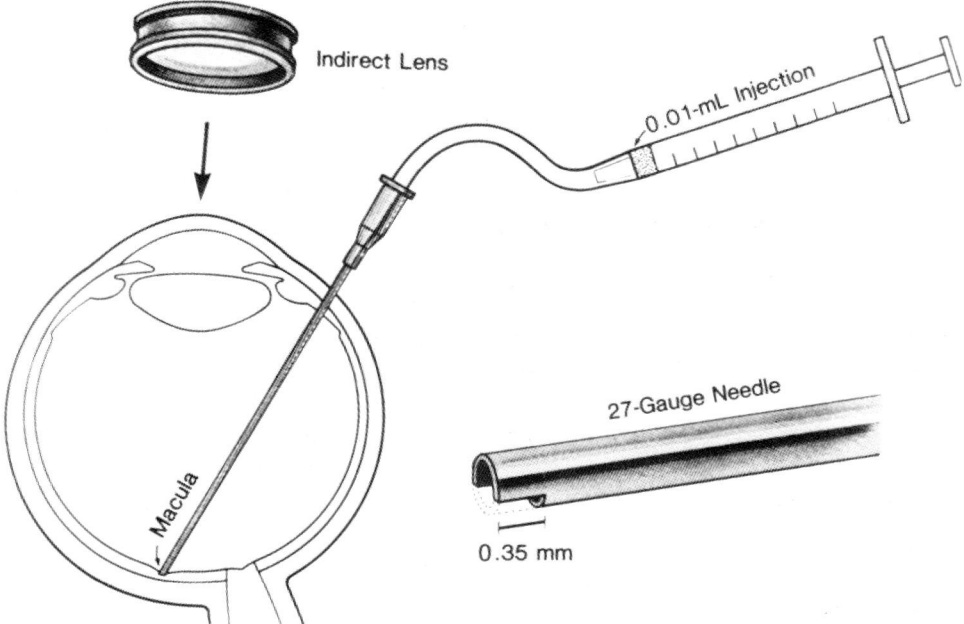

Figure 9-1. Technique for intraocular inoculation of toxoplasma organisms in nonhuman primates. (From Culbertson, W. W., Tabbara, K. F., and O'Connor, R. G., Experimental ocular toxoplasmosis in primates, *Arch Ophthalmol*, 100:323, 1982. Copyright 1982, American Medical Association.)

penetrates lipid barriers better than any other tetracycline. It also passes the blood-brain barrier (and presumably the blood-retina barrier) better than any other anti-*Toxoplasma* drug thus far produced, with the possible exception of the sulfonamides. When used in combination with sulfonamides, it promises to provide a very effective treatment for toxoplasmosis.

Because a toxoplasmic retinochoroiditis of a type very similar to that of man can be produced in the monkey model, it appeared to satisfy most of the criteria established for an ideal model of the disease. The lesions were produced in an eye anatomically similar to that of man and the animal's immunologic responses closely resemble those of man. One disadvantage of this animal model is that monkeys are expensive.

Recent Studies on Experimental Ocular Toxoplasmosis in the Monkey

Newman et al.[15] attempted to determine the role of hypersensitivity to *Toxoplasma* antigens in recurrent ocular toxoplasmosis in primates. Having induced focal retinochoroiditis in monkeys by the intraretinal inoculation of living RH strain *Toxoplasma gondii* organisms, they allowed the lesions to heal without further therapy. Four months thereafter *Toxoplasma* antigens in the form of heat-killed RH strain tachyzoites were injected into the right internal carotid artery. No exacerbation of the previously established retinochoroiditis was produced. Five weeks after this, a suspension of heat-killed *Toxoplasmas* was injected into the left retina through a needle inserted into the pars plana area. Within 24–48 hours all eyes developed edema at the site of retinal injection, but this subsided within a few days. In every eye injected with nonliving *Toxoplasma* antigens, retinal edema developed around the site of injection, but focal necrotizing retinitis was not observed in any of the animals.

From these studies the authors concluded that recurrent focal retinitis is probably related to proliferation of *Toxoplasma* parasites released when cysts break down in the retina. They also concluded that focal retinitis is probably not related to the sudden appearance of *Toxoplasma* antigens in the retina. They could neither confirm nor deny a theory promulgated by Nussenblatt et al.[16] that hypersensitivity to retinal autoantigens might be responsible for some of the damage seen in recurrent focal retinochoroiditis. This theory suggests that patients subjected to multiple recurrences of toxoplasmic retinochoroiditis become sensitized to retinal autoantigens as a result of destruction of rod outer segments. The destruction of even a few retinal cells by proliferating *Toxoplasmas* is thought to represent an adequate stimulus for autoimmune reactions in the retina that might contribute to the prolonged course of recurrent retinochoroiditis.

Challenging Issues for Future Investigation

It is entirely possible that antigens other than those present in heat-killed *Toxoplasma* tachyzoites might be responsible for recurrent *Toxoplasma* retinochoroiditis. Upon rupture, cysts liberate bradyzoites, a slowly proliferating form of the parasite. It may be that these forms are antigenically different from tachyzoites, and such differences could probably be established by the use of monoclonal antibodies. Furthermore, suspensions of cysts could be prepared (by special floatation techniques) from the minced brain tissue of chronically infected mice. Such cysts, ruptured by freezing or ultrasonication, might provide a more suitable stimulus for recurrent retinochoroiditis in a nonhuman primate model.

It is possible that heat-killing of *Toxoplasma* tachyzoites alters them in such a way that their antigens are no longer representative of organisms that might appear in the retina. Ultrasonication or treatment of the organisms with dilute formalin or phenol might provide antigens more characteristic of the parasite.

Reactions to autoantigens have yet to be identified in experimentally induced toxoplasmic retinochoriditis. Nussenblatt et al.[16] have shown that peripheral lymphocytes from patients with recurrent ocular toxoplasmosis respond to S-antigen (soluble retinal autoantigen) by lymphocytoblastic responses in tissue culture, but the activity of these stimulated lymphocytes in the retinal lesions has not yet been identified. This should be possible through the use of monoclonal antibodies as markers.

Of all the animal models of experimental ocular toxoplasmosis that have thus far been described, that produced by the direct inoculation of living *Toxoplasma* organisms into the monkey retina seems to be most applicable to human disease. It is likely that additional manipulations of this model will yield the information that is ultimately desired.

Summary

A series of animal models of ocular toxoplasmosis has been described, beginning with Hogan's model of toxoplasmic retinochoroiditis in the rabbit (1950). Additional models were later produced in the pigeon and in the hamster. All of these early models had serious shortcomings: they affected inappropriate tissues of the eye in some cases; they caused premature death of the animal in others.

Later work with a rabbit model of ocular toxoplasmosis produced retinal lesions that were morphologically similar to those seen in man. However, the rabbit's retina is not supplied with blood vessels in the same manner as man's retina, and its immunological defenses against *T. gondii* are quite different from those of man.

Direct inoculation of the monkey retina by living *Toxoplasma* organisms appears to be the best method of producing lesions comparable to those of man. The monkey's eye is anatomically similar to that of man, and its immunologic defenses against the parasite are comparable. Future manipulations of this model may yield important information about the relative roles of infection and hypersensitivity in recurrent toxoplasmic retinochoroiditis.

REFERENCES

1. Hogan, M. J.: *Ocular Toxoplasmosis*. New York, Columbia University Press, 1951.
2. Frenkel, J. K.: Host, strain, and treatment variation as factors in the pathogenesis of toxoplasmosis. *Am J Trop Med Hyg*, 2:390–415, 1953.
3. Beverley, J. K. A., Beattie, C. P., and Fry, B. A.: Experimental toxoplasmosis of the uveal tract. *Brt J Ophthalmol*, 38:489–496, 1954.
4. Frenkel, J. K.: Ocular lesions in hamsters with chronic Toxoplasma and Besnoitia infection. *Am J Ophthalmol*, 39:203–225, 1954.
5. Frenkel, J. K.: Pathogenesis of toxoplasmosis with a consideration of cyst rupture in Besnoitia infection. *Surv Ophthalmol*, 6:799–825, 1961.
6. Nozik, R. A., and O'Connor, G. R.: Experimental toxoplasmic retinochoroiditis. *Arch Ophthalmol*, 79:485–489, 1968.
7. O'Connor, G. R., and Nozik, R. A.: Studies on factors influencing the recurrence of ocular toxoplasmosis. Proc XXI Int'l Cong Ophthalmol. *Excerpta Med*, 222:1411–1415, 1971.
8. Nozik, R. A., and O'Connor, G. R.: Studies on experimental ocular toxoplasmosis in the

rabbit. I. The effect of antigenic stimulation. *Arch Ophthalmol, 83*:724–728, 1970.
9. Nozik, R. A., and O'Connor, G. R.: Studies on experimental ocular toxoplasmosis in the rabbit. II. Attempts to stimulate recurrences by local trauma, epinephrine, and corticosteroids. *Arch Ophthalmol, 84*:788–791, 1970.
10. Nozik, R. A., and O'Connor, G. R.: Studies on experimental ocular toxoplasmosis in the rabbit. III. Recurrent inflammation stimulated by systemic administration of anti-lymphocyte serum and normal horse serum. *Arch Ophthalmol, 85*:718–722, 1971.
11. Tabbara, K. F., Nozik, R. A., and O'Connor, G. R.: Clindamycin effects on experimental ocular toxoplasmosis in the rabbit. *Arch Ophthalmol, 92*:244–247, 1974.
12. Rollins, D. F., Tabbara, K. F., Ghosheh, R., and Nozik, R. A.: Minocycline in experimental ocular toxoplasmosis in the rabbit. *Am J Ophthalmol, 93*:361–365, 1982.
13. Tabbara, K. F., O'Connor, G. R., and Nozik, R. A.: Effect of immunization with *Mycobacterium bovis* on experimental toxoplasmic retinochoroiditis. *Am J Ophthalmol, 79*:641–647, 1975.
14. Culbertson, W. W., Tabbara, K. F., and O'Connor, G. R.: Experimental ocular toxoplasmosis in primates. *Arch Ophthalmol, 100*:321–323, 1982.
15. Newman, P. E., Ghosheh, R., Tabbara, K. F. O'Connor, G. R., and Stern, W.: The role of hypersensitivity reactions to *Toxoplasma* antigens in experimental toxoplasmosis in non-human primates. *Am J Ophthalmol, 94*:159–164, 1982.
16. Nussenblatt, R. B., Gery, I., Ballintine, E. J., and Wacker, W. B.: Cellular immune responsiveness of uveitis patients to retinal S-antigen. *Am J Ophthalmol, 89*:173–179, 1980.

Chapter 10

THE NINE-BANDED ARMADILLO (*DASYPUS NOVEMCINCUTUS L.*) AS A MODEL FOR LEPROSY (HANSEN'S DISEASE)

H. BRUCE OSTLER, M.D.

Introduction

In 1971, Kircheimer and Storrs reported the experimental production of lepromatoid leprosy in a nine-banded armadillo.[1] In this animal they found over a thousandfold increase of acid-fast bacteria at the inoculation sites, and great numbers of the same bacillus in skin sites remote from the areas of inoculation. Histological studies from the animal revealed a severe disseminated infection involving skin, lymph nodes, bone marrow, liver, spleen, lung, meninges, and eye.[2] The findings of intracellular organisms, bacillary invasion of nerves, the appearance of "lepra cells," and the presence of small and giant globi all suggested lepromatous leprosy. Clinically, large palpable granulomata were found at the sites of inoculation (abdomen and ear lobes). However, there were features that were atypical for lepromatous leprosy including lung and esophageal involvement, leprotic meningitis, and widespread bone marrow infection. In addition, there was no characteristic "free zone" separating the basal layer of the epidermis from the infiltrate of the dermis as is typically seen on biopsy of skin lesions in human lepromatous leprosy.

That the organism isolated from the armadillo was *Mycobacterium leprae* is suggested by the findings that the organism was capable of oxidizing D-dopa, that it did not grow on artificial media, but that it did multiply in the foot pads of mice.[1,2]

Since the initial reports by Kircheimer and Storrs, other armadillos have been studied. These animals have been successfully infected with material obtained from lepromatous patients, from other infected armadillos, and from the infected foot pads of mice.[3] The methods of inoculation have included intradermal abrasion, and the subcutaneous and intravenous routes.[3,4] All of these methods have been successful. Areas of inoculation have included the abdomen, the ears, between the bands on the abdomen, and in the foot pads.[5]

Description

The nine-banded armadillo (*Dasypus novemcincutus* L.) is a primitive mammal that looks much like a small pig covered with armor. It is found exclusively in the western hemisphere and has been identified in northern Argentina and all successive contiguous countries of the Andes, up to and including the southern United States. In the United States, the armadillo is found in Texas, Oklahoma, Arkansas, Georgia, and the Carolinas.[5]

The armadillo weighs from 50 to 150 grams at birth and reaches three to five kilograms in weight as an adult. The animal has very poor eyesight and depends upon its senses of hearing and smell for guidance and protection. Its teeth have poorly developed enamel, making the animal safe to handle. Its legs, often used for burrowing, are short and very powerful and when alarmed the animal can run with considerable speed. Armadillos are brownish black with markings of yellow above and yellowish white beneath. On the underside of the body there are sparse tufts of coarse hair. Their "armor" (a leathery carapace) protects the dorsal surface from cacti and thorny scrubs. The carapace is comprised of three main sections: the upper, a large scapular shield covering the head and shoulders; a central section consisting of nine movable bands, covering the abdomen and thoracic region; and a large dorsal section, covering the upper hips, pelvic area, and upper tail. The three sections of the carapace and the nine movable bands are joined by folds of skin. The nine bands are each composed of 50 to 75 scutes, which are somewhat similar to fish scales. (Anomalous changes in the scute and band patterns are not uncommon and consist of doubling or interruption of scute patterns or the occurrence of an additional band or a partial band.)

The female normally bears a litter of quadruplets which, since the animals are monozygous, are all identical. The young are born with their eyes open and are ambulatory. The carapaces are fully developed at birth but are soft and gradually become harder and more leathery with age. The newborns remain in seclusion for up to six weeks before venturing out with the mother to forage for food.

The armadillo is nocturnal and its food consists primarily of insects (75%); animal material (amphibians, reptiles, birds, eggs, and mammals) (15%); and vegetable matter (roots, fruit) and dirt (10%). The animals can be adapted to dog or cat chow supplemented with vitamins and minerals, although they will also eat eggs, liver, chicken and other meat, and some fruits, including bananas and melon. (Storrs has suggested combining the food and water in one dish to make a gruel so the armadillo will learn to eat out of a pan while in captivity.[5])

With an ambient temperature of 25°C the body temperature varies 30–36° (rectal). If the ambient temperature is lowered, the skin temperature also goes down but the rectal temperature increases. At high ambient temperatures both the skin and rectal temperatures increase. These findings suggest that the thermostatic control for body temperature is quite primitive.

The cellular elements of the blood of armadillos are only slightly different morphologically from those of the human. The red blood cells are smaller, the platelets variable in size, and the megakaryocytes have one multilobed nucleus. The macrophages of man and armadillo are similar.

Clinical Findings in the *M. leprae* Infected Armadillo Eye

Bacilli are found in varying numbers in every ocular tissue except the lens, the retina, the aqueous, or the vitreous. The organisms are most numerous in the iris, ciliary body, and the choroid. *M. leprae* are also found in large numbers within the eyelids, the palpebral and bulbar conjunctiva, the limbus, and in the cornea. The organisms are also found within the endoneural zones of the small branches of the periocular nerves. Within the cornea, the organisms are found just below the epithelium and within the stroma. Within the choroid they are located within the pigmented cells.

The only evidence of cell-mediated immune response to the infection within the eye is the host macrophage. There is no evidence of polymorphonuclear leukocytic response nor is there evidence of a vasculitis.

As in the human, most organisms are found within the anterior segment of the armadillo's eye, but unlike the human, the organisms may be found in the choroid of the armadillo.

Value of Armadillos as a Model for Hansen's Disease[1,2,4,5]

Advantages

Among the advantages of the armadillo model of leprosy is that large quantities of acid-fast bacilli (*M. leprae*) can be recovered when a susceptible armadillo is injected with the organism. The quantities of bacilli produced in the tissue are in the order of 10^{10} to 10^{12} organisms per gram of tissue and up to 3.5 grams of organism can be obtained from one animal.[1]

Almost 90 percent of armadillos develop infection when small doses of *M. leprae* are injected,[6] and almost 100 percent are susceptible to infection when several hundred million organisms are injected intravenously.[7]

The lower temperature of the armadillo simulates the lower temperatures of those parts of the human body where the *M. leprae* are found in large numbers. Such low temperatures probably aid in the growth of the organism or serve to depress lymphocyte transformation.

The fact that armadillos produce four monozygous offspring is useful to investigators because it allows them to eliminate variable genetic factors, especially those dealing with immunity. This greatly enhances the investigation of the role of the immune system in Hansen's disease. Moreover, the immune system need not be manipulated for an infection to occur.

Because of the slow multiplication rate of the *M. leprae* organism, several years are often necessary before clinical disease is apparent in the human or experimental animal, thus an animal with a long life span such as the armadillo (12 to 15 years) is desirable.

Armadillos are easy to handle, hardy, and appear to be plentiful in their natural habitat.

Disadvantages

The armadillo has not been successfully bred in captivity. Their eyes are small and the corneal epithelium is keratinized and vascularized to its center.[8] The location of the organism in the eye and the body of the armadillo does not correspond to the location of the organism in the human. Furthermore, only the lepromatous form of the disease has been noted, while the tuberculoid form has not been recognized.

The majority of the animals are susceptible to the organism, whereas the majority of humans are resistant, suggesting that there may be a different mode of immune deficiency in the armadillo when compared to humans.

Summary

As a model for the study of Hansen's Disease, the armadillo will prove to be very useful in helping to determine the role of genetic factors and the role of the immune system in the production of the disease. The animal is abundant, easy to handle, and has a life span suitable for studying the natural course of the disease and the pathogenesis of infection.

REFERENCES

1. Kirchheimer, W. F., and Storrs, E. E.: Attempts to establish the armadillo (*Dasypus novemcincutus* Linn.) as a model for the study of leprosy. 1. Report of lepromatoid leprosy in an experimentally infected armadillo. *Int J Lep Mycobact Dis, 39*:693–701, 1971.
2. Kirchheimer, W. F., Storrs, E. E., and Binford, C. H.: Attempts to establish the armadillo (*Dasypus novemcincutus* Linn.) as a model for the study of leprosy II. Histopathologic and bacteriologic postmortem findings in lepromatoid leprosy in the armadillo. *Int J Lep Mycobact Dis, 40*:229–242, 1972.
3. Binford, C. H., Storrs, E. E., and Walsh, G. P.: Disseminated infection in the nine-banded armadillos (*Dasypus Novemcincutus*) resulting from inoculation with *M. leprae*. Observations made on 15 animals studied at autopsy. *Int J Lep Mycobact Dis, 44*:80–83, 1976.
4. Hobbs, H. E., Harman, D. J., Rees, R. J. W., and McDougall, A. C.: Ocular histopathology in animals experimentally infected with *Mycobacterium leprae* and *M. lepraemurium*. *Brt J Ophthalmol, 62*:516–524, 1978.
5. Storrs, E. E.: The nine-banded armadillo: A model of leprosy and other biomedical research. *Int J Lep Mycobact Dis, 39*:703–714, 1971.

6. Kirchheimer, W. F., Sanchez, R. M., Pascua, J. P., and Walsh, T.: Quantitative aspects of experimental infection of armadillos with *Mycobacterium leprae. Int J Lep Mycobact Dis,* 46:109, 1978.
7. Kirchheimer, W. F., and Sanchez, R. M.: Intraspecies differences of resistance against leprosy in nine-banded armadillos. *Lep in India,* 53:525–530, 1981.
8. Duke-Elder, S.: System of ophthalmology. In *The Eye in Evolution,* vol. I. London, Kimpton 1958, pp 456–457.

Chapter 11

ANTIBIOTICS IN THE TREATMENT OF EXPERIMENTAL BACTERIAL ENDOPHTHALMITIS

CAREEN YEN-LOWDER, M.D., PH.D.

Introduction

Endophthalmitis is one of the most dreaded complications of intraocular surgery. Management of infectious endophthalmitis continues to be a challenge to ophthalmologists, since treatment success as measured by useful vision is still poor. The study of various treatment modalities in the rabbit model has provided the basis for the rational management of human bacterial endophthalmitis.

In this chapter I will provide an overview of laboratory studies performed in the rabbit model and discuss the evolution of therapy for human bacterial endophthalmitis based on the results of those studies.

Recoverability of Organisms

In 1955, Maylath and Leopold[1] demonstrated that the rabbit's anterior chamber resisted an infectious agent better than its vitreous. Inoculation of 700 organisms of *Staphylococcus aureus* or *Escherichia coli* into the anterior chamber consistently resulted in a sterile aqueous humor. Although hypopyons developed after inoculation, they were not severe and cleared without specific therapy. When the same number of organisms were introduced into the vitreous, cultures taken from the vitreous at 48 hours were still positive in all of them, while those taken from the anterior chamber were negative in one-third of the cases. Cultures documented that extension of infection from the anterior chamber to the vitreous was less rapid than the converse. The ability of the anterior chamber to resist an infectious agent was attributed to the circulation of aqueous fluid, the availability of inflammatory cells from the uveal blood vessels, and the phagocytic properties of the endothelial cells. In contrast, the vitreous is an avascular, acellular immunologically compromised gel.

Systemic and Periocular Antibiotic Treatment

Antibiotic Levels in the Normal Rabbit Eye

In the 1950s and 1960s the prognosis for visual recovery following bacterial endophthalmitis was poor.[2,3] Therapy consisted of systemic and topical antibiotics in combination with cycloplegia. In 1945, Von Sallman and other investigators reported the use of intravitreal penicillin, but both the procedure and the drug were found to be unsafe.[4]

Between 1965 and 1975 there were a great number of studies using many different antibiotics and various routes of administration to measure the concentrations that could be achieved in the normal rabbit eye.[5-15] These studies produced some interesting results. It was found that, in general, the same dose of antibiotic given intravenously achieves a higher level of concentration in the aqueous humor than those produced by intramuscular injections, whereas antibiotics administered through the conjunctiva penetrate more effectively than those given by intravenous injection. Subconjunctival injections produced effective inhibitory concentrations in the aqueous humor but not in the vitreous. In subconjunctival injections, a gradient of antibiotic concentration is produced that decreases with increasing distance from the injection site.

With intravenous injections of antibiotics, ocular penetration was found to be dependent on the chemical properties of the antibiotic—properties such as lipid solubility and plasma protein binding. Oxacillin, for example, was found to have poor intraocular penetration since 92 percent of the drug is protein-bound.[16] This drug is thus not available for diffusion outside the intravascular space.

Antibiotic Level in the Inflamed Rabbit Eye

The presence of local inflammation alters the permeability of the capillaries. The blood-aqueous barrier is disrupted. Drug penetration studies performed in the noninfected eye, therefore, may not be applicable. Barza et al. studied the effect of infection on the ocular penetration of antibiotics.[13] They injected 50 *Pseudomonas aeruginos* organisms into the vitreous of healthy albino rabbits through the pars plana, and twenty-four hours later a moderately severe endophthalmitis was seen. The intraocular penetration of several dosages of carbenicillin given intravenously and subconjunctivally was then compared in the normal and infected rabbit eye. It was found that the penetration into uninflamed rabbit aqueous by intravenously administered carbenicillin is similar to that of penicillin G[6] and ampicillin.[14] Inflammation, on the other hand, markedly increased the penetration of carbenicillin into aqueous and tissue concentration of iris and cornea. Inflammation increased the levels of tissue concentration in the choroid-retina and vitreous; levels remained suboptimal when the antibiotic was given intravenously. On the other hand, inflammation did not increase penetration when antibiotics were given via the subconjunctival route. This result was attributed to the inflammatory effect of the injection and to the extremely high local concentrations achieved. These high concentrations were considered sufficient to overcome the barriers to diffusion present in an avascular gel. Low vitrous levels of subconjunctival antibiotics were confirmed in studies using cefazolin and cefamandole in the treatment of *Staphylococcus aureus* endophthalmitis in the rabbit.[16]

Retrobulbar versus Subconjunctival Routes

Retrobulbar and subconjunctival injections of antibiotic in the normal rabbit eye were compared to rabbit eyes infected intravitreally with *Staphylococcus aureus* 72 hours before therapy.[17] Subconjunctival administration produced concentrations of gentamicin in the cornea, sclera, choroid, and retina of the infected rabbit eye that were higher than those produced by retrobulbar injections. Subconjunctival injections also produced levels in the vitreous, posterior sclera, and choroid-retina of the normal eye that were higher than those produced by retrobulbar injections. On the other hand, concentrations in the inflamed vitreous were similar in the two routes. The vitreous levels were low by either periocular route.

Studies evaluating the two modes of periocular administration using the rabbit model may not represent the human response because the rabbit has a large vascular orbital plexus that may absorb the retrobulbar antibiotic.

Combination of Systemic and Subconjunctival Therapy

In most of the studies mentioned, ocular penetration of antibiotic was evaluated using one route of administration. It was not until 1980 that Barza et al.[18] used a rabbit model of endophthalmitis to evaluate the clinical practice of giving systemic and periocular antibiotics together. In this experiment, rabbit eyes were infected intravitreally with 500 colony-forming units of *Staphylococcus aureus*. Intraocular antibiotic levels were determined after treatment with oxacillin given subconjunctivally, intravenously, or both. Combined therapy added little to the very high levels of oxacillin achieved in the cornea and aqueous humor following subconjunctival injection. The choroid-retina complex showed that the use of the two routes had an additive effect. Concentrations in the vitreous were about 2 percent of the serum level with either route or with both routes combined. Fifteen minutes after subconjunctival injection of 100 mg of oxacillin, the serum level was 41.1 μg/ml and the vitreous concentration was 0.8 μg/ml. The continuous infusion of 40 mg/kg/hr of exacillin produced a serum level of 32.4 μg/ml and a vitreous level of 0.4 μg/ml. Following combined therapy, the serum level was 78.1 µg/ml and the vitreous level was 1.5 µg/ml. These results suggest that the systemic circulation may contribute significantly to the antibiotic level in the inflamed vitreous, even in the periocular mode of administration. However, this study also showed that the levels achieved in the vitreous with combined therapy are suboptimal for the treatment of rabbit endophthalmitis.

Intravitreal Injection of Antibiotics

Because poor drug penetration makes it difficult to achieve bactericidal antibiotic levels in the vitreous, Peyman[19-24] was prompted to reevaluate the safety of intravitreally injected antibiotics. This approach is useful only when antibiotics are injected into the vitreous at a nontoxic but therapeutic level. Several criteria were used in evaluating the toxicity of intravitreal antibiotics. Not all of the criteria were used in each study.[19-23,25] Toxicity evaluations were performed in noninfected rabbit eyes by injecting various doses of antibiotics in 0.1 ml volume through the pars plana into the anterior vitreous under direct visualization. The eyes were examined at intervals with the indirect ophthalmoscope following injection and enucleated for histologic examination. Electroretinograms were performed on some eyes both before and at intervals after administration of antibiotics. Clearance and half-life of the intravitreal antibiotics were determined in the normal rabbit eye.

Peyman et al.[22] found that the intravitreal level of 0.5 mg of gentamicin was not toxic to the normal rabbit eye. Zachary and Forster[26] found, contrary to Peyman, that the intravitreal level of 0.5 mg of commercially available gentamicin was unsafe. The electroretinogram (ERG) was completely extinguished in all eyes treated with 0.4 mg.[26] Even at the 0.1 mg level, only three of ten eyes had normal ERG, while three out of ten had extinguished ERG. Although the discrepancy between the two studies has not been resolved because the effect of preservatives was not determined, Peyman and others still insist that safe intravitreal levels of many antibiotics have been established. They point out that electroretinography is the most sensitive indicator of drug-induced retinal toxicity. Minimal histologic changes may be seen in the retina when the electroretinogram is completely extinguished.[26]

The Efficacy of Intravitreal Antibiotic

The efficacy of intravitreal administration of antibiotics was demonstrated in several studies of rabbit endophthalmitis. One study showed that 2 mg of intravitreal methicillin sterilized the vitreous when given up to 24 hours after intravitreal inoculation of 10,000 *Staphylococcus aureus*.[25] A direct relationship between onset of therapy, severity, and sequelae of infection was found. When treatment was delayed for ten hours, all eyes retained large, oval vitreous opacities. Anterior chamber damage was manifested by synechiae formation. Although vitreous cultures were negative in eyes treated 24 hours after inoculation, these eyes developed severe uveitis and progressed to phthisis bulbi.

Intravitreal Injections of Antibiotics in the Infected Rabbit Eye

Until 1981, all of the studies evaluating the safety and vitreous levels of intravitreal injections of antibiotics concentrated on normal rabbit eyes. An interesting study by Kane et al.[27] examined the effect of infection and pigmentation on the levels of intravitreal antibiotics. Five hundred colony-forming units of *Staphylococcus aureus* were injected intravitreally in Dutch belted (pigmented) and New Zealand white (albino) rabbits. About 48 hours later, the red reflex was lost and 50 μg of gentamicin was injected into the vitreous through the pars plana. Uninfected eyes were used as controls. This study showed that infection dramatically reduced the half-life of gentamicin from 24 hours to 10 hours. There was no difference between pigmented and albino rabbits in the levels of gentamicin in the aqueous, cornea, and vitreous. Levels of gentamicin were much lower in the choroid, retina, and sclera of pigmented animals.

Studies performed on the normal rabbit eye may overestimate the peak and sustained antibiotic levels in the infected vitreous. Thus, the likelihood of toxicity with a given dose may be less in the infected eye. The shortened half-life might necessitate repeated intravitreal injections to maintain effective drug levels.

Efficacy of Periocular and Intravenous Administration Compared to Intravitreal Injection of Antibiotics

The efficacy of intravitreal injection of antibiotics in eradicating infection was compared to subconjunctival combined with intravenous injections in several studies of experimental endophthalmitis.[21,23,24]

In one report, negative cultures were obtained when 0.25 mg of cephaloridine was given intravitreally six hours after inoculation of 500–1000 *E. coli* organisms. At that time, the eyes had congested conjunctival and iris vessels; the corneae were edematous and the vitreous cloudy. Infected eyes treated at six hours with either 50 mg injected subconjunctivally or with 750 mg of cephaloridine injected intravenously were destroyed by uncontrolled infection. Unfortunately, there was no report on the results of cultures taken from eyes treated by these two methods.[23]

Studies using intravitreal cephalothin[20] confirmed the results obtained with methicillin[25] and cephaloridine.[23] Intravitreal injection of 2 mg cephalothin eliminated infection without any residual clinical signs for up to ten hours after inoculation of 2000–2500 *Staphylococcus aureus* into the vitreous of rabbit eyes. The eyes treated after ten hours had various degrees of residual vitreous opacities, which ranged from pinpoint size to total vitreous clouding, directly proportional to the delay in treatment. Intravitreal injection eradicated intraocular organisms, and all of the eyes treated with subconjunctival injections of antibiotics continued to be culture positive. These studies show that intravitreal antibiotics can sterilize experimental endophthalmitis and that a delay in treatment will cure the infection but will result in an eye without visual function because of residual vitreous opacities.

Effect of Vitrectomy Compared to Intravitreal Antibiotics in the Treatment of Bacterial Endophthalmitis

Cottingham and Forster[28] examined the results of vitreous cultures after treatment with either a vitrectomy procedure or with intravitreal antibiotics, or with a combination of both. When 10^4 *Staphylococcus epidermidis* were inoculated into the vitreous cavity of pigmented rabbits, 0.1 mg intravitreal gentamicin given at 24 hours rendered all eyes culture negative. Of the 11 eyes treated by a vitrectomy procedure alone, six were culture negative. A vitrectomy was performed on two of these 48 hours after inoculation. All eyes treated with the combined procedure were culture negative. Intravitreal gentamicin (0.1 mg) produced negative cultures in infections caused by 30–100 organisms of *Staphylococcus aureus* if given prior to 24 hours after inoculation. Therefore, the effect of vitrectomy on culture results was evaluated at 25–31 hours after infection, intravitreal gentamicin rendered 33 percent of the culture negative, whereas combined vitrectomy and intravitreal gentamicin rendered 88 percent of the culture negative. In the group evaluated 40–49 hours postinfection, cultures were negative in 50 percent of the eyes treated with intravitreal antibiotic and in 100 percent of the group treated with combined therapy. These results were statistically significant and demonstrated that a combination of vitrectomy and intravitreal injection of antibiotic offers substantial advantage in eliminating infection after 24 hours, especially infection caused by pathogenic bacteria.

The above study was performed in phakic rabbit eyes. Several years later, McGetrick and Peyman[29] performed similar studies using an aphakic rabbit model. The lenses of all of the experimental animals were extracted in order to simulate more closely the human postoperative condition. Immediately after lens extraction, 40–65 *Staphylococcus aureus* organisms were inoculated into the anterior vitreous through the sutured limbal incision. In addition to comparing vitrectomy and intravitreal antibiotic injection, the combined efficacy of subconjunctival and intramuscular injections of gentamicin was evaluated. The investigators found that all eyes treated 20 hours after inoculation were destroyed regardless of treatment. Of the ten eyes treated with 20 mg gentamicin subconjunctivally and 4 mg/kg/day intramuscularly, only one eye recovered. Treatment of this eye began at eight hours postinoculation. Of the ten eyes that received 0.2 mg intravitreal gentamicin in addition to systemic therapy, eight recovered. The two eyes that became phthisical were treated 24 hours postinoculation. Cultures were negative for all ten eyes. Only the eyes treated at 8–12 hours were histologically normal. Similar results were obtained with the group treated with vitrectomy containing 8 µg/ml gentamicin in the infusion fluid in addition to systemic therapy. These investigations showed that intravitreal injection combined with systemic therapy or vitrectomy combined with systemic therapy were equally effective in eradicating infection. The difference between the vitrectomy group and the group of eyes that received intravitreal antibiotics was in the clarity of the vitreous.

Although in these two studies[28,29] similar numbers of *Staphylococcus aureus* organisms were injected into the vitrous, different criteria were used for determining the success of treatment. Both studies clearly demonstrated, however, that a combination of intravitreal antibiotics and vitrectomy is effective in sterilizing the vitreous. This combination produces negative cultures in cases where treatment is delayed. However, when the success of treatment is measured not only by culture results but also by clinical and histologic appearance, as in the second study, it is apparent that the visual outcome of an infected eye depends upon the early initiation of treatment. The infectious agent may be eliminated but the residual vitreous opacities and retinal damage secondary to the inflammatory process prevent useful vision. The reasons for performing a vitrectomy would be to allow more diffusion of antibiotic in the vitreous cavity; to remove the bulk of the infectious organisms and any sequestered infectious pockets; and to eliminate toxic products that may continue to damage ocular structures even after the infection has been stopped by antibiotics.

Effect of Corticosteroids in Bacterial Endophthalmitis

As early as 1955, Maylath and Leopold[1] showed that the addition of subconjunctival cortisone to antibiotic therapy improved the results of therapy in *Staphylococcal* endophthalmitis in rabbits. Baum et al.[30] demonstrated that retrobulbar corticosteroids were beneficial when used in combination with subconjunctival antibiotics. Clarity of the vitreous and histologic examination of the treated eyes were the basis of this evaluation. Graham and Peyman[31] evaluated the intravitreal injection of dexamethasone in combination with an antibiotic in the treatment of experimental endophthalmitis. In combination with 0.5 mg gentamicin, 0.36 mg dexamethasone significantly reduced intraocular inflammation induced by inoculation of 20,000 pseudomonas into the vitreous of rabbit eyes. In eyes treated within five hours of inoculation, there was less retinal destruction and a reduction in the exudate in the anterior and posterior chambers and vitreous. When treatment was delayed for more than five hours, the eyes treated with dexamethasone had less retinitis and choroiditis, but destruction was not prevented.

Summary

Studies of bacterial endophthalmitis using the rabbit eye have provided a great deal of insight into the treatment of human bacterial endophthalmitis.[32-39] They have shown that although subconjunctival injection of antibiotics produces more than adequate levels in the anterior segment, those levels are not sufficient to sterilize the vitreous cavity in the phakic eye. Intravitreal antibiotics were shown to be safe and effective in sterilizing the vitreous if given early in the course of infection. Vitrectomy was shown to be effective in producing negative cultures, and the combination of intravitreal antibiotics and a vitrectomy procedure was more effective in treating endophthalmitis after a delay in treatment.

Further studies are indicated to determine optimum management of postsurgical bacterial endophthalmitis in humans. How long are effective levels of intraocular antibiotics sustained in the infected eye? Does aphakia influence the pharmacokinetics and toxicity of antibiotics in the infected eye? How do prophylactic antibiotics influence the course of experimentally induced endophthalmitis? Ultimately, these questions will have to be answered by carefully designed experiments in the animal model.

REFERENCES

1. Maylath, F. R., and Leopold, I. H.: Study of experimental intraocular infection. *Am J Ophthalmol, 40:*86-11, 1955.
2. Allen, H. F., and Mangiaracine, A. B.: Bacterial endophthalmitis after cataract extraction: A study of 22 infections in 20,000 operations. *Arch Ophthalmol, 72:*454-462, 1964.
3. Allen, H. F., and Mangiaracine, A. B.: Bacterial endophthalmitis after cataract extraction. *Arch Ophthalmol, 91:*3-7, 1974.
4. von Sallman, L: Penicillin therapy of infections of the vitreous. *Arch Ophthalmol, 33:*455-462, 1945.
5. Abel, R., Boyle, G., Furman, M., and Leopold, I. H. L. Intraocular penetration of cefazolin sodium in rabbits. *Am J Ophthalmol, 78:*779-787, 1974.
6. Bloome, M. A., Golden, B., and McKee, A. P.: Antibiotic concentration in ocular tissues. *Arch Ophthalmol, 83:*78-83, 1970.
7. Faris, B., and Uwayday, M.: Intraocular penetration of semi-synthetic penicillin. *Arch Ophthalmol, 92:*501-505, 1974.
8. Golden, B., and Coppel, S.: Ocular tissue absorption of gentamicin. *Arch Ophthalmol, 84:*792-796, 1970.
9. Litwack, K. D., Pettit, T., and Johnson, B. L.: Penetration of gentamicin. *Arch Ophthalmol, 82:*687-693, 1969.
10. Records, R. E.: Intraocular penetration of cephalothin. *Am J Ophthalmol, 66:*436-443, 1968.

11. Tabbara, K., and O'Connor, R.: Ocular tissue absorption of clindamycin phosphate. *Arch Ophthalmol, 93*:1180–1185, 1975.
12. Barza, M., and Baum, J.: Penetration of ocular compartments by penicillins: Analysis of factors affecting intraocular concentration and half-life. *Surv Ophthalmol, 18*:71–82, 1973.
13. Barza, M., Baum, J., Birkby, B., and Weinstein, L.: Intraocular penetration of carbenicillin in the rabbit. *Am J Ophthalmol, 75*:307–313, 1973.
14. Records, R. E., and Ellis, P. P.: The intraocular penetration of ampicillin, methicillin, and oxacillin. *Am J Ophthalmol, 64*:135–143, 1967.
15. Records, R. E.: Intraocular penetration of cephaloridine. *Arch Ophthalmol, 81*:331–335, 1969.
16. Barza, M., Kane, A., and Baum, J. L.: Intraocular levels of cefamadole compared with cefazolin after subconjunctival injection in rabbits. *Invest Ophthalmol Vis Sci, 18*:250–255, 1979.
17. Barza, M., Kane, A., and Baum, J. L.: Regional differences in ocular concentration of gentamicin after subconjunctival and retrobulbar injection in the rabbit. *Am J Ophthalmol, 83*:407–413, 1977.
18. Barza, M., Kane, A., and Baum, J. L.: Oxacillin for bacterial endophthalmitis: Subconjunctival, intravenous, both or neither? *Invest Ophthalmol Vis Sci, 19*:1348–1354, 1980.
19. Baum, J. L., and Peyman, G. A.: Antibiotic administration in the treatment of bacterial endophthalmitis. *Surv Ophthalmol, 21*:332–346, 1977.
20. Rutgard, J. J., Berkowitz, R. A., and Peyman, G. A.: Intravitreal cephalothin in experimental Staphylococcal endophthalmitis. *Annals of Ophthalmol, 8* 293–298, 1978.
21. Peyman, G. A., and Sanders, D. R.: *Advances in Uveal Surgery, Vitreous Surgery, and the Treatment of Endophthalmitis.* New York, Appleton-Century-Crofts, 1975.
22. Peyman, G. A., May, D. R., Ericson, E. S., and Aple, D.: Intraocular injection of gentamicin. *Arch Ophthalmol, 92*:42–47, 1974.
23. Graham, R. O., Peyman, G. A., and Fishman, G.: Intravitreal injection of cephaloridine in the treatment of endophthalmitis. *Arch Ophthalmol, 93*:56–61, 1975.
24. Fisher, J. P., Viviletto, S. E., and Forster, R. E.: Toxicity, efficacy and clearance of intravitreally injected cefazolin. *Arch Ophthalmol, 100*:650–652, 1982.
25. Daily, M. J., Peyman, G. A., and Fishman, G.: Intravitreal injection of methicillin for treatment of endophthalmitis. *Am J Ophthalmol 76*:343–350, 1973.
26. Zachary, I. G., and Forster, R. K.: Experimental intravitreal gentamicin. *Amer J Ophthalmol, 82*:604–611, 1976.
27. Kane, A., Barza, M., and Baum, J. L.: Intravitreal injection of gentamicin in rabbits. *Invest Ophthalmol Vis Sci, 20*:593–397, 1981.
28. Cottingham, A. J., and Forster, R. K.: Vitrectomy in endophthalmitis. *Arch Ophthalmol, 94*:2078, 1976.
29. McGetrick, B. S., and Peyman, G. A.: Vitrectomy in experimental endophthalmitis: Part II—Bacterial endophthalmitis. *Ophthalmic Surgery, 10*:87–92, 1979.
30. Baum, J. L. Barza, M., Lugar, J., and Origman, P.: The effect of corticosteroids in the treatment of experimental bacterial endophthalmitis. *Amer J Ophthalmol, 80*:513–517, 1975.
31. Graham, R. O., and Peyman, G. A.: Intravitreal injection of dexamethasone. *Arch Ophthalmol, 92*:149–154, 1974.
32. Kanski, J. J.: Treatment of late endophthalmitis associated with filtering blebs. *Arch Ophthalmol, 91*:339–343, 1974.
33. Allen, H. F., and Mangiaracine, A. B.: Bacterial endophthalmitis after cataract extraction. *Arch Ophthalmol, 91*:3–8, 1974.

34. Forster, R. K., Zachary, I. G., Cottigham, A. J., and Norton, E. W.: Further observations on the diagnosis, cause and treatment of endophthalmitis. *Am J Ophthalmol, 81*:52–56, 1976.
35. Vastine, D. W., Peyman, G. A., and Guth, S. B.: Visual prognosis in bacterial endophthalmitis treated with intravitreal antibiotics. *Ophthalmic Surg, 10*:76–83, 1979.
36. Forster, R. K., Abbot, R. L., and Gelender, H.: Management of infectious endophthalmitis. *Ophthalmol, 87*:313–319, 1980.
37. Peyman, G. A., Raichand, M., and Bennett, T. O.: Management of endophthalmitis with pars plana vitrectomy. *Br J Ophthalmol, 64*:472–475, 1980.
38. Diamond, J. G.: Intraocular management of endophthalmitis: a systematic approach. *Arch Ophthalmol, 99*:96–99, 1981.
39. Peyman, G. A., Carroll, C. P., and Raichand, M.: Prevention and management of traumatic endophthalmitis. *Ophthalmol, 87*:320–324, 1980.

Chapter 12

OCULAR LISTERIOSIS

MASAO OKUMOTO, M.A.

Introduction

Ocular listeriosis is a relatively rare disease although the causative organism, *Listeria monocytogenes,* is commonly encountered in nature. Several studies indicate that many cases of listeriosis are occurring, but most of these are too mild to be recognized or are entirely unapparent or latent.[1]

Since the original report by Murray, Webb, and Swan in 1926,[2] this organism has been extensively investigated, and as clinicians and microbiologists have become more aware of this bacterium, more cases are being reported. Immunosuppressive therapy, particularly with corticosteroids, is a major factor in the development of human listeriosis.[3]

The Organism

L. monocytogenes is a small, gram-positive rod with one to four flagella that endow the organism with a peculiar type of motility. This bacterium can be cultured on blood agar and most other noninhibitory isolation media. On blood agar, small translucent colonies with a narrow zone of beta-hemolysis can be seen within 48 hours. A unique property of *L. monocytogenes* is that it can sometimes resist isolation from tissue specimens unless it has been kept under refrigeration for from several days to three months.[4] The exact mechanism for this property, known as "cold enrichment," is still unknown. Another curious feature concerning the isolation of *L. monocytogenes* is the organism's sensitivity to saline in low populations.[4] Yet, this bacterium is reported to be capable of growing in sodium chloride concentrations of 10%.[5]

The statement is often made that *L. monocytogenes* can be mistaken for diphtheroids and discarded as insignificant. Anyone who has seen cultures of this organism is not likely to make this mistake. Colonies of *Listeria* are smooth and translucent, in contrast to diphtheroid colonies that appear dry and opaque. *Listeria* also produce a hemolysin that results in a narrow zone of beta-hemolysis around each colony, whereas diphtheroids are all nonhemolytic. Most distinctive is the tumbling motility of *L. monocytogenes,* best seen in cultures incubated at room temperature. Diphtheroids, on the other hand, are all nonmotile. In scrapings or smears, *L. monocytogenes* evoke a marked inflammatory response, in contrast to the diphtheroids, which are associated with keratinized epithelial cells. The rods of *Listeria* are usually short, but long forms may be seen. These are generally symmetrical with parallel sides and stain evenly. *Listeria* are often intracellular in PMNs and monocytes, or they may be seen attached to healthy epithelial cells. Diphtheroids on the other hand are extracellular, pleomorphic and stain irregularly.

Ocular Manifestations

Human Studies

At the Francis I. Proctor Foundation we have had the rare opportunity to study two cases of *Listeria* endophthalmitis.[6,7] In both cases the patients presented with poor vision and uveitis of unknown etiology. One of the patients complained of pain. The cornea in both patients was edematous but nonulcerated. The anterior chamber of one patient showed a 4+ flare with an occasional cell, whereas in the other patient it was 40 percent filled with hypopyon. The patients were first treated with corticosteroids, but their failure to respond and their worsening condition prompted a detailed laboratory investigation, resulting in the isolation of *L. monocytogenes* from the aqueous in the first case and from the vitreous in the second. In both patients the endophthalmitis responded to intensive treatment with various antibiotics, principally penicillin and ampicillin. The infectious agent was eradicated, but final visual acuity was poor due to debris on the lens in one patient and a chronic stromal corneal edema with recurrent breakdown of the epithelium in the second patient.

Subsequently, three more reports of *Listeria* endophthalmitis have appeared in the recent ophthalmic literature.[8,9,10] Abbot and associates[9] have published an excellent tabulation of the pertinent features of four cases. A modified, updated version is presented here summarizing these four cases and an additional case from the more recent literature (Table 12-I).

These cases have been in individuals ranging in age from 57 to 76. All had anterior uveitis that, in four of the five, was accompanied by a hypopyon. All patients had uniformly high intraocular pressure, but in two cases the pressure eventually returned to normal, and in the remaining three patients, one still had glaucoma, and another a final pressure of 16. In the last case, the intraocular pressure was not stated.

No history of previous trauma or surgical manipulation was reported in any of the five patients, but all cases had had corticosteroid therapy. Since it appears that the endophthalmitis was endogenously acquired, a bilateral infection would be a possibility, but all cases were unilateral.

TABLE 12-I
SUMMARY OF FIVE CASES OF LISTERIA ENDOPHTHALMITIS

	1. Goodner & Okumoto	2. Bagnarello et al.	3. Snead et al.	4. Abbott et al.	5. Ballen et al.
Age, Sex	76, M	68, M	62, M	68, F	57, F
Gen. health	Good	Good	Good	Good	Carcinoma of the breast
Prev. trauma	None	None	None	None	None
Initial visual acuity	6/60	L.P.	H.M.	H.M.	L.P.
Final visual acuity	6/60	H. M.	6/120	6/1200	6/60
Initial diagnosis	Anterior uveitis & corneal edema	Anterior uveitis & corneal edema	Anterior uveitis & corneal edema	Pigmented hypopyon & corneal edema	Anterior unveitis & corneal edema
Hypopyon	Absent	Dense hypopyon	40% hypopyon	Pigmented hypopyon	3 mm hypopyon
Initial intra-ocular pressure	43	68	44	52	46
Final intra-ocular pressure	Normal	6	Glaucoma	46	Not stated
Steroid therapy	Depot & topical steroid	Predisolon-acetate	0.1% Dexamethasone	Sub-conj beta methasone & Triamcinolone	Prednisolone acetate
Antibiotic therapy	Penicillin Tetracycline Chloramphenicol	Ampicillin Gentamicin Methicillin	Bacitracin Gentamicin Methicillin	Cephalothin Penicillin Gentamicin Cephaloridine	Methicillin Gentamicin Neosporin Ampicillin
Specimen for culture	Aqueous humor	Aqueous humor	Vitreous humor	Aqueous humor	Aqueous humor
Antibiotic sensitivity test results	*Sensitive to:* Penicillin Tetracycline Chloramphenicol	Not stated	*Sensitive to:* Ampicillin Gentamicin *Resistant to:* Penicillin Methicillin	Not stated	*Sensitive to:* Gentamicin Penicillin Ampicillin Cephalothin Tetracycline Chloramphenicol Erythromycin *Resistant to:* Clindamycin Novobiocin

In four of the five cases the organism was isolated from the aqueous humor, suggesting that *L. monocytogenes* has a predilection for the anterior chamber. It seems prudent therefore to do diagnostic anterior chamber taps in cases of acute anterior uveitis with a possible bacterial etiology, and to defer a vitreous aspiration, unless there is a good indication for it.

Although conjunctivitis was one of the earliest recorded manifestations of listeric infection in man, only a few confirmed cases of conjunctivitis are to be found in the medical literature. Several Russian authors reported some 50 cases of conjunctivitis in children and adults but unfortunately all diagnoses were based solely on serological evidence.[4] It is well known that *L. monocytogenes* cross-reacts with a number of commonly occurring bacteria, particularly *Staphylococcus aureus*. Gray and Killinger have stated that the diagnosis of infection can only be made by the isolation of *L. monocytogenes*. Listeric conjunctivitis in man is mentioned often but seldom actually observed. Available information indicates that it is one of the rarest manifestations of listeric infection.[4]

Animal Studies

Ocular listeriosis is probably more common in animals than in man. Kummeneje and Mikkelsen have reported a number of cases of naturally occurring keratoconjunctivitis in cattle and sheep from which *L. monocytogenes* was isolated.[11]

A useful test for identifying this organism is the so-called Anton's eye test. Classically, a severe keratoconjunctivitis results following inoculation of the conjunctiva in a rabbit or guinea pig. This reaction is unique to *L. monocytogenes*. This test was discovered independently by Anton in Austria and Morris and Julianelle in the United States almost simultaneously, but Anton's test is the commonly used designation.[5]

As a part of the laboratory work-up on Case One with listeric endophthalmitis, a rabbit was subjected to the Anton test by simple conjunctival instillation of the strain of *Listeria* isolated from this patient. The rabbit developed a severe purulent conjunctivitis on day 2, an edematous cornea on day 4, and a pannus involving the entire peripheral half of the cornea by day 15 (Fig. 12-1). To obtain additional information regarding this test, five more rabbits were inoculated by conjunctival instillation of the *Listeria* isolated from Case Two. This was accomplished by rolling a cotton-tipped applicator over a 24-hour culture of this organism grown on blood agar and gently rubbing the swab over the lower palpebral conjunctiva. In two rabbits both eyes were inoculated, and only the right eye in three rabbits. The rabbits were examined daily for 15 days, and cultures and scrapings were taken from the lower conjunctiva. They were all bled every day for the first seven days and periodically thereafter. The blood was cultured for isolation of the organisms, and a drop placed on a slide for a differential blood count. These rabbits were observed for 19 days.

On day 2, 4, and 8, aqueous and vitreous were aspirated from one of the rabbits, using a different animal each time. These specimens were used for

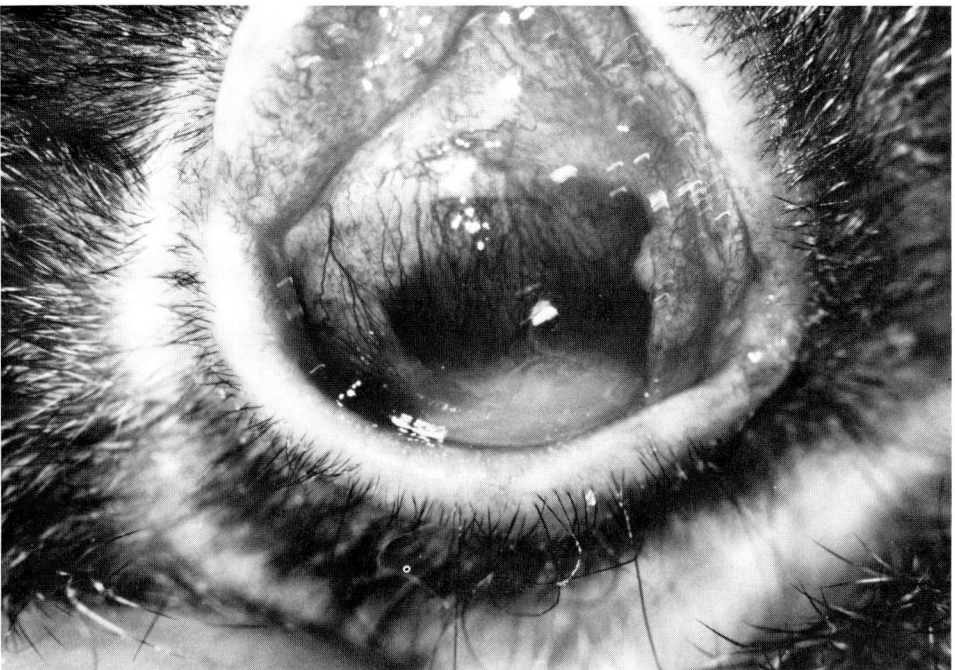

Figure 12-1. Experimental listeriosis: Severe keratoconjunctivitis in a rabbit eight days after inoculation.

cultures and cytologic examination. All inoculated eyes developed a mild to moderate conjunctivitis within 24 hours with slight to moderate discharge. By 48 hours, the conjunctivitis increased in severity and was accompanied by a profuse purulent discharge. The cornea remained clear until day 4, when small areas of opacity resembling infiltrates and haze covering most of the cornea were noted. On day 6 the corneas were so cloudy that the iris could not be seen clearly and a superior pannus extended approximately a millimeter into the cornea. On day 4 a mild to moderate iritis was noted, but thereafter the cloudy cornea obscured visual examination of the anterior chamber. By day 10 there was 360° pannus extending to approximately half of the cornea. By day 14 the pannus had extended into the visual axis but many of the vessels had cleared and the cornea between the vessels was becoming transparent.

The conjunctival cultures taken prior to inoculation showed occasional colonies of *Micrococcus sp.*, diphtheroids, and in one rabbit, rare colonies of *Pasteurella multocida*-like organisms. Conjunctival cultures taken 24 hours after inoculation showed many colonies of *L. monocytogenes*, and continued to do so until day 6 when the number of colonies decreased slightly. By day 10 colonies were seen only rarely. On day 13 all conjunctival cultures were negative for *L. monocytogenes*. Cultures of the aqueous and vitreous were all negative. A blood culture taken from one of the rabbits on day 2 was positive, but all subsequent cultures were negative, as were blood cultures from all the other rabbits. One of the rabbits was found dead in its cage on day 4 (Seeliger has mentioned that instillation of *Listeria* into the conjunctiva may be followed by listeriosis of the central nervous system, but most animals recover[5]). It is probable that there was dissemination of the organism in the dead rabbit, and possibly in some of the others. The blood cultures were all negative except in one instance, and very likely more positive cultures would have resulted if the cold enrichment technique had been used.

Three guinea pigs were inoculated in similar fashion with *L. monocytogenes* and observed for four weeks. At regular intervals the conjunctiva was cultured on blood agar and a scraping taken for Giemsa staining. The clinical course and culture results in the guinea pigs were similar to that of the rabbits, except for a more rapid onset of keratitis and a more pronounced vascularization of the cornea. As in the rabbits, the keratoconjunctivitis, severe as it was, eventually healed and the cornea was normal in three weeks. However, rare colonies of *L. monocytogenes* could still be cultured at three weeks, but by four weeks the cultures were all negative. The conjunctival scrapings from the guinea pigs showed most of the *Listeria* attached to normal appearing conjunctival epithelial cells. Zimianski, Dawson, and Togni have shown with the light and electron microscopy that *L. monocytogenes* is phagocytosed by the conjunctival epithelial cells of the guinea pig as early as 15 minutes after inoculation.[12] The inflammatory cell type was predominantly polymorphonuclear, but monocytes were more prominent than in the rabbit. The monocytosis associated with *L. monocytogenes* is best demonstrated in the peripheral blood following intravenous inoculation of the organism.

Therapy

Penicillin and ampicillin are considered to be the drugs of choice based on clinical experience.[13] Scheld and associates have shown, using an experimental rabbit model of meningitis, that the addition of gentamicin to either penicillin or ampicillin significantly enhanced their bactericidal activity *in vivo*. Recently, Winslow and Pankey were able to demonstrate the *in vitro* effectiveness of trimethoprim combined with sulfamethoxazole in a ratio of 1:19 against 26 clinical isolates of *L. monocytogenes*.[14]

In spite of the effectiveness of antimicrobial agents, an intact host defense system is important. Bakker-Woudenberg et al. have reported on the failure of ampicillin to eradicate *Listeria* in nude mice with T-cell deficiency, even with ampicillin doses twenty times that needed to effect a cure in normal mice.[15]

REFERENCES

1. Gregorio, S. B., and Eveland, W. C.: Isolation of *L. monocytogenes* from inapparent sources in Michigan. In Woodbine, M. (Ed.): *Problems of Listeriosis.* Leicester, England, Leicester University Press, 1975, pp. 87–93.
2. Murray, E. G., Webb, R. A., and Swann, M. B.: A disease of rabbits characterized by a large mononuclear leucocytosis, caused by a hitherto undescribed bacillus, *Bacterium monocytogenes* (N. sp.) *J Path Bact, 29*:407–439, 1926.
3. Nieman, E. R., and Lorber, E.: Listeriosis in adults: A changing pattern. Report of eight cases and review of the literature. 1968–1978. *Rev Inf Dis, 2*:207–229, 1980.
4. Gray, M. L., and Killinger, A. H.: *Listeria monocytogenes* and Listeric infections. *Bact Rev, 30*:309–382, 1966.
5. Seeliger, H. P. R.: *Listeriosis,* 2nd ed. New York, Hafner Publishing Co., 1961.
6. Goodner, E. K., and Okumoto, M.: Intraocular listeriosis. *Am J Ophthalmol, 64*:682–686, 1967.
7. Snead, J. W., Stern, W. H., Whitcher, J. P., and Okumoto, M.: *Listeria monocytogenes* endophthalmitis. *Am J Ophthalmol, 84*:337–339, 1977.
8. Bagnarell, A. G., Berlin, A. J., Weinstein, A. J., McHenry, M. C., and O'Connor, P. S.: *Listeria monocytogenes* endophthalmitis. *Arch Ophthalmol, 95*:1004–1005, 1977.
9. Abbott, R. L., Forster, R. K., and Rebell, G.: *Listeria monocytogenes* endophthalmitis with a black hypopyon. *Am J Ophthalmol, 86*:715–719, 1978.
10. Ballen, P. H., Loffredo, F. R., and Painter, B.: *Listeria* endophthalmitis. *Arch Ophthalmol, 97*:101–102, 1979.
11. Kummeneje, K., and Mikkelsen, T.: Isolation of *Listeria monocytogenes* type 04 from cases of keratoconjunctivitis in cattle and sheep. *Nord Vet Med, 27*:144–149, 1975.
12. Zimianski, M. C., Dawson, C. R., and Togni, B.: Epithelial cell phagocytosis of *Listeria monocytogenes* in the conjunctiva. *Invest Ophthalmol, 13*:623–626, 1974.
13. Tuazon, C. V., Shamsuddin, D., and Miller, H.: Antibiotic susceptibility and synergy of clinical isolates of *Listeria monocytogenes. Antimicrob Ag Chem, 21*:525–527, 1982.
14. Winslow, D. L., and Pankey, G. A.: In vitro activities of trimethoprim and sulfamethoxazole against *Listeria monocytogenes. Antimicrob Ag Chem, 22*:51–54, 1982.
15. Bakker-Woudenberg, I. A. J. M., de Bos, P., Van Leeuwen, W. B., and Michel, M. F.: Efficacy of ampicillin therapy in experimental Listeriosis in mice with impaired T-cell-mediated immune response. *Antimicrob Ag Chem, 19*:76–81, 1981.

Chapter 13

ANIMAL MODELS OF BACTERIAL CORNEAL ULCERS

GARY BARTH, M.D.

Introduction

Experimental animals have been used extensively as subjects for the study of bacteria that produce corneal ulcers in humans. Rabbits have been the animals most studied, followed by guinea pigs and mice. This article will review the work that has been done on these animals for the past ten years. Attention will focus on the successful attempts to establish animal models of ulcers that occur following corneal injury or in the compromised host.

The intact cornea is extremely resistant to experimental infections. In rabbits, guinea pigs, and mice, the local defense mechanisms of tear production, lysozyme, antibodies, and epithelial desquamation prevent direct corneal invasion by all bacteria except for virulent strains of *Shigella flexneri*.[1] Even with induced corneal trauma, only the most virulent bacteria are able to establish corneal ulcers. Consequently, the successful experimental models have been largely limited to the use of *Pseudomonas aeruginosa* infections.

The use of animal experimental models for corneal ulcers has been successful for the study of the more virulent bacterial infections, most notably *Staphylococcus aureus*, *Pseudomonas aeruginosa*, *Serratia marcescens*, and *Shigella flexneri*. Limited success has been achieved with uncommon human bacterial infections such as *Proteus mirabilis*,[2] *Pasteurella multocida*,[3] *Clostridium perfringins*,[4] and *Bacteroides fragilis*.[5]

These experiments have greatly enhanced our knowledge of cellular and noncellular defense mechanisms, bacterial infectivity, bacterial toxins, altered states of immunodefense, and the various treatments available for fighting the infections.

Unfortunately, experimental animal models have been unsuccessful in establishing infections with some common ocular pathogens such as *Pneumonococcus*, *S. epidermidis*, *Moraxella lacunata*, and some of the more serious but rare infections such as *N. gonococcus*, *Nocardia asteroides*, and *Mycobacterium fortuitum* (see Table 13-I). Because negative results are rarely published, it is difficult to know how extensively investigators have tried to infect animal corneas with these organisms, but personal communication with Mas Okumoto suggests that the attempts have been both numerous and ingenious.

TABLE 13-I
**MOST COMMON CAUSES OF BACTERIAL CORNEAL ULCERS
AT THE PROCTOR FOUNDATION**

Pneumococcus
Staphylococcus
Moraxella sp.
Pseudomonas sp.
Alpha streptococcus
Nocardia

To initiate bacterial ulcers or to test bacterial toxic substances three methods have been used:

1. The Cignetti technique of scraping the cornea with a toothed chalazion curette filled with inoculum.[2]
2. Corneal scratch with a needle or scalpel followed by a drop of inoculum.[6]
3. Intracorneal injection of small amounts of inoculum. (In some pseudomonas experiments, for instance, as little as 10 organisms[7] or 0.0005 milligrams of exotoxin have been used.[8])

Normal Host Response

Through the use of animal models for bacterial corneal ulcers, the mechanisms of nonimmunological cellular responses have become better understood. Mondino and co-workers[9] used intracorneal injections of *Pseudomonas aeruginosa* and heat-inactivated *Pseudomonas* and *E. coli* to produce a corneal ring in rabbits. Immunofluorescence staining demonstrated the presence of C3 complement and properdin along with polymorphonuclear cells (PMNs). No immunoglobulin was discovered. The authors hypothesized that the bacterial endotoxin stimulated the alternate complement pathway, causing an early chemotactic response that brought in PMNs before an immunological response could be mounted.

The polymorphonuclear response has been studied using transmission and scanning electron microscopic evaluations of corneas soon after inoculation.[10] Such studies in rabbits have shown that at four hours, the earliest PMNs enter the corneal ulcer from the tears. It is only at 48 hours that significant numbers of PMNs come in from the limbal cornea.[6] Phagocytosis and digestion occurred as early as eight hours after inoculation. In the case of an overwhelming infection with *Pseudomonas aeruginosa*, completely degranulated PMNs have been shown to contain intact bacteria within their cytoplasm.[10]

Numerous investigators have looked at the role PMNs play causing corneal damage. Recent scanning and transmission electron microscopic work by

Van Horn et al.[10] failed to show collagen breakdown with bacteria alone or with heat-inactivated bacteria. The earliest collagen breakdown occurred well after the buildup of *Pseudomonas* organisms and was always associated with the influx and degranulation of PMNs. The collagen destruction was first seen at 8–16 hours and did not become significant until 24 hours after infection. The keratocytes and adjacent epithelial basement membranes were damaged and digested early in the infection.[6] Kessler et al.[11] demonstrated that corneal destruction in *Pseudomonas aeruginosa* infections relies on both the PMNs and the *Pseudonomas* organisms.

Bacterial Toxins

Experiments have been designed to analyze the effect on the cornea of the various substances released by the infecting bacteria.[12-16] The extracellular hemolysins of *Pneumococcus* and *Pseudomonas* have been extensively studied in rabbits by Johnson and Allen.[17-19] These predominantly phospholipidase substances are able to lyse erythrocytes and other cells. Their role in corneal destruction seems less significant than that of the proteases or classic exotoxins.[20]

The bacterial proteases have been examined for the presence of true collagenase. Gray and Kreger[21] used electron microscopic analysis and histochemical studies of *C. histolyticum* rabbit infections to demonstrate abnormal collagen fibrils consistent with the activity of a true collagenase. The same authors failed to find collagenase activity with *Pseudomonas* or its toxin. Morihara[22] and Berman[23] demonstrated that *Pseudomonas* secretes proteases that are nonspecific collagenases.

Lyerly, Gray, and Kreger used rabbits to study the protease of *Serratia marcescens*.[24] Intracorneal injections of the purified protease and the intact organisms caused the ground substance of the cornea to be solubilized. The *Serratia* proteases created necrosis of the cornea without any true collagenase activity.

The role of elastase was analyzed in mouse *Pseudomonas* infections.[25] A mutant strain, deficient in elastase, was found to damage the cornea as extensively as the nonmutant strains. Endotoxin has also been evaluated and found to be relatively unimportant in producing corneal damage.[20]

The most devastating extracellular product is the exotoxin A of *Pseudomonas aeruginosa*. Exotoxin A is a heat-labile substance that inhibits protein synthesis in all tested mammalian cells.[13] It works on the NAD system in a manner identical to diphtheria toxin.[14] This toxin has also been shown to inhibit phagocytosis of the bacteria by PMNS. Iglewski, Burns, and Gipson[26] demonstrated that intrastromal injection of exotoxin A destroyed rabbit epithelial, endothelial, and keratocyte cells. Destruction was prevented when exotoxin

A was neutralized by antitoxin A. Hazlett et al.[15] also found that this damage could be induced by topical application of 15 micrograms of toxin to the nonpenetrated wounded epithelium of the mouse cornea.

Experiments with Compromised Hosts

Neonatal mice have been used as models of immunocompromised subjects. Hazlett and co-workers[27] infected newborn mice by using a nontraumatic injection of inoculum under the fused eyelids. These animals died from severe keratitis and septicemia. Successively older mice developed resistance to a nontraumatic inoculation. Similar results showing increased resistance with age were found when the experiment was done with exotoxin A.[15] This animal model correlated with the experience of Burns in the fatal keratitis of infants that sometimes follows *Pseudomonas* keratitis in the nursery.[28]

The immature mouse model was also used to study the penetration of *Pseudomonas* organisms into the uninjured cornea.[29] Scanning and transmission electron microscopy showed that *Pseudomonas* organisms were able to attach to epithelial cells, partially digest the younger appearing cells, and invade the stroma. This occurred within 15 minutes of inoculation. This type of invasion and the resulting corneal ulcer could not be induced in 30-day-old animals.

Response to Therapy

The most common reason for using experimental animals has been to study the response to antibiotic therapy.[30-42] After having been infected with known amounts of bacteria, the corneas are analyzed by clinical observation and laboratory analysis to determine the success of therapy. The most reliable methods involve removing the infected cornea, homogenizing the corneal substance in a bacterial media, and then plating out the colonies that grow.[15] In this manner, quantitative results can be analyzed. In more than one study the corneas appeared clear and the subsequent cultures were positive for *Pseudomonas aeruginosa*.[43]

Animal models have been used not only to investigate various antibiotics, but also to examine routes of administration.[6,31,44-46] Treatment schedules involving topical, subconjunctival, and combined methods have been used in looking for a superior method. The most recent data by Hyndiuk[6] and by Kupferman and Liebowitz[45] have suggested that topical treatment with fortified antibiotics offers the most effective and least painful method.

Numerous animal studies have examined the adverse effects of corticosteroid drops in the treatment of bacterial corneal ulcers.[47-50] In some experiments, steroids were used alone or in combination with antibiotics. In general, steroid use did not interfere with the treatment by appropriate antibiotics. In a study using gentamicin-resistant *Pseudomonas aeruginosa*, animals given both steroids and gentamicin had significantly more bacteria recovered from their corneas than those treated only with the antibiotic.[50] Whether or not steroids reduced corneal scarring is difficult to determine from these experimental models.

The role of idoxuridine (IDU) was examined in rabbits treated with IDU four times a day.[51] On day 6 of treatment, the rabbits were inoculated with *S. aureus* using the Cignetti technique. The animals treated with IDU were then continued on their IDU therapy for four more days, after which time they were found to be significantly more infected. The authors attributed the adverse effect of the IDU to its local immunosuppressive effect.

Cryosurgery was also tested as a treatment of *Pseudomonas aeruginosa* corneal ulcers in guinea pigs.[43] Six strains of virulent *Pseudomonas* were individually tested by injecting them into the corneas of guinea pigs. The corneas were treated for six seconds with a brass probe that had been immersed in liquid nitrogen. The freeze proved to be immediately bactericidal and significantly improved the efficacy of topical antibiotic therapy. The results, however, were not supported by *in vitro* experiments in which the same bacteria were subjected to six seconds of similar freezing in cold acetone.

Summary

Studies of experimental animal models have successfully simulated the traumatic etiology of most human corneal ulcers. These studies have also shed light on bacterial infection in the compromised host. The human cornea, however, is affected by bacteria other than *Pseudomonas, Serratia,* and *Staphylococcus*, and by other conditions that can predispose to corneal infections, such as the use of soft contact lenses, infection by herpes virus, and keratitis sicca.[4] Future studies of bacterial ulcers in animals will be directed at studying the attachment and penetration of bacteria in corneas compromised in ways other than by immunosuppression or corneal injury.

REFERENCES

1. Cross, W. R., and Nakamura, M.: Analysis of virulence of *Shigella flexneri* by experimental infection of the rabbit eye. *J Infect Dis, 122*:394–400, 1970.
2. Okumoto, M., Smolin, G., Belfort, R., Kim, H., and Siverio, C. E.: *Proteus* isolated from human eyes. *Am J Ophthalmol, 81*:495–501, 1976.
3. Purcell, J. J., and Krachmer, J. H.: Corneal ulcer caused by *Pasteurella multocida*. *Am J Ophthalmol, 83*:540–542, 1977.
4. Stern, G. A., Hodes, B. L., and Stock, E. L.: *Clostridium perfringens* corneal ulcer. *Arch Ophthalmol, 97*:661–663, 1979.
5. Stern, G. A., and Stock, E. L.: Experimental *Bacteroides fragilis* keratitis. *Arch Ophthalmol, 96*:2264–66, 1978.

6. Hyndiuk, R. A.: Experimental *Pseudomonas* keratitis. *Trans Am Ophth Soc, 79*:541–624, 1981.
7. Davis, S. D., Sarff, L. D., and Hyndiuk, R. A.: Experimental *Pseudomonas* keratitis in guinea pigs: Therapy of moderately severe infections. *Br J Ophthalmol, 63*:436–439, 1979.
8. Bernstein, H. N., and Maddox, Y. T.: Corneal pathogenicity of *Serratia marcescens* in the rabbit. *Trans Am Acad Ophthalmol Otol, 77*:432–440, 1973.
9. Mondino, B. J., Rabin, B. S., Kessler, E., Gallo, J., and Brown, S. I.: Corneal rings with gram-negative bacteria. *Arch Ophthalmol, 95*:2222–2225, 1977.
10. Van Horn, D. L., Davis, D. S., Hyndiuk, R. A., and Pederson, H. J.: Experimental *Pseudomonas* keratitis in the rabbit: Bacteriologic, clinical and microscopic observations. *Invest Ophthalmol, 20*:213–221, 1981.
11. Kessler, E., Mondino, B. J., and Brown, S. I.: The corneal response to *Pseudomonas aeruginosa. Invest Ophthalmol Vis Sci, 16*:116–125, 1977.
12. Berk, R. S., Iglewski, B. H., and Hazlett, L. D.: Age-related susceptibility of mice to ocular challenge with *Pseudomonas aeruginosa* exotoxin A. *Infect and Immun, 33*:90–94, 1981.
13. Lui, P. V.: Extracellular toxins of *Pseudomonas aeruginosa. J Infect Dis, 130*:594–599, 1974.
14. Iglewski, B. H., Lui, P. V., and Kabat, D.: Mechanism of action of *Pseudomonas aeruginosa* exotoxin A adenosine diphosphate ribosylation of mammalian elongation factor in vitro and in vivo. *Infect and Immun, 15*:138–144, 1977.
15. Hazlett, L. D., Berk, R. S., and Iglewski, B. H.: Microscopic characterization of ocular damage produced by *Pseudomonas aeruginosa* exotoxin A. *Infect and Immun, 34*:1025–1035, 1981.
16. Pavlovskis, O. R., Callahan, L. T., and Meyer, R. D.: Characterization of exotoxin of *Pseudomonas aeruginosa. J Infect Dis, 130*:100–102, 1974.
17. Johnson, M. K., and Allen, J. H.: The role of cytolysin in pneumococcal ocular infection. *Am J Ophthalmol, 80*:518–521, 1975.
18. Johnson, M. K., and Allen, J. H.: Ocular toxin in *pneumococcus. Am J Ophthalmol, 72*:175, 1971.
19. Johnson, M. K., and Aultman, K. S.: Studies on the mechanism of action of oxygen labile hemolysins. *J Gen Micro, 101*:27–41, 1977.
20. Jones, D. M.: Pathogenesis of bacterial and fungal keratitis. *Trans Ophthalmol Soc U K, 98*:367–71, 1978.
21. Gray, L. D., and Kreger, A. S.: Rabbit corneal damage produced by *Pseudomonas aeruginosa* infection. *Infect and Immun, 12*:419–432, 1975.
22. Morihara, K.: Pseudomonas aeruginosa proteinase. *Biochem Biophys Acta, 73*:113–124, 1963.
23. Berman, M.: Regulation of collagenase. *Trans Ophthalmol Soc U K, 98*:397, 1978.
24. Lyerly, D., Gray, L., and Kreger, A.: Characterization of rabbit corneal damage produced by *Serratia* keratitis and by a *Serratia* protease. *Infect Immun, 33*:927–32, 1981.
25. Ohman, D. E., Burns, R. P., and Iglewski, B. H.: Corneal infections in mice with toxin A and elastase mutants of *Pseudomonas aeruginosa. J Infect Dis, 142*:435–442, 1980.
26. Iglewski, B. H., Burns, R. P. and Gipson, I. K.: Pathogenesis of corneal damage from *Pseudomonas* exotoxin A. *Invest Ophthalmol, 16*:73–76, 1977.
27. Hazlett, L. D., Rosen, D. D., and Berk, B. S.: Age-related susceptibility to *Pseudomonas aeruginosa* ocular infections in mice. *Infect Immun, 20*:25–29, 1978.
28. Burns, R. P.: *Pseudomonas aeruginosa* keratitis: Mixed infections of the eye. *Am J Ophthalmol, 67*:257–262, 1969.
29. Hazlett, L. D., Wells, P., Spann, B., and Berk, R. S.: Penetration of the unwounded immature mouse cornea and conjunctiva by *Pseudomonas*: SEM–TEM analysis. *Invest Ophthalmol, 19*:694–697, 1980.

30. Ahmad, A., Smolin, G., Okumoto, M., and Ohno, S.: Ticarcillin in the treatment of experimental *Pseudomonas* keratitis. *Br J Ophthalmol*, 61:92–95, 1977.
31. Baum, J. L., Barza, M., Shushan, D., and Weinstein, L.: Concentrations of gentamicin in experimental corneal ulcers: Topical versus subconjunctival therapy. *Arch Ophthalmol*, 92:315, 1974.
32. Belfort, R., Smolin, G., Okumoto, M., and Kin, H. B.: Nebcin in the treatment of experimental *Pseudomonas* keratitis. *Br J Ophthalmol*, 59:725, 1975.
33. Davis, S. D., and Chandler, J. W.: Experimental keratitis due to *Pseudomonas aeruginosa*: Model for evaluation of antimicrobial drugs. *Antimicrob Ag Chemo*, 8:350, 1975.
34. Davis, S. D., Sarff, L. D., and Hyndiuk, R. A.: Topical tobramycin therapy in experimental *Pseudomonas* keratitis: An evaluation of some factors that potentially enhance efficacy. *Arch Ophthalmol*, 96:123–5, 1978.
35. Davis, S. D., Sarff, L. D., and Hyndiuk, R. A.: Therapeutic effect of topical antibiotic on untreated eye in experimental keratitis. *Can J Ophthalmol*, 13:273–6, 1978.
36. Davis, S. D., Sarff, L. D., and Hyndiuk, R. A.: Bacteriologic cure of experimental *Pseudomonas* keratitis. *Invest Ophthalmol*, 17:916–8, 1978.
37. Davis, S. D., Sarff, L. D., and Hyndiuk, R. A.: Comparison of therapeutic routes in experimental *Pseudomonas* keratitis. *Am J Ophthalmol*, 87:710–716, 1979.
38. Davis, S. D., Sarff, L. D., and Hyndiuk, R. A.: Relative efficacy of the topical use of amikacin, gentamicin and tobramycin in experimental pseudomonas keratitis. *Can J Ophthalmol*, 15:28–29, 1980.
39. Hansen, K. D., and Meyer, R. F.: Amikacin treatment of *Pseudomonas* caused corneal ulcer. *Arch Ophthalmol*, 98:199–102, 1980.
40. Kupferman, A., and Liebowitz, H. M.: Topical antibiotic therapy of *Pseudomonas* keratitis. *Arch Ophthalmol*, 97:1699–1702, 1979.
41. Smolin, G., Okumoto, M., and Wilson, F. M.: The effect of tobramycin on *Pseudomonas* keratitis. *Am J Ophthalmol*, 76:555–560, 1973.
42. Wilkie, J., Smolin, G., and Okumoto, M.: The effect of rifampicin on *Pseudomonas* keratitis. *Can J Ophthalmol*, 7:309–313, 1972.
43. Alpren, T. V., Hyndiuk, R. A., Davis, S. D., and Sarff, L. D.: Cryotherapy for experimental *Pseudomonas* keratitis. *Arch Ophthalmol*, 97:711–714, 1979.
44. Davis, S. D., Sarff, L. D., and Hyndiuk, R. A.: Failure of subconjunctival antibiotics in experimental *Pseudomonas* keratitis. *Invest Ophthalmol*, 17:228, 1978.
45. Kupferman, A., and Liebowitz, H. M.: Antibiotic therapy of bacterial keratitis: Topical application or periocular injection. *Invest Ophthalmol*, 19:112, 1981.
46. Sloan, S. H., Petit, T. H., and Litwack, K. D.: Gentamicin penetration in the aqueous humor of eyes with corneal ulcers. *Am J Ophthalmol*, 73:750–753, 1972.
47. Behrems-Bauman, W., Paul, H. H., and Ansorg, R.: The influence of cortisone in the treatment of *Pseudomonas aeruginosa* keratitis: An animal experimental study. *Klin Monatsbl Augenheilkd*, 178:200–202, 1981.
48. Bohigian, G. M., and Foster, C. S.: Treatment of *Pseudomonas* keratitis in the rabbit with antibiotic-steroid combinations. *Invest Ophthalmol*, 16:553–6, 1977.
49. Liebowitz, H. M., and Kupferman A.: Topically administered corticosteroid effect on antibiotic-treated bacterial keratitis. *Arch Ophthalmol*, 98:1287–1290, 1980.
50. Stern, G. A., Okumoto, M., Friedlaender, M., and Smolin, G.: The effect of combined gentamicin-corticosteroid treatment on gentamicin-resistant *Pseudomonas* keratitis. *Ann Ophthalmol*, 12:1011–1014, 1980.
51. Yamaguchi, K., Okumoto, M., Stern, G., Friedlaender, M., and Smolin, G.: Idoxuridine and bacterial corneal infection. *Am J Ophthalmol*, 87:202–205, 1979.

Chapter 14

EXPERIMENTAL BACTERIAL ENDOPHTHALMITIS

IRA G. WONG, M.D.

Introduction

Infectious endophthalmitis is a devastating complication of ocular surgery or of a penetrating injury to the eye. Endophthalmitis often results in blindness in spite of intensive and appropriate antibiotic therapy. The treatment of endophthalmitis has produced generally poor results because of the rapidity with which the eye can become irreparably damaged from the infectious process and because the penetration of antibiotics into the eye is relatively poor.

Because endophthalmitis is an uncommon condition, and because no case of endophthalmitis is exactly the same as another, the relative efficacy of our diagnostic and therapeutic techniques has been difficult to evaluate. Cases may differ in terms of the origin of the infection, the virulence of the infecting agent, the appropriate time to begin therapy and the type of antibiotic needed. Thus, it has become essential to develop an experimental model of endophthalmitis in order to evaluate, under controlled situations, the diagnostic and therapeutic measures used in the clinical situation.

The experimental model allows us to control certain variables such as the type of infectious agent and the temporal course of the infection. It also allows us to manipulate variables such as the antibiotic dosage. Outcome can be more precisely measured in terms of *in vivo* antibiotic levels and histopathologic damage to the model—data that are generally unavailable in the clinical setting.

Despite these advantages, there are potential hazards and pitfalls when it comes to translating information from the experimental model of endophthalmitis to the clinical situation. My purpose here is to describe some experimental models of endophthalmitis and the research designs used to study this condition. The advantages and limitations of the experimental model are described in order to determine how we can better apply experimental results to this difficult clinical condition.

Animal Models of Endophthalmitis

The most frequently studied animal model of endophthalmitis uses the vitreous of the albino rabbit eye infected with bacteria. After 8–48 hours, the eye is treated with an antibiotic and its effect evaluated.

The rabbit is commonly used because the animal and its eye are a convenient size and because of the rabbit's characteristic docility, availability, and relative low cost. The rabbit eye, however, has significant anatomic and physiologic differences from the human or primate eye that may affect the course of an infection and the response to antibiotics. These differences have resulted in differing conclusions about the efficacy of various routes of antibiotic administration. In studies of the rabbit by Barza,[1] antibiotics injected into the subconjunctival space produced a higher vitreous level than when injected into the retrobulbar space. When this study was repeated in the squirrel monkey, no significant difference was noted in antibiotic penetration of the vitreous, regardless of whether injection was via the subconjunctival or the retrobulbar route. The author proposed that the findings in the rabbit and the monkey experiments were different because of the greater vascularity of the rabbit orbit, which allowed more of the antibiotic into the systemic circulation.

Other anatomic differences between the rabbit and the primate eye may affect the study of the treatment of endophthalmitis. For example, the rabbit retina is less vascularized than that of the primate, so that relatively less antibiotic may be delivered to these areas. The sclera is thinner in the rabbit than in the primate, and the irritation of a subconjunctival injection may thus lead to greater absorption of antibiotic. Last, tearing and blinking rates are much slower in the rabbit than in the primate, and this affects the absorption of topical antibiotics.

Factors in Experimental Design

In the animal model of endophthalmitis, a number of experimental design factors directly affect the outcome of the study and must therefore be considered before beginning an experiment. For example, the site and size of the infectious inoculum are important. Our own studies[2] have shown that a much larger inoculum of bacteria is needed to cause endophthalmitis when the bacteria are injected into the anterior chamber rather than into the vitreous. We found that about 100,000 colony-forming units (cfu) of *Pseudomonas* or *Pneumococcus* had to be injected into the anterior chamber of the phakic rabbit eye to obtain a 100 percent infection rate. In comparison, from 50–100 cfu of the same organisms were needed to achieve the same results in the vitreous. Our *in vitro* studies[2] showed that the aqueous had a capacity identical to the vitreous for supporting bacterial growth, and that there was no apparent inhibiting factor in the aqueous to prevent growth. We believe that the rapid turnover, the presence of immunoglobulins, and the lack of nutrients may prevent bacterial infection, thus protecting the anterior segment of the eye from infection. We can speculate that endophthalmitis occurring after filtering operations for glaucoma may result in part from reduced outflow facility and in part from the presence of a fistula. Many studies of experimental endophthalmitis have overwhelmed the vitreous with inoculations of 10,000–20,000 organisms, creating an infection so rapidly progressive that it requires antibiotic treatment earlier than normal.

Another factor that must be considered in the experimental design is if the experimental animal is phakic, because the presence of an intact lens-zonule diaphragm can affect the spread of bacteria within the eye. We have shown experimentally that the lens-zonule forms a physical barrier to confine bacteria within the separate compartments.[2] If 1 million cfu of *Pneumococcus* are injected into the anterior chamber, the number of organisms found 48 hours later will be 100,000 times greater in the anterior chamber than in the vitreous. If a thousand organisms are injected into the vitreous, the concentration of organisms in the vitreous 48 hours later will be 10,000 times greater than in the anterior chamber.

We have found, on the other hand, that if the lens is removed, the concentration of bacteria is the same in the anterior chamber as in the vitreous, regardless of whether the bacteria are introduced in the anterior chamber or in the vitreous.

The iris-lens-zonule diaphragm may also affect the level of antibiotics in the aqueous. Peyman,[3] using the rabbit model, found that when gentamicin was administered subconjunctivally, aqueous levels of gentamicin were higher in the aphakic than in the phakic eye.

In the experimental design, inflammation is another factor that greatly affects the results of antibiotic studies. In the noninflamed eye, the blood-ocular barrier is intact. The capillary system is nonfenestrated, and the anterior uveal and retinal epithelium have tight junctions. Inflammation disrupts these barriers and enhances the intraocular penetration of drugs into the eye. The study by Barza[1] found that antibiotic penetration in noninflamed rabbit and monkey eyes differed when the eyes were infected. The difference in antibiotic penetration between animal species was much less when eyes were infected. The subconjunctival and retrobulbar routes were found to be equivalent in the inflamed eyes but not in the noninflamed eyes.

The study of Barza[1] emphasizes the need to investigate the inflamed eye if study results are to be clinically relevant. Most studies of antibiotic penetration, however, are of normal eyes. When antibiotic studies are performed in infected eyes, clinical and histologic examinations are done but intraocular antibiotic levels are not measured.

In developing the model of experimental endophthalmitis, selection of the infectious agent is critical to the outcome of the experiment. The virulence of the organism, for example, has a direct effect on outcome. A highly virulent organism may replicate to induce rapid destruction of ocular tissue, or a virulent organism may release large amounts of exotoxin and proteolytic enzymes. Vastin and associates[4] have shown that the visual outcome in their clinical cases of bacterial endophthalmitis was directly related to the level of exotoxin and proteolytic enzyme activity of the infecting bacteria.

Whether the experimental animal is pigmented or albino also affects drug studies of endophthalmitis.[1] The pigmentation of the eye may bind some antibiotics tightly, rendering them less available to kill bacteria. Intraocular gentamicin levels were found to differ between pigmented and albino rabbits, as the pigmentation appeared to make less gentamicin available. Binding effects differ from one antibiotic to another and an *in vitro* study shows that gentamicin is bound by synthetic melanin much more than clindamycin.[5]

Experimental Factors in Antibiotic Studies of Endophthalmitis

Of great interest in studying endophthalmitis are the effects of antibiotics on the condition. Major questions concern which antibiotics to give and which routes of administration are the most effective and safest. Antibiotics, by the nature of their molecular structure, display different pharmacologic behavior in the eye. Some antibiotics, such as chloramphenicol and some tetracyclines, are lipophilic molecules that readily pass through the blood-ocular barrier. Others, such as penicillin, the cephalosporins, and aminoglycosides, are hydrophilic and do not penetrate well across the blood-ocular barrier. A few antibiotics, such as penicillin, are actively transported by the ciliary body epithelium into the eye.

A considerable body of literature compares various routes of antibiotic administration. Some have argued for the use of intravitreal injection,[6] others for the subconjunctival route.[7] Many questions remain unanswered, however, because of the lack of attention to some of the variables described here.

In antibiotic studies using the experimental model of endophthalmitis, the method of measuring antibiotic levels is important: different methods may give different results. Radioactive assays are among the most convenient and accurate techniques for determining the total concentration of a drug, and results from this type of measurement may be useful in evaluating the toxicity of antibiotics.

As I have mentioned, not all of the antibiotic that penetrates into the eye is readily available for destroying bacteria. How do we determine the available proportion? In studies of endophthalmitis, equilibrium dialysis or ultracentrifuge techniques have sometimes been used to answer this question. To approximate the concentration of freely available antibiotic, Barza and associates[8] used a trephine-disk bioassay to detect readily available antibiotic.

The amount of antibiotic that diffused out of the trephined ocular tissue was compared with that which diffused out of a filter paper disk soaked with known amounts of antibiotic. The study of readily available antibiotic may help us to compare more precisely the efficacy of various drugs.

In our study of experimental endophthalmitis, we have been evaluating alternative ways of measuring the severity of infection. Most commonly, a clinical assessment of the eye is made, electroretinography may be done, and the histopathologic sections are evaluated. Less often, bacterial colony counts are obtained. We have been interested in measuring bacterial antigen concentration and the metabolic consumption of glucose in the aqueous and vitreous. The concentration of pneumococcal polysaccharide capsular antigen gives us an approximation of the number of killed and viable *Pneumococci*.[9] The glucose concentration in the aqueous and vitreous declines in the presence of an active bacterial infection.[10] The level of glucose has provided us with a way to assess the activity of the bacteria *in vivo*. We believe that these techniques offer another quantitative tool for following the course of endophthalmitis and for allowing us to compare the severity of infection and the effects of an antibiotic on infection.

As we probed into the variables of the experimental model of endophthalmitis, many questions were raised and we were able to appreciate the complexity of the model. Nonetheless, by continuing our investigation of these questions, we hope to treat our clinical cases of endophthalmitis more effectively.

REFERENCES

1. Barza, M.: Factors affecting the intraocular penetration of antibiotics: the influence of route, inflammation, animal species and tissue pigmentation. *Scand J Infect Dis* (Suppl), *14*:151–9, 1978.
2. Wong, I. G., Ostler, H. B., and Swan, I. S.: Intraocular spread of bacteria endophthalmitis (in preparation).
3. Peyman, G. A., May, D. R., Homer, P. I., and Kasbeer, R. T.: Penetration of gentamicin into the aphakic eye. *Ann Ophthalmol*, *9*(7):871–80, 1977.
4. Vastine, D. W., Peyman, G. A., and Guth, S. B.: Visual prognosis in bacterial endophthalmitis treated with intravitreal antibiotics. *Ophthalmic Surg*, *10*:76–83, 1979.
5. Tabbara, K. F., and O'Connor, G. R.: Ocular tissue absorption of clindamycin phosphate. *Arch Ophthalmol*, *93*:1180–1185.
6. Baum, J. L.: Viewpoints: Antibiotic administration in the treatment of bacterial endophthalmitis. I. Periocular injections. *Surv Ophthalmol*, *21*(4):332–339, 1977.
7. Peyman, G. A.: Viewpoints: Antibiotic administration in the treatment of bacterial endophthalmitis. II. Intravitreal injections. *Surv Ophthalmol*, *21*(4):332; 339–346, 1977.
8. Barza, M., Baum, J. L., and Kane, A.: Comparing radioactive and trephine-disk bioassays of dicloxacillin and gentamicin in ocular tissues in vitro. *Am J Ophthalmol*, *83*:530–9, 1977.

9. Wong, I. G., Ostler, H. B., and Swan, I. S.: Counterimmunoelectrophoresis for the early detection of endophthalmitis (in preparation).
10. Wong, I. G., Ostler, H. B., and Swan, I. S.: Reduced intraocular glucose in bacterial endophthalmitis (submitted for publication, *Arch Ophthalmol*).

SECTION II
NEOPLASTIC DISEASES

Chapter 15

OCULAR FINDINGS IN CUTANEOUS MALIGNANT MELANOMAS IN SWINE

Robert P. Burns, M.D.; Lynette Feeney-Burns, Ph.D.; Kathy Lentz, M.D.;
Kent Loeffler, B.S.; Reuel R. Hook, Jr., Ph.D.; Jane Berkelhammer, Ph.D.;
Ronald W. Oxenhandler, M.D.; Charles C. Middleton, D.V.M.

Introduction

The pig is an excellent animal for biomedical research. It has an anatomy and physiology quite similar to the human being and can be bred easily. Pigs are intelligent and docile. However, because investigators are accustomed to using smaller laboratory animals such as the mouse, rat, and rabbit, the pig has not been used often. Another reason is that most medical research facilities are located in large cities where it is undesirable to maintain a herd of pigs. However, in a rural area, where adequate space and veterinary help are available, the swine is an excellent research animal.

Knowing this, the Hormel Meat Packing Company of Austin, Minnesota, some years ago started breeding for miniature size in swine to make them more acceptable for scientific research. A fully grown ordinary pig for the food market may reach the unmanageable size of 600 to 800 pounds, but the Hormel strain of miniature swine matures at around 100 to 200 pounds, making them comparable in size to human beings. At the University of Missouri-Columbia, the Sinclair Comparative Medicine Research Farm established a breeding herd of these Hormel miniature swine. These pigs are mostly black.

In 1967, a cutaneous melanoma was noticed in one of these Sinclair Farm pigs.[1] This discovery led to an examination of all the miniature swine born in the Missouri herd. By 1968, it was recognized that 11 percent of the miniature swine had protruding skin tumors and that 15 percent had flat, deeply pigmented melanin spots.[2]

We thank Werner K. Noell, M.D. for his generous help with the electroretinography. This research was aided in part by grants EY 03680, CA 28230, and CA 25718 from the National Institutes of Health, from Research to Prevent Blindness, and from the Eye Research Foundation of Missouri.

These swine were given gross examinations at approximately one month intervals for a year. The color, shape, and size of both the elevated tumors and pigmented flat spots were recorded. Biopsy studies were done on the lesions.

Classification of Lesions

Lesions were classified into three distinct types:[3] (1) flat black spots, (2) raised black tumors, and (3) blue tumors. The first type consisted of heavily pigmented spots or dark black spots in the skin that were usually oval to circular, of variable size, and flat. The texture did not appear to differ from the adjacent unaffected skin. Histologic examination of the biopsies showed that the epidermis had moderate thickening with elongation of rete pegs. The epidermis contained excess melanin pigment throughout each layer, but melanin was especially dense in the basal layer of epidermis of the elongated rete pegs. Frequently, there were clumps of melanin-containing cells in the superficial dermis subjacent to the hyperpigmented epidermis.

With Masson's trichrome, after bleaching the melanin, it was seen that the lesions consisted of many clear cells along the basal layer of epidermis corresponding in position to the heavily pigmented sites. Presumably, these cells were melanocytes, originating from the neural crest.

The second type of lesion was a raised black tumor (Fig. 15-1). These lesions varied in size; their color ranged from deep black to a lighter bluish black. They had discrete edges and were elevated and firm on palpation. The surface varied from smooth to rough with deep cracks and occasional ulcerations that were shiny and jet black.

Histologically, the raised black tumors were similar to the pigmented spots in that they contained melanin in both epidermis and dermis. The epidermis frequently contained nests of heavily pigmented cells at the dermal-epidermal junction. These lesions contained a much larger number of melanin-laden cells in the dermis, which formed a mass causing an elevation of the overlying epidermis. These masses were somewhat circumscribed. Again, after melanin bleaching and Masson's staining, many clear cells were found. They were polyhedral with a large amount of cytoplasm and a relatively small nucleus, often located eccentrically. These cells varied in size and some were multinucleated. There was no mitotic activity and the cells were thought to be melanin-filled macrophages.

The third type of lesion identified in early studies was a slightly raised blue tumor. These lesions differed from the black tumors in color and were not elevated as much as the black tumors. The blue color can be described by analogy with a blue iris, which has the same pigment, but in different amounts and at different depth, as a black iris. The skin adjacent to these tumors occasionally became depigmented, forming a white halo around the

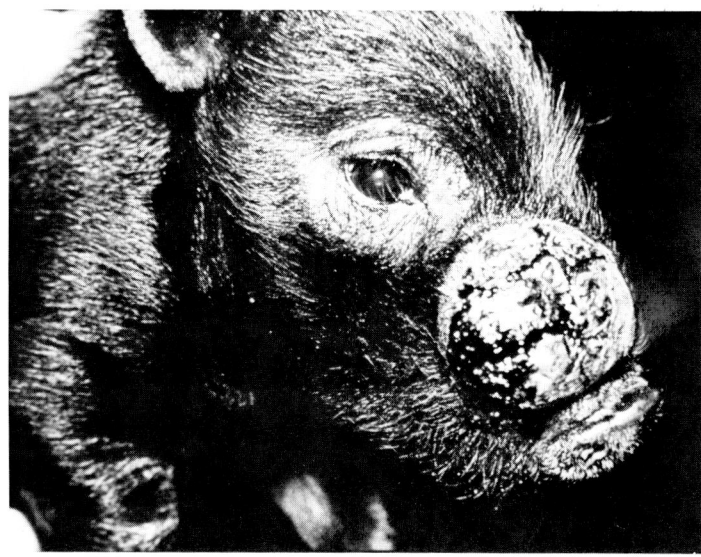

Figure 15-1. Baby Sinclair swine, black skin and hair, with large, black, cracked-surface malignant melanoma arising from snout. This animal died from ulcerative necrosis of the tumor and airway obstruction.

blue tumor. Histologically, they were similar to the blue-black lesions but the epidermis and adjacent dermis contained no melanin. Melanin in these tumors was widely dispersed in the middle and deeper parts of the dermis in small clumps of cells frequently orientated around blood vessels.

Overall, the three classifications of skin lesions suggested a transition of the melanotic lesions with time; they appeared to progress from heavily pigmented spots to raised black tumors and then to slightly raised blue tumors. During these studies it was further noted that some of the hair in the normally black coat of the Hormel Miniature Swine becomes depigmented even in nontumor areas, resulting in a mixture of black and white hair.

These early studies suggested that the Sinclair Miniature Swine might be a better animal in which to study the spontaneous development of malignant melanomas than the only previously known animal model— the old grey horse. (As grey horses pass middle age, they often have depigmentation of the hair and they occasionally develop malignant melanomas.[4]) Therefore, it was decided to study further these melanomas in miniature swine.

The next step was a more detailed dermatologic classification of the lesions. The pigmented lesions in the swine were classified and compared with their human counterparts.[5]

These comparisons are as follows:

Swine Lesions	Human Counterparts
Flat lesions	Junctional nevus
Elevated lesion	Human compound nevus
Raised blue tumors	Blue nevus
Peripheral depigmentation	Vitiligo
Regressing lesions	Sutton's halo nevus
Ulcerative tumors	Melanoma
Systemic pigmented tumors	Metastasis of melanoma
Congenital tumors	Bathing trunk-congenital nevus

The morphologic stages of these tumors were compared with their histology. The age of the animal at the times when different tumor stages develop also varies progressively.

During the histologic study, it was found that although the skin of the pig differs notably from human skin, as noted by Montagna,[6] the tumors resemble their human counterparts. Histologic studies were difficult at first because the large amount of melanin in the cells obscured cellular detail. However, electron microscopy and bleaching with the potassium permanganate technique made visualization easier.

There is a marked difference between these animal tumors, which regress spontaneously, and human tumors, which usually have a progressive course and are often lethal. This difference has raised the question of whether the animal melanoma is truly malignant.

Necropsy Studies

Our next study consisted of a necropsy of 60 pigs that were part of a carefully planned breeding program.[7] The results of this study showed that the flat lesions were like junctional nevi with melanocytes migrating into the epidermis and along the rete ridges of the epidermis. Nevi composed of cytologically malignant cells were seen. These cells had a large nucleus to cytoplasm ratio. However, the large raised lesions invariably showed an invasive malignant melanoma with frequent central ulceration. There was occasional loss of cell cohesion. Mitoses were common, varying from 1 to 3 percent per high power field. Vascular invasion of the melanomas was seen occasionally, although it was more common to find pigment-laden macrophages in vein walls.

The host inflammatory response leading to regression of the cutaneous tumor was quite similar to that seen occasionally in human melanoma. A series of cellular events preceded depigmentation and scar formation. Extensive lymphocytic infiltrates occurred following a plateau of rapid tumor growth. This dense lymphocytic infiltrate contributed significantly to the gross bulk of the tumor.

In this 1979 necropsy study of 60 pigs, 15 or 25 percent had metastatic disease.[7] All of the animals with metastases had deeply invasive, malignant skin melanoma. As in human melanoma, the highest incidence of metastases was to lymph nodes, lungs, and liver. Only one-third of the animals had metastases to multiple organ systems. No other primary neoplasia were identified.

By now the correspondence between the skin tumors of Sinclair pigs and the Clark system of classification of human malignant melanoma became apparent. The pigs with metastatic disease displayed cutaneous invasion into the deep reticular dermis or into the panniculus (Clark's Levels 4 and 5).[8] Further studies were begun to document the inheritance of the melanomas.

Inheritance Pattern

A breeding study was published in 1979,[9] which showed that the incidence of melanomas at birth was highest (54%) in newborn pigs derived from mating of melanoma-carrying females to melanoma-bearing males. If normal females were mated to melanomic males, there was a 22 percent incidence of tumor. When melanomic females were mated to normal males the incidence was 21 percent, whereas the mating of non-tumor-bearing females and males resulted in only a 2 percent incidence of melanoma. The non-tumor-bearing animals were from the main herd of Hormel swine. These differences are highly significant statistically.

During this study, it was further observed that there was an increased frequency of melanomas by one year of life. This showed that the melanomas continued to develop after birth. The rate of development of the tumors varied with the different breeding groups. This was an important observation—that tumor development decreases as age of swine increases—because it suggests that control of tumor development might be acquired with age. Control of tumor growth was also suggested by the high incidence of tumor regression observed in this model system.

Etiologic factors other than a genetic predisposition were not found, although the role of viruses and other biological agents has not been studied. Ultraviolet radiation is a common cause of human malignant melanomas; but these melanoma swine had only limited access to sunlight, as opposed to the main swine herd that was maintained in an external environment and that has low incidence of melanomas.

It is well known that melanomas are rare in humans with black skin. Therefore, the development of melanomas in black swine, almost exclusively, is a reversal of the human situation. Melanomas in predominantly white swine are rare.

Immunologic Studies

The striking fact of melanoma regression in these swine prompted an investigation of lymphocyte reactivity to soluble tumor extracts.[10] Lymphocytes of melanomic swine, normal swine, swine sensitized to tuberculin, and swine sensitized to DNCB–BSA were studied using an *in vitro* rosette assay. The ability of each group's lymphocytes to form rosettes with sheep red blood cells was measured. An increase in active rosette-forming cells after incubation with each of nine separate allogeneic melanoma extracts indicated that the ability to stimulate lymphocyte reactivity was not limited to a single melanoma. Therefore, it was felt that the tumor-related immune response that occurs in melanomic swine is directed toward a tumor-associated antigen or antigen-like substance.

The next investigation of this model sought to simplify the complexity of *in vivo* tumor regression by putting the melanoma cells in tissue culture and subjecting them to long-term growth.[11] The morphology of cultured melanoma cells ranges from dendritic to cuboidal, and thus it is similar to that of human melanoma cells. Doubling times of swine melanoma cells were also similar to those of human melanoma cells *in vitro*. DOPA positive cells were detected by light microscopy; melanin and premelanosomes were detected by electron microscopy. Cell cultures could be propagated from progressing, partially regressed, and primary cutaneous lesions, as well as from visceral metastases. More than 70 percent of the melanoma specimens cultured grew progressively. Eight specimens were propagated 8–14 months *in vitro* with 19–46 passages being done. Therefore, it seems that the factor or factors operating *in vivo* to cause regression of melanoma cells within two to three months do not operate *in vitro*. Karyotype analysis revealed diploid cell cultures with 38 chromosomes, the normal chromosome number for domestic swine.

In another study, specimens from seven Sinclair Swine melanomas were transplanted to the cheek pouches of Syrian golden hamsters that were pretreated with cortisone.[12] The specimens were taken from young swine that had either raised tumors at birth or tumors that developed shortly after birth from melanocytic lesions. All seven specimens grew in the hamster cheek pouch. One was subcultured in subsequent passages through other hamster cheek pouches. Histologically, the cheek pouch growth appeared to be very similar to the primary swine melanoma. The cortisone treatment rendered the hamster susceptible to infection, which sometimes resulted in the death of the animal, but metastases were not observed. Human melanomas have also been transplanted to the hamster cheek pouch, but only about 10 percent of them will grow, whereas 100 percent of the Sinclair Swine melanomas grew in the hamster cheek pouch.[12]

Next, a visual microcytotoxicity technique was used to evaluate the activity of melanoma swine leukocytes against allogeneic swine melanoma target cells.[13] Peripheral blood leukocytes were collected during the *in vivo* growth and regression of the tumor and in liquid nitrogen. The sequential samples of leukocytes were thawed and tested on the same day against melanoma tissue culture cells.

Comparison of longitudinal leukocyte reactivity with *in vivo* tumor volume indicated that swine with regressing melanomas exhibited increased leukocyte reactivity during tumor regression. Swine with maximum tumor volumes less than 30,000 cubic millimeters exhibited patterns of leukocyte reactivity that paralleled the patterns of *in vivo* tumor growth and regression. However, swine with maximum tumor volumes greater than 30,000 cubic millimeters demonstrated increased *in vitro* leukocyte reactivity at the time of maximum *in vivo* tumor volume.

Histopathologic analysis revealed that increase in tumor volume was frequently a result of host inflammatory cells, particularly pigment-laden macrophages, infiltrating the tumor. Thus, at the time of maximum tumor volume, malignant melanocytes were proportionately decreasing in number while pigment-laden macrophages were proportionately increasing. These studies provide additional evidence that the spontaneous tumor cell regression of swine melanoma is associated with immunologic events, and that assays of leukocyte activity are useful *in vitro* correlates of host antitumor immunity. It is of interest, by contrast, that human melanoma patients receiving either autologous or allogeneic irradiated melanoma cells plus BCG exhibit increased leukocyte reactivity against allogeneic melanoma cells. However, this increase in reactivity does not correlate with clinical response to immunotherapy in human beings.[14]

In a further study, 55 black tumors from 23 Sinclair Melanoma Swine were studied by sequential punch biopsies and tumor volume correlations.[15] ("Tumor" is used in the classic sense to mean "swelling.") These swine were developed from melanomic female and melanomic male matings. Cutaneous tumor volume was calculated as a volume of a cylinder, and 104 punch biopsies were done. These studies further showed that tumors developing from normal skin reached maximum tumor volume in 100 days, those from congenital flat lesions in 56 days, and those from congenital raised lesions in 28 days. However, the time for the relation of the tumors to regress, as pigment-laden macrophages entered the tumors, was approximately the same for all origins.

Resemblance to Human Melanoma

Thus it appears that the Sinclair Swine Melanoma model has many features in common with its human counterpart:[16]

1. Tumors develop spontaneously.
2. Swine and humans possess a wide spectrum of benign melanocytic lesions capable of malignant transformation.
3. Histopathologically, melanomas in pigs resemble superficial spreading melanomas in humans.
4. Metastatic disease is correlated with deeply invasive cutaneous tumors.
5. The pattern of metastatic spread is analogous to the distribution of metastases in human melanoma.
6. The histopathology of cutaneous regression is similar.
7. Tumor-related immune response occurs in the host.
8. A genetic component is readily apparent and is comparable to the genetic component of some melanomas in man.

However, there are three features that differentiate swine and human melanomas:

1. Melanomas do not occur in white swine.
2. Tumor development in swine is not related to ultraviolet radiation.
3. Tumor regression occurs in most of the swine.

Although these differences may somewhat limit the types of studies that can be performed with this animal, complete tumor regression is a feature that can be exploited. Additionally, several swine melanoma lesions can progress and regress simultaneously in the natural history of swine melanoma. This has also been suggested in human melanomas and may partly account for the mixed reaction of multiple metastases to chemotherapy. The ability to perform sequential biopsies in a single lesion is an advantage afforded by the large size of the swine melanomas.

Sex hormones do not seem to play a role in swine melanoma. Despite the recognized proliferation of human melanocytes in puberty and pregnancy, there is no difference in the melanomas of male and female Sinclair swine.[17] Also, despite some evidence that there may be a relationship between pregnancy and malignant choroidal melanomas in humans,[18] Sinclair swine are usually in a state of tumor regression when they become sexually mature, and pregnancy has not been identified as a factor in melanoma growth.[17]

Ocular Studies

It seems logical to study the eyes of these pigs: it has been noticed that the iris also depigments as the skin and melanomas whiten,[19] and some animals exhibited blind behavior after ocular depigmentation; nevertheless, a thorough study of the eyes had not been done before 1980.[20,21]

We therefore conducted a longitudinal study of the eyes of 30 melanomatic pigs using clinical, histopathologic, immunologic, and electrophysiological techniques. In our initial study, we correlated the phenomena of cutaneous tumor regression and depigmentation with histologic ocular events, notably, the simultaneous invasion of the uveal tract by mononuclear cells. We soon found that visual impairment was caused by multiple factors, including a reduction in the transparency of ocular tissues and a decrease in photoreceptor function.

Thirty Sinclair swine were examined every two to four weeks under general anesthesia with halothane. Pupils were dilated with 1% tropicamide. External eye examinations, slit lamp examinations with a Kowa SL-5 portable slit lamp, indirect ophthalmoscopy, and fundus photography with a Kowa RC-2 camera were performed as needed to illuminate the ocular vascular beds and transmission defects.

Coloration of the iris, overall fundus, and the superior-temporal quadrant of each eye was graded on a scale of 0 to 4, 4 being normal pigmentation and 0 marked depigmentation. Pigs were followed as early as three weeks of age up to one year. Records of tumor development and regression were kept. In addition, 70 other pigs were given fundus examinations to look for possible choroidal melanomas; none has been found so far.

Enucleations were done randomly and also to select certain pathological stages. In several animals one eye was enucleated at one time and the other at a later stage in order to follow the sequence of depigmentation. Globes were immediately immersed in aldehyde fixative (2% glutaraldehyde, 1% formaldehyde, in cacodylate buffer pH 7.2). Eyes were bisected in a superior-temporal to inferior-nasal plane. Half eyes were embedded in paraffin and sectioned at 6 microns. Sections were stained with Wright's stain, periodic acid-Schiff (PAS), and hematoxyline and eosin (H&E). For Wright's staining the sections were deparaffinized in xylene and rehydrated, stained 3.5 minutes in diluted (1:1 with H_2O) Wright's stain solution, then destained in 0.1% acetic acid for 15 seconds. The other half of selected eyes was cut into small blocks, post-fixed in osmic acid, and embedded in epoxy resin for electron microscopy. One micron thick sections were stained with toluidine blue 0. Selected areas of the tissue were thin-sectioned, stained with uranyl and lead salts, and photographed in a Philips 300 electron microscope.

In the normal pig eye the iris is dark brown (Fig. 15-2) and the fundus is slate blue (Fig. 15-3). The superior-temporal quadrant of the fundus was always lighter in very young animals and is therefore considered to be the normal condition. The cornea is egg-shaped and the optic nerve oval. A specific pattern of depigmentation was observed in the animals undergoing tumor regression. By two months of age, 50 percent of all irides had started to depigment, becoming less than 4+ and eventually becoming pinkish white (Fig. 15-4). By 16 weeks, 82 percent of the superior-temporal quadrants and 40 percent of overall fundi were less than 4+. Fundus depigmentation was first isolated to the superior-temporal quadrant. Depigmentation then spread to the rest of the fundus; the orange choroidal vasculature became increasingly visible. Depigmentation patterns varied, being diffuse, tigroid (striped), mottled, in patches, and in fingerprint patterns. Occasionally, white specks were observed in depigmented eyes (Fig. 15–5); fluorescein angiography identified these starlike spots as pigment epithelial window defects (Fig. 15-6). The irides and fundi eventually progressed to 0/4 (or lack of all normal pigmentation) in four animals. In the other 26, degrees of depigmentation varied from very little to almost total depigmentation. Eye and skin depigmentation progressed at varied rates.

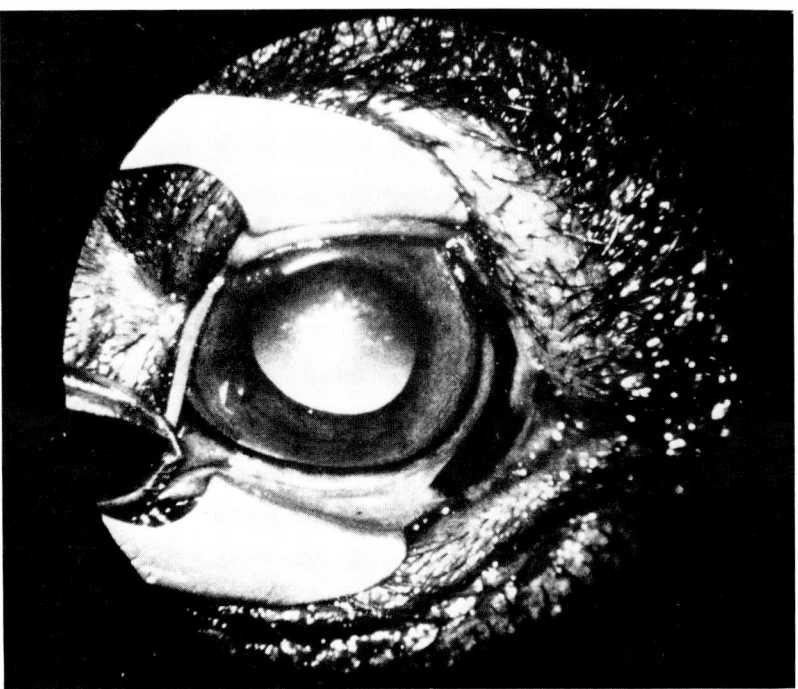

Figure 15-2. Normal deeply pigmented iris of young black pigs. For color differences in Figures 2 to 10, see color plates in Lentz et al.[21]

Frequently, iris hyperemia developed during iris depigmentation. Occasionally, posterior synechia and cataracts formed. With long-standing inflammation, corneal band keratopathy was seen.[22] No cells or flare was ever seen in the anterior chamber with a portable slit lamp.

The normal Sinclair swine eye is more richly pigmented than the human eye. Specifically, the conjunctiva terminates at the limbus with a ring of

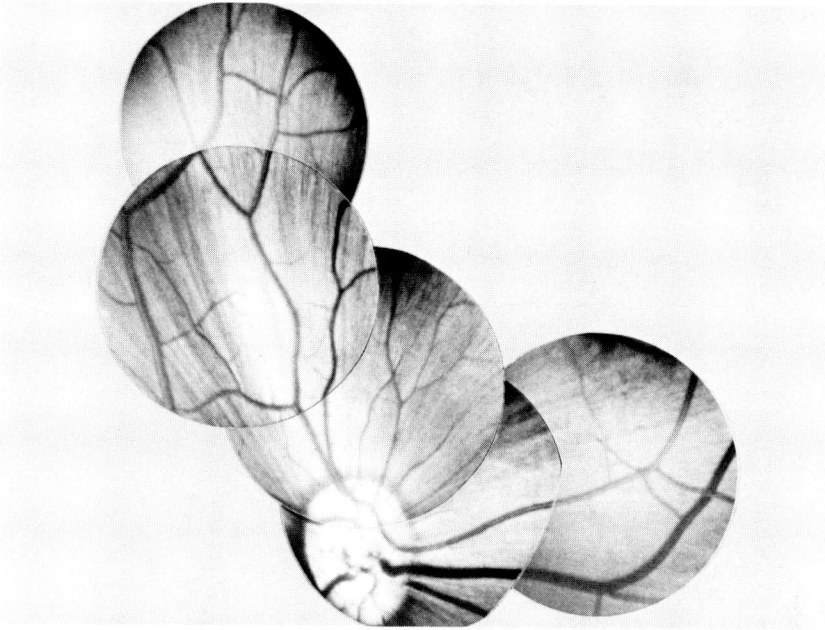

Figure 15-3. Montage of slate blue-gray fundus of young black pig. Normal oval shape of optic nerve; note prominent nerve fiber layer.

multilayered melanin-containing cells; the sclera, trabecular meshwork, and lamina cribrosa also contain many melanocytes. The uveal tract contains evenly dispersed branching melanocytes throughout the choroid and iris stroma (Fig. 15-7, 15-8). The superior-temporal coloration of the normal fundus is lighter due to fewer melanin granules in the retinal pigment epithelium (RPE) in that region. This may be an evolutionary hangover of a tapetal RPE, although modern inbred swine have no tapetum lucidum. Other histologic features of the normal swine eye pertinent to this study are the unusually thin, delicate Bruch's membrane and the high ratio of cone to rod photoreceptors.

Eyes enucleated during the progressive stages of cutaneous tumor regression present a sequence, representing (1) uveal invasion by mononuclear cells, (2) melanocyte destruction, (3) macrophage sequestration of melanocyte cytoplasmic components, and (4) migration of engorged macrophages to the walls of veins (Figs. 15-7, 15-8 normal uvea; 15-9, 15-10 depigmented uvea). This redistribution of melanin from its normal dispersed location within branching melanocytes to round macrophages densely clustered near blood vessels accounts for the lightening of the fundus coloration and its tigroid pattern (Fig. 15-5).

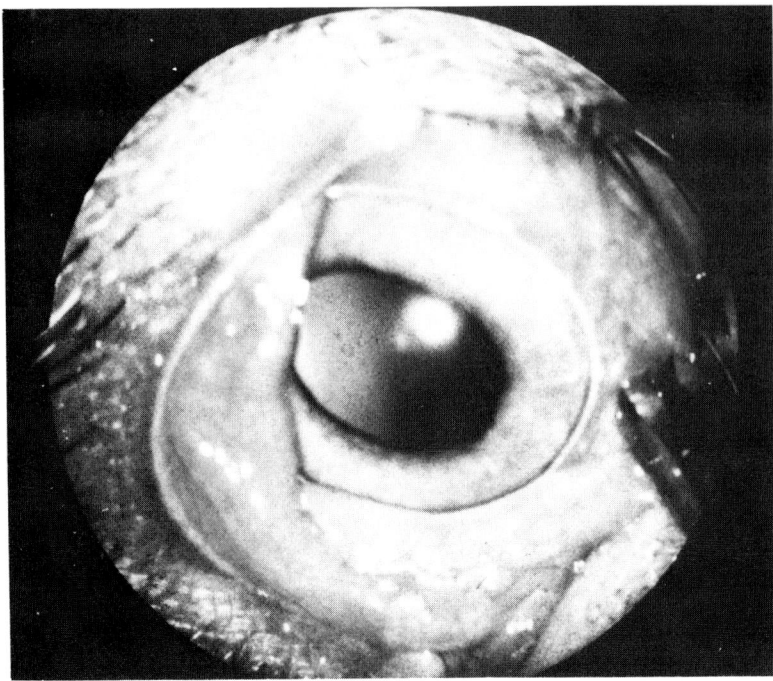

Figure 15-4. White iris and almost white eyelid skin and hair of older, fully depigmented swine.

Mononuclear cells that have migrated outside the blood vessels are flattened by connective tissue so that their characteristic morphology, e.g. nuclear shape, nuclear-cytoplasmic ratio, becomes distorted. Most of the cells are lymphocytes, judging from Wright staining and ultrastructural features that show a paucity of organelles and monoribosomes (Fig. 15-11). A small percentage of the cells that have more cytoplasm, a larger Golgi complex, and lysosomelike granules may be monocytes (e.g. nonphagocytosing mononuclear cells[23]) or early macrophages. No plasma cells have been seen.

The iris presents a similar histopathology that may precede or follow events in the choroid (Fig. 15-9). Melanocyte destruction in the iris occurs simultaneously with engorgement of iris vessels. Rarely, proteinaceous fluid was found in the anterior chamber of eyes removed after extensive depigmentation of the iris, posterior synechia, and cataract development. A full-blown anterior uveitis initiates numerous other secondary phenomena: anterior and posterior synechia formation, deposition of calcium phosphate in the cornea,[22] and disruption of lens epithelium and cortical fibers (i.e. cataract formation).

Occasional variations in this pattern were encountered. Three eyes with

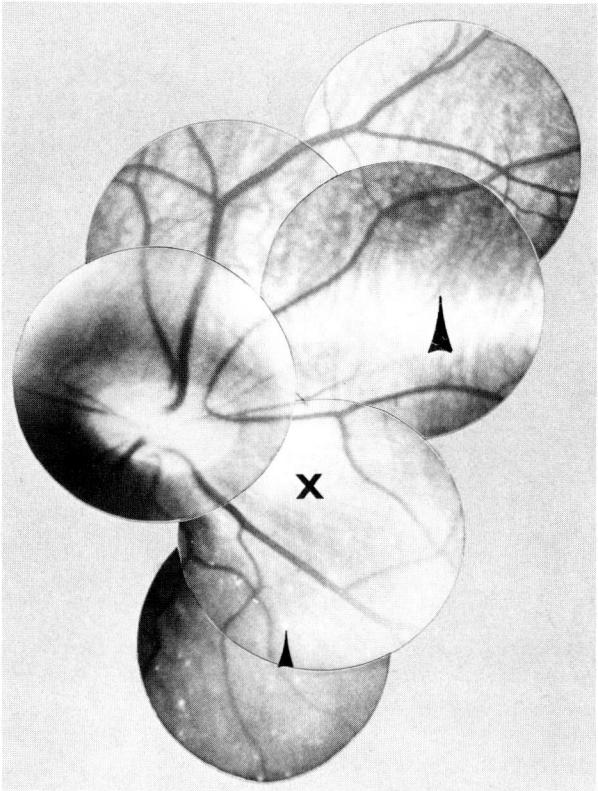

Figure 15-5. Montage of fully depigmented fundus of older swine. Note starlike pigment epithelial defect (small arrow) and prominent choroidal vessels surrounded by perivascular pigment streaks (large arrow). Nerve fiber bundles (X) barely visible.

scattered starlike window defects in the fundus on clinical examination had a histopathologic examination, revealing focal accumulations of lymphocytes that disrupted Bruch's membrane and lifted several overlying pigment epithelial cells (Fig. 15-12). At these sites the RPE changed from their normal cuboidal shape to a rounded shape and progressively lost their anchorage to Bruch's membrane. RPE cells at these sites were almost amelanotic. In one extreme case the RPE duplicated itself to form a 1 mm wide placoid folded triple-layered lesion. Also, patches of retinal photoreceptors at these sites had pyknotic nuclei; however, similar patchy degeneration of the retina has been found in normal eyes, so the significance of this finding needs further evaluation.

Electroretinograms (ERG) were obtained using a PS11 Photic Simulator positioned over the dilated pupil, 27 cm above the cornea. A Burian-Allen corneal electrode was used as the positive, the lid retractor as the reference electrode, and a ground electrode was applied to a shaved ear with conducting

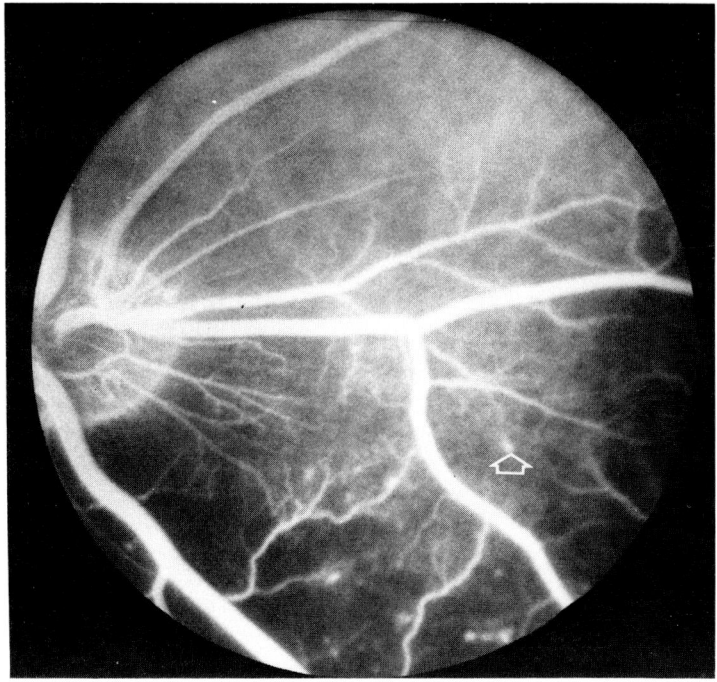

Figure 15-6. Fluorescein angiogram (late venous phase) of fundus of pig shown in Figure 15-5. Window defects (open arrows) seen during choroidal flush.

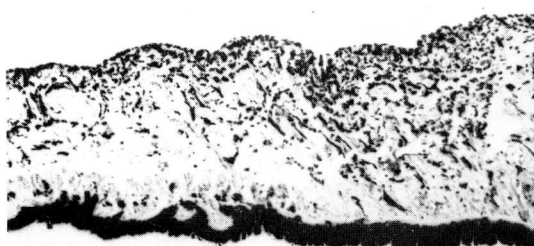

Figure 15-7. Iris of normal pig. Melanocytes are evenly dispersed in anterior border layer and through stroma fibroblasts. Few other cells are seen in stroma. × 88

paste.[24] ERGs were recorded using a Grass amplifier, Dagan averager, and Tektronix oscilloscope and camera.

After dark adaptation for 25 minutes, the animals were anesthetized with halothane. The pigs were placed on their side with their heads held in the same position for every ERG. Pupils were dilated with 1% tropicamide. Normal saline drops kept the electrode in good contact with the cornea. Light flashes of near maximum intensity were used at 3 hertz (flashes/sec). Sixteen responses were averaged for each record.

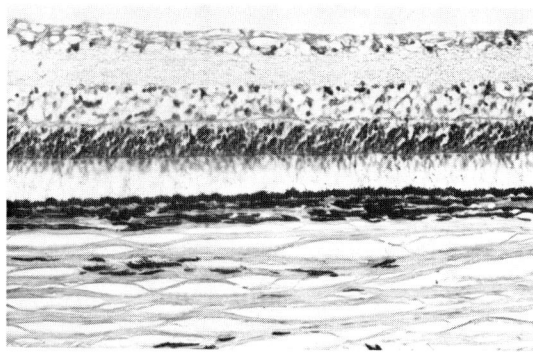

Figure 15-8. Choroid and retina of normal pig eye. Note evenly branched melanocytes of the choroid. Paraffin section, Wright's stain, ×140.

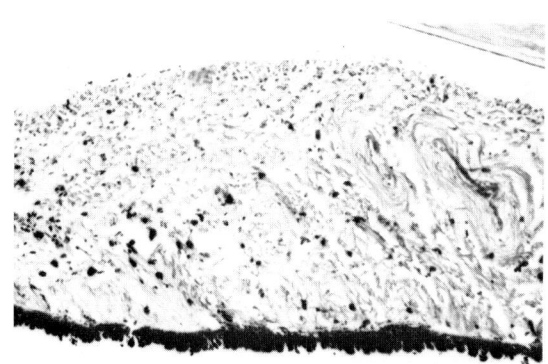

Figure 15-9. Iris of pig undergoing tumor regression and depigmentation. Melanocytes are gone. Melanin is gathered into macrophages. Stroma contains many round mononuclear cells. ×88.

The normal pig electroretinogram (ERG) is very similar to the human; a and b waves and oscillatory potentials can be identified (Fig. 15-13). In a depigmented animal, matched to the normal for age and sex, the morphology of the ERG was similar to that of the control, but electrical activity was decreased. The light-adapted electroretinograms revealed a peak-to-peak amplitude of 212, 5 V in the control eye with a b wave latency of 29.7 msec. In the depigmented animal, the right eye peak-to-peak amplitude was 85 V, while the latency remained identical to the normal. In the left eye, the peak-to-peak amplitude was 45 V, while the b wave latency was 14.36 msec. Thus, the uveitis eyes differed from each other in b-wave amplitude by 47 percent but differed from the normal pig's b-wave amplitude by 60 and 79 percent.

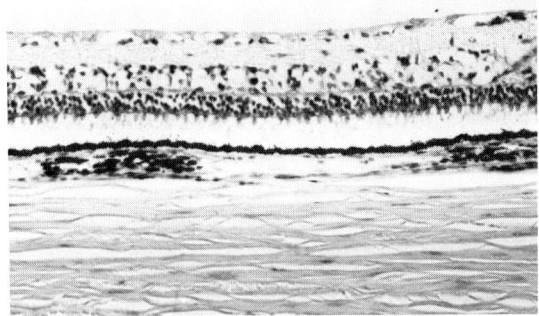

Figure 15-10. Choroid and retina of pig during rapid phase of depigmentation and tumor regression. Melanin is concentrated within macrophages located around dilated blood vessels. Paraffin section, Wright's stain, ×140.

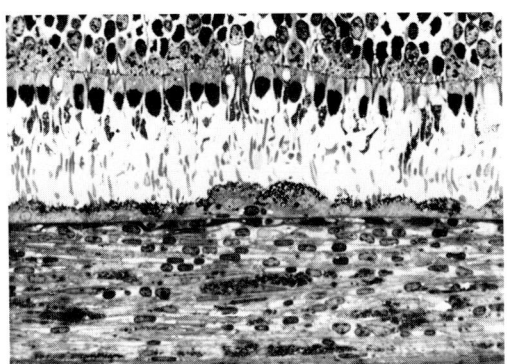

Figure 15-11. Histologic section of window defect shown in Figures 15-5 and 15-6. Note lymphocytic invasion of Bruch's membrane and swelling of a few pigment epithelial cells. Toluidine blue stain, ×480.

Previously established tissue-cultured allogeneic Sinclair swine cutaneous melanoma cells[11] were used as the target cells to test lymphocytes of selected pigs. Whole blood of animals with moderate tumor load and with signs of depigmentation was fractionated on a Ficoll-Hypaque gradient and white blood cells from these samples were cryopreserved until a complete temporal sequence of samples was ready for testing.[13] The thawed, washed leukocytes ($1 \times 10^5/10^1$) were added to tumor cells in MicroTest plates and incubated for 48 hours at 37°C. Tumor cells without leukocytes served as controls. After incubation, the leukocytes were removed and the remaining tumor cells were fixed with acetone-alcohol and stained with Giemsa stain. Surviving tumor cells were counted using a 25× objective. The survival

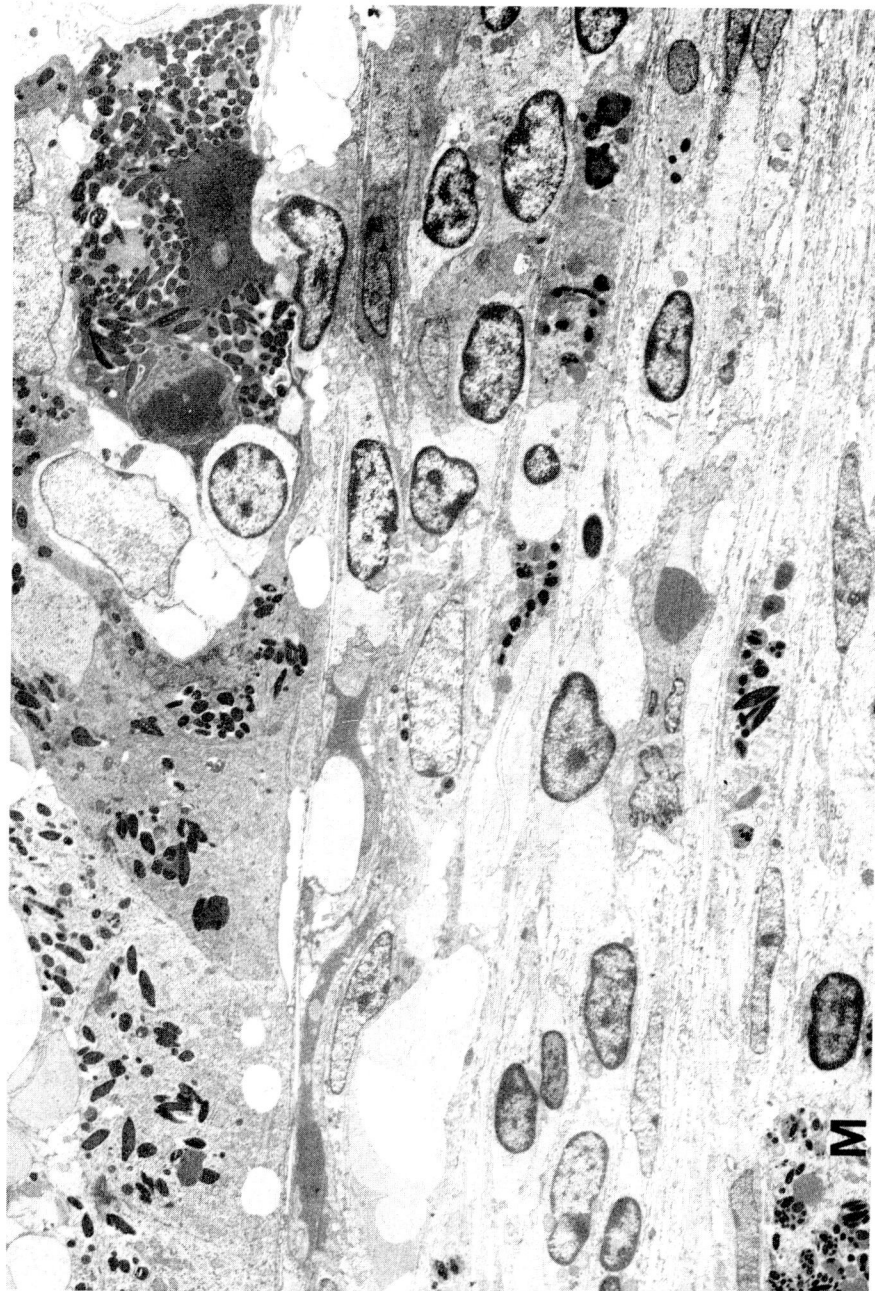

Figure 15-12. Electron micrograph of choroid showing lymphocytic invasion. Macrophages (M) contain phagocytized remnants of melanocytes.

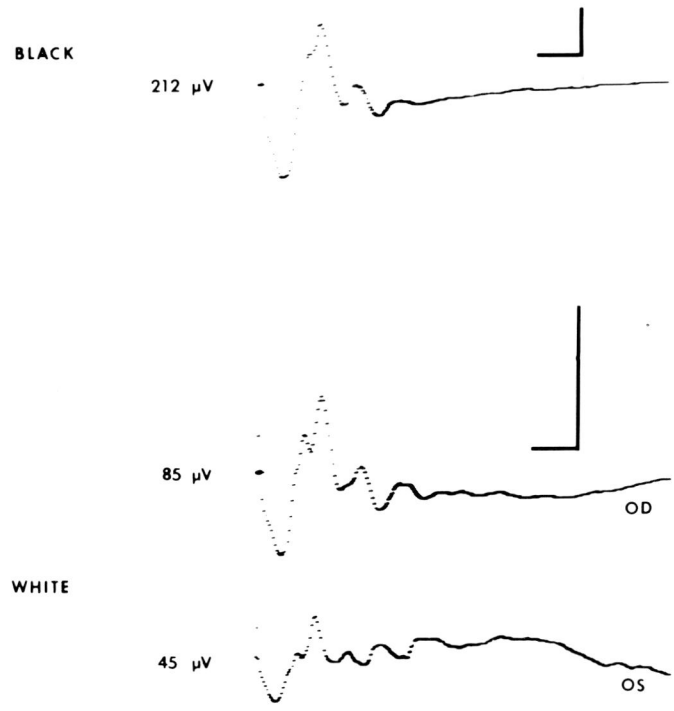

Figure 15-13. Electroretinogram of normal black pig (top) and depigmented, uveitis pig (bottom).

fractions were determined by dividing the mean number of tumor cells remaining in the wells that contained leukocyte by the mean number in the control wells.

The result of sequential cytotoxicity assays on one pig is shown in Figure 15-14. Leukocytes of this pig were seldom able to kill swine cutaneous melanoma cells *in vitro* when the ocular fundus was normal (Fig. 15-3). As the fundus began to depigment, however, we could demonstrate increasing cytotoxic activity of this pig's leukocytes against the tissue cultured melanoma cells. By 80 days of age, when the fundus was markedly depigmented (Fig. 15-5), the animal's leukocytes killed 100 percent of the test melanoma cells.[13]

These studies have now been expanded to a longitudinal examination of leukocyte cytotoxicity in nine animals followed for four to eleven months with assessment of skin depigmentation, iris depigmentation, tumor burden, and leukocyte reactivity. The iris depigmentation correlated more closely with leukocyte reactivity than total tumor mass or skin color.[25]

The histopathologic findings and the cytotoxicity studies indicate that the

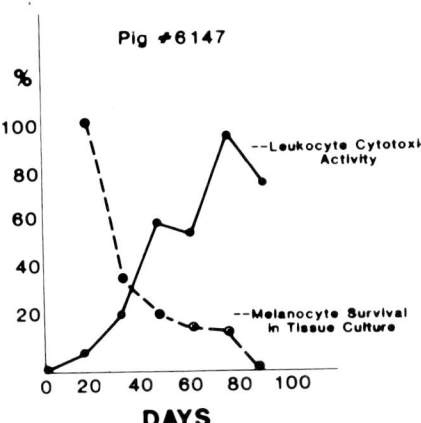

Figure 15-14. Sequential cytotoxicity assays on a pig whose fundus had rapidly depigmented by 80 days of age. Blood lymphocytes of this pig destroyed 100 percent of the cultured melanoma cells in vitro when its uvea was undergoing rapid depigmentation.

ocular disease in these melanomatous animals results from a systemic immunologic process. Our investigation indicates that the destructive attack on the uveal tract is directed against normal melanocytes, not melanoma cells, since ocular melanomas have not been detected in examination of more than 100 animals. The nature of the antigen(s) and the identity of participating immunoglobulins and immune cells remains to be determined. The predictable development of the ocular disease in animals undergoing active tumor regression and the consistent reproducibility of the clinical and histopathologic findings show that the pig is an excellent animal model for further study of immunogenic uveitis.

Since ocular changes are the first clue to tumor regression, the eye provides a window through which we can observe the mobilization of systemic immunologic activity. Tumor regression at cutaneous sites is difficult to assess because the invasion of tumors by leukocytes and the engorgement of tissue by macrophages masks the loss of tumor mass in the early, and most significant, phases of tumor lysis.[15] Therefore, because it is clearly visible, ocular depigmentation within the thin flat sheet of choroid or iris can be used as an indicator for estimating the most appropriate times for sampling blood and for performing tests of the early immune response to melanomas.

Although two types of melanin-containing cells are to be found in the eye—pigment epithelial cells and melanocytes—only the latter are destroyed by the immunologic response. This indicates that melanin per se can probably be ruled out as the antigen recognized by the immune cells. It seems most likely that antigens common to the surface of both the malignant skin melanocyte and the normal uveal melanocytes, cells with a common neural crest origin, are the initial basis for a cross-reacting "innocent bystander" immune response. The possibilities that lysed melanocytes release a variety of "foreign" antigens to cause a cascade of immune responses must also be considered as later epiphenomena.[26]

Late in the disease process when severe anterior uveitis and other secondary phenomena occur (e.g. glaucoma, cataract, band keratopathy), the pigment epithelial cells of the iris, ciliary body, and retina may also be destroyed by the massive inflammatory response; this, however, is not part of the antitumor phenomenon. Similarly, the starlike window defects in the retinal pigment epithelium are secondary to activities of immune cell infiltrates in the choriocapillaris and Bruch's membrane. This stimulus on one occasion caused a discoid benign duplication of the RPE.

The pilot electroretinography study showed a 60–80 percent decrease in the amplitude of the b-wave of the ERG in the eyes of an animal with advanced depigmentation of the uveal tract. This decreased photoreceptor electrical activity undoubtedly contributes to the visual impairment of these animals. However, other disturbances in the transparency of the ocular media (i.e. band keratopathy, cataract) seem to be the major cause of the blind behavior observed in the depigmented animals.

Human uveitis is divided into granulomatous and nongranulomatous types. Clinically, granulomatous uveitis is more chronic. It can involve both the posterior and anterior uvea and is associated with anterior and posterior synechiae, and iris nodules. The protein content in the anterior chamber is greatly increased but not the cellularity of the aqueous humor. Clinically, uveitis in Sinclair pig's eyes has a chronic course, but there are few anterior and posterior synechiae, and only rarely have eyes been found with high protein content in the aqueous or vitreous. Iris nodules have never been seen. The histopathology of granulomatous uveitis specifically includes epithelioid cell clumps surrounded by lymphocytic infiltrates, giant cells, and fibrocytic proliferation. Swine uveitis, by contrast, has a lymphocytic infiltrate and perivascular macrophages but does not form granulomas nor are giant cells present. Therefore, it seems that the melanomatous swine uveitis cannot readily be classified as either granulomatous or nongranulomatous.

The cutaneous depigmentation seen in the common human disease vitiligo[27] is at times associated with iritis[28] and chorioretinitis.[29,30] Some vitiligo patients have antibodies to melanin-producing cells[31] and both uveitis and vitiligo have been associated with BCG treatment of malignant melanoma.[32] Much remains to be learned of the relationship between uveitis and ocular tumors.[33] Immunology of other chorioretinal disorders such as sympathetic ophthalmia and Vogt-Koyanagi-Harada syndrome, both of which may be associated with skin depigmentation, needs further study.[34,35] This swine model of the immunologic destruction of melanocytes provides an opportunity to find the mechanism(s) of cell death and to develop a strategy for its prevention.

REFERENCES

1. Shaffers, A. D., Dommert, A. R., and Tumbleson, M. E.: Melanoma in a miniature piglet. *Mo Vet*, 16:19, 1967.
2. Flatt, R. E., Middleton, C. C., Tumbleson, M. E., and Perez-Mesa, C.: Pathogenesis of benign cutaneous melanomas in miniature swine. *J Am Vet Med Ass*, 153:939, 1968.
3. Millikan, L. E., Hook, R. R., Jr., and Manning, P. J.: Immunobiology of melanoma. *Yale J Biol Med*, 46:631–645, 1973.
4. Lerner, A. B., and Cage, G.: Melanomas in horses. *Yale J Biol Med*, 46:646–649, 1973.
5. Millikan, L. E., Boylon, J. L., Hook, R. R., and Manning, P. J.: Melanoma in Sinclair swine: A new animal model. *J Invest Derm*, 62:20–30, 1974.
6. Montagna, W., and Tun, J. S.: The skin of the domestic pig. *Invest Dermatol*, 43:11–21, 1964.
7. Oxenhandler, R. W., Adelstein, E. H., Haigh, J. P., Hook, R. R., Jr., and Clark, W. A., Jr.: Malignant melanoma in the Sinclair miniature swine: an autopsy study of 60 cases. *Am J Pathol*, 96:707–720, 1979.
8. Clark, W. H., Jr., Ainsworth, A. M., Bernardine, E. A., and Mihm, M. C., Jr.: The histogenesis and biologic behavior of primary human malignant melanomas of the skin. *Cancer Res*, 29:705–727, 1969.
9. Hook, R. R., Jr., Aultman, M. D., Adelstein, E. H., Oxenhandler, R., Millikan, L. E., and Middleton, C. C.: Influence of selective breeding on the incidence of melanomas in Sinclair miniature swine. *Int J Cancer*, 24:668–682, 1979.
10. Aultman, M. D., and Hook, R. R., Jr.: In vitro lymphocyte reactivity to soluble tumor extracts in Sinclair Melanoma Swine. *Int J Cancer*, 24:673–678, 1979.
11. Berkelhammer, J., Caines, S. M., Dexter, D. L., Adelstein, E. H., Oxenhandler, R. W., and Hook, R. R., Jr.: Adaptation of Sinclair swine melanoma cells to long term growth in vitro. *Cancer Res*, 39:4960–4964, 1979.
12. Berkelhammer, J., and Hook, R. R., Jr.: Growth of Sinclair swine melanoma in the hamster cheek pouch. *Transplantation*, 29:193–195, 1980.
13. Berkelhammer, J., Ensign, B. M., Hook, R. R., Jr., Hecker, C. J., Smith, G. D., and Oxenhandler, R. W.: Growth and spontaneous regression of swine melanomas: relationship of in vitro leukocyte reactivity. *J Nat Cancer Int*, 68:461–468, 1982.
14. Berkelhammer, J., Mastrangelo, M. J., Bellet, R. E., Berd, D., and Prehn, R. T.: Chemoimmunotherapy increases the lymphocyte reactivity of melanoma patients. *Eur J Cancer*, 15:197–204, 1979.
15. Oxenhandler, R. W., Berkelhammer, J., Smith, G. D., and Hook, R. R., Jr.: Growth and regression of cutaneous melanomas in Sinclair miniature swine. *Am J Pathol*, in press, 1983.
16. Hook, R. R., Jr., Berkelhammer, J., and Oxenhandler, R. W.: Animal model of human disease: Sinclair swine melanoma. *Am J Pathol*, 108:130–133, 1982.
17. Hook, R. R., Jr.: Personal communication.
18. Seddon, J. M., MacLaughlin, D. T., Albert, D. M., Gragoudas, E. S., and Ferenie, M.: Uveal melanomas presenting during pregnancy and the investigation of oestrogen response in melanomas. *Br J Ophthalmol*, 66:695–705, 1982.
19. Hook, R. R., Jr., Aultman, M. D., Millikan, L. E., and Hutcheson, D. P.: The biology of

cutaneous exophytic melanomas in Sinclair (S-1) miniature swine. *Am Assoc Cancer Res,* *18*:46, 1977.
20. Lentz, K. J., Burns, R. P., Loeffler, K., Berkelhammer, J., and Hook, R. R., Jr.: Malignant melanoma regression with uveal melanocyte destruction and blindness. *Invest Ophthalmol Vis Sci Suppl, 22*:261, 1982.
21. Lentz, K. J., Burns, R. P., Loeffler, K., Feeney-Burns, L., Berkelhammer, J., and Hook, R. R., Jr.: Uveitis caused by cytotoxic immune response to cutaneous malignant melanoma in swine: Destruction of uveal melanocytes during tumor regression. *Invest Ophthalmol Vis Sci,* in press, 1983.
22. Burns, R. P., Lentz, K. J., Hook, R. R., Jr., and Berkelhammer, J.: Spontaneous animal model of band keratopathy in the pig. *Invest Ophthalmol Vis Sci Suppl, 22*:20, 1982.
23. Roubin, R., Cesarini, J. P., Fridman, W. H., Pavie-Fischer, J., and Peter, H. H.: Characterization of the mononuclear cell infiltrate in human malignant melanoma. *Int J Cancer, 16*:61–73, 1975.
24. Zangalli, A. L., Ghizoni, M., and Dantas, A. U.: As ondas do electroretinogram do proco como modelo experimental. *Rev Bras Oftalmol, 39*:105–110, 1980.
25. Crane, J. L., and Berkelhammer, J.: Relationship of leukocyte reactivity to depigmentation phenomena during spontaneous regression of Sinclair Swine melanoma. Submitted for publication.
26. Malaty, A. H. A., Rahi, A. H. S., and Garner, A.: Ostensible antimelanoma antibodies in patients with nonmalignant eye disease. In Silverstein, A. M., and O'Connor, G. R. (Eds.): *Immunology and Immunopathology of the Eye.* New York, Masson Press, 1979, pp. 216–219.
27. Lerner, A. B., and Nordlund, J. J.: Vitiligo: What is it? Is it important? *JAMA, 239*:1183–1187, 1978.
28. Albert, D. M., Sober, A. J., and Fitzpatrick, T. B.: Iritis in patients with cutaneous melanoma and vitiligo. *Arch Ophthalmol, 96*:2081–2084, 1978.
29. Albert, D. M., Nordlund, J. J., and Lerner, A. B.: Ocular abnormalities occurring with vitiligo. *Ophthalmol, 86*:1145–1160, 1979.
30. Gass, J. D. M.: Vitiliginous chorioretinitis. *Arch Ophthalmol, 99*:1778–1787, 1981.
31. Hertz, K. C., Gazze, L. A., Kirkpatrick, C. H., and Katz, S. I.: Autoimmune vitiligo detection of antibodies to melanin-producing cells. *New Engl J Med, 297*:634–637, 1977.
32. Donaldson, R. C., Canaan, S. A., Jr., McLean, R. B., and Ackerman, L. V.: Uveitis and vitiligo associated with BCG treatment for malignant melanoma. *Surgery, 76*:771–778, 1974.
33. Char, D. H.: *Immunology of Uveitis and Ocular Tumor.* New York, Grune and Stratton, 1978.
34. Corwin, J. M., and Weiter, J. J.: Review: Immunology of chorioretinal disorders. *Surv Ophthalmol, 25*:287–305, 1981.
35. Char, D. H.: Vogt-Koyanagi-Harada Syndrome and sympathetic ophthalmia: Clinical and immunologic characteristics. In Helmsen, R. J., Suran, A., Gery, I., and Nussenblatt, R. B. (Eds.): *Immunology of the Eye: Workshop II.* Sp Suppl Immunol Abst, 1981, pp. 67–75.

Chapter 16

IMMUNOTHERAPY FOR RABBIT LID PAPILLOMAS

GILBERT SMOLIN, M.D.; MASAO OKUMOTO, M.A.;
MITCHELL FRIEDLAENDER, M.D.; RICHARD CYR

Virus-induced papillomas present a management problem for ophthalmologists. The excision, incision, or cryotherapy of the tumors is often followed by their recurrence, sometimes in a more extensive form. In an attempt to find a better alternative, immunotherapy has been tried. The method is to sensitize the host to a skin-sensitizing agent and then to paint the tumors with the agent. Dinitrochlorobenzene (DNCB) has been used for this purpose, despite its toxicity.[1]

Materials and Methods

ANIMALS. The experimental animals were eight New Zealand white adult rabbits weighing five to six pounds each.

VIRUS. The Shope papilloma virus (papovavirus), a wild strain, was obtained from the American Type Culture Collection. The virus was recovered from wild cottontail rabbit papillomas but can produce tumors in other types of rabbits. The incubation period varies from 7 to 42 days.

VIRUS PROPAGATION. After removing the papilloma tissue from the shipping vial and placing it in a small mortar, we rinsed it twice with 10 ml potassium phosphate (KPO) buffered saline solution and then discarded the solution. With a pestle we then triturated the tissue with 3 gm of silicon carbide (GRID 120) and 5 ml of buffered saline solution, transferred the fluid to a centrifuge tube, and added more KPO buffered saline solution until the volume was 10 ml. We centrifuged this material at 500 rpm for five minutes and removed the supernatant fluid for application to the skin.[2]

The lower lids of all eight rabbits were shaved and clipped. In each area we abraded the epidermis with a No. 64 beaver blade, placed four or five drops of the supernatant fluid on the abraded areas, and injected the areas intradermally with 0.1 ml of the fluid.

SENSITIZATION AND CHALLENGE WITH OXAZOLONE. When the tumors had reached a moderately large size, the right ear of each rabbit received six drops of a 6% solution of oxazolone in ethyl alcohol on two successive days. Seven days later, four drops of a 6% solution of oxazolone in olive oil were placed on the left ear; eight drops of this solution were placed on the right lower lid; and eight drops of olive oil alone were placed on the tumor on the left lower lid.

The tumors were examined and measured three times a week. Any signs of inflammation were recorded. The animals were killed three weeks after the applications of oxazolone, and the tumor sites were examined histologically.

Results

Three weeks after the inoculation of virus, tumors had developed on 13 of the 14 lids (Fig. 16-1) and when untreated for two months had increased in size (Fig. 16-2). The initial application of oxazolone to the right ear produced no sign of inflammation, but the challenge dose applied to the left ear produced erythema and induration that reached maximum intensity at 48 hours. All animals exhibited some degree of this type of reaction, indicating the presence of cell-mediated immune hypersensitivity to oxazolone in all of the animals.

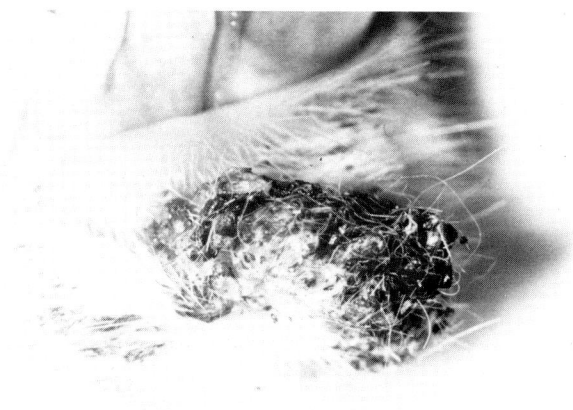

Figure 16-1. Papilloma of lower lid three weeks after viral inoculation. ×2. (From *Annals of Ophthalmology* 13:101–103, January 1981. Reproduced with permission.)

The application of oxazolone to the tumors produced inflammation that resulted in dermatitis and loss of hair. By postapplication day 10, the tumors also began to regress, and after two weeks six of seven had regressed significantly (Mann-Whitney statistical analysis) (Table 16-I, Fig. 16-3). They had not recurred when the animals were killed on postapplication day 21.

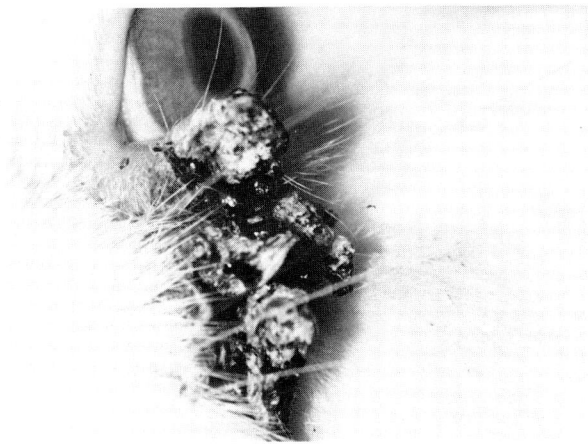

Figure 16-2. Papilloma eight weeks after viral inoculation. ×2. (From *Annals of Ophthalmology* 13:101–103, January 1981. Reproduced with permission.)

TABLE 16-I
RABBIT LID PAPILLOMAS TREATED WITH OXAZOLONE OD AND OLIVE OIL OS

Rabbit	Tumor Size (Square Millimeters)							
	Day 0		Day 5		Day 10		Day 15	
	OD	OS	OD	OS	OD	OS	OD	OS
1	50	40	45	38	15	40	2	42
2	28	32	28	32	14	34	9	38
3	32	24	34	28	16	30	9	30
4	9	21	10	24	0	26	0	26
5	16	24	16	24	12	24	14	26
6	18	18	18	22	10	22	4	24
7	—[a]	16	—	18	—	18	—	18
8	24	40	24	40	24	44	4	48

[a] No tumor

From *Annals of Ophthalmology*, 13:101–103, January 1981. Reproduced with permission.

Histologic examination of the oxazolone-treated tumors indicated severe inflammation of the dermis with sparing of the epidermis (Fig. 16-4). The cells were predominantly lymphocytes, but there were some polymorphonuclear leukocytes and plasma cells (Fig. 16-5). Perivascular cuffing (Fig. 16-6) and occlusive vasculitis were prominent features of the dermal pathology.

The tumors treated with olive oil alone did not regress; after two weeks most of them were in fact slightly larger. There was no clinical or histologic evidence of inflammation associated with the application of olive oil alone.

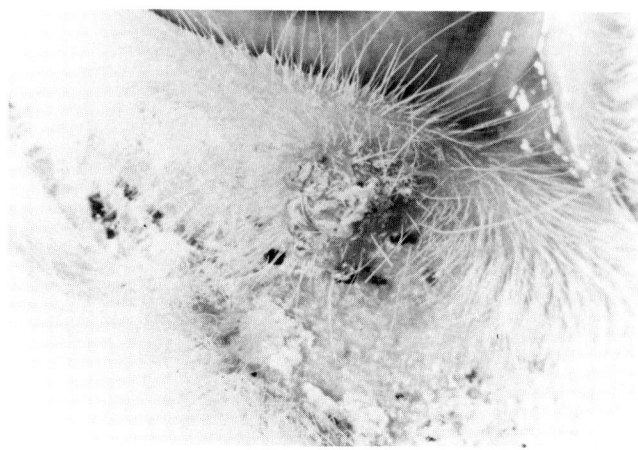

Figure 16-3. A significantly regressed oxazolone-treated tumor. Note dermatitis and hair loss. ×2. (From *Annals of Ophthalmology* 13:101–103, January 1981. Reproduced with permission.)

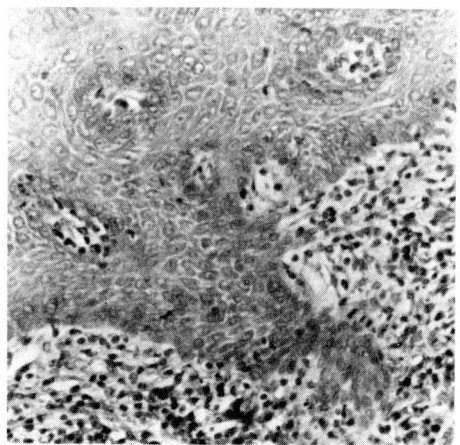

Figure 16-4. Inflammation of dermis underlying oxazolone-treated tumor. ×40. (From *Annals of Ophthalmology*, 13:101–103, January 1981. Reproduced with permission.)

Discussion

We used the Shope papilloma virus in this study because it shares antigenic determinants with some human papilloma viruses. For this reason the results may have some human clinical application.[3] The cell-mediated immune systems of patients with warts are known to be somewhat depressed,[4]

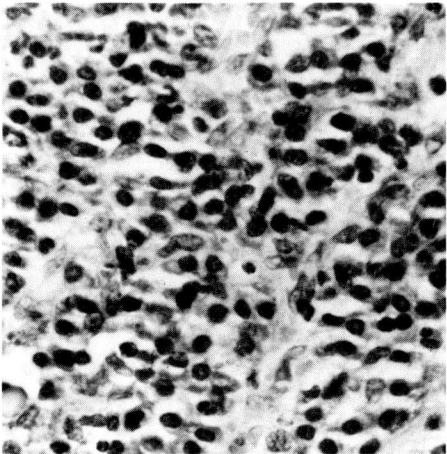

Figure 16-5. Dermal inflammatory cells are predominantly lymphocytes. ×100. (From *Annals of Ophthalmology* 13:101–103, January 1981. Reproduced with permission.)

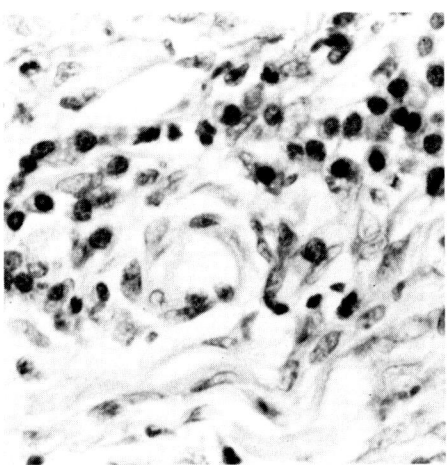

Figure 16-6. Perivascular cuffing in dermis underlying oxazolone-treated tumor. ×150. (From *Annals of Ophthalmology,* 13:101–103, January 1981. Reproduced with permission.)

and some of these patients show spontaneous regression of the papillomas, possibly due to some immunologic surveillance mechanism. These virus-induced tumors may thus be especially susceptible to immunotherapy.

DNCB has been shown to cause regression of verruca vulgaris,[1] but in view of the drug's toxicity, we used the much less toxic skin sensitizer, oxazolone. Oxazolone can sensitize the host in a few days.[5]

Our results showed that oxazolone was not toxic for the sensitized ear; when we also placed ten drops of our preparation mixed with olive oil into the inferior cul-de-sac of four eyes of unsensitized rabbits, there were no signs of either toxicity or inflammation.

Oxazolone caused the tumor masses to regress. The mechanism has not yet been determined, but the reports in the literature, and both the perivascular cuffing and the occlusive vasculitis under the treated tumors, point to an immunologic mechanism. Studies designed to test this suspicion are underway.

Despite the promising results of this study, one must reflect soberly on the following possible complications of the use of oxazolone: there could be (1) hypersensitivity reactions to cross-reacting substances; (2) associated dermatitis and hair loss; and (3) late recurrences.

REFERENCES

1. Buckner, D., and Price, N. M.: Immunotherapy of verrucae vulgares with dinitrochlorobenzene. *Br J Ophthalmol, 98*:451–455, 1978.
2. Shope, R. E.: Immunization of rabbits to infectious papillomatosis. *J Exp Med, 65*:219–231, 1937.
3. Orth, G., Breitburd, F., and Faure, M.: Evidence for antigenic determinants shared by the structural polypeptides of rabbit papillomavirus and human papillomavirus type 1. *Virology, 91*:243–255, 1978.
4. Chretien, J. H., Esswein, J. G., and Garagusi, V. F.: Decreased T-cell levels in patients with warts. *Arch Dermatol, 114*:213–215, 1978.
5. Venetianer, A., Aranyi, P., Bosze, Z. S., and Fachet, J.: Sensitivity to glucocorticoids of lymph node cells stimulated in vivo by oxazolone. *Scand J Immunol, 8*:325–326, 1978.

Chapter 17

BOVINE OCULAR SQUAMOUS CELL CARCINOMA

LEIGH WEST-HYDE, V.M.D.

Introduction

Ocular squamous cell carcinoma (OSCC), occurs in man, dogs, horses, cats, sheep, swine, and cattle. The condition is particularly common in cattle, especially the Hereford breed.[1-3] In the United States, the estimated incidence of the disease in cattle is 0.8 to 1.6 percent, and in some areas as high as 5 percent.[2,4,5] Bovine OSCC accounts for 88 percent of all cattle condemned for neoplasia by meat inspectors. Death from the disease, weight loss, and reduced sale price cause additional economic losses.[2] Aside from its economic importance, bovine OSCC offers an attractive model for comparative oncologists who wish to study a spontaneous, superficial carcinoma that is readily available and easily observable.

Pathology and Pathogenesis

Before progressing to carcinomas, most cases of bovine OSCC develop through a series of nonmalignant precursor lesions, called "epidermal plaques." About 25 percent of all lesions occur in the palpebral conjunctiva, nictitating membrane, and eyelid skin.[5] The remaining 75 percent of lesions affect the bulbar conjunctiva and cornea primarily in the limbal region.[6] The clinical and histologic appearance of these lesions has been described elsewhere.[1,2,6]

The plaque, papilloma, noninvasive carcinoma (carcinoma *in situ*), and invasive carcinomas have an incidence of 11, 7, 3, and 79 percent, respectively.[6] Not all plaques progress to form papillomas, nor do all papillomas give rise to squamous cell carcinomas. Precursor lesions have reported regression rates of 26–50 percent. Spontaneous regression of ocular squamous cell carcinoma is a very rare event. The time required for malignant transformation of benign lesions varies from three months to two years.[2]

Both invasiveness and the tendency to metastasize vary with the location of the tumor. Local invasion may involve the globe, the orbital bones, maxilla, and orbital part of the frontal bones. Lesions of the eyelid skin, palpebral conjunctiva, and nictitating membrane have a greater tendency to metastasize than do limbal and corneal lesions. The parotid lymph node is the first site of metastasis via the lymphatic route, with progression to the chain of head and neck lymph nodes enroute to the thoracic duct and venous circulation. Hematological spread to the visceral organs, without involvement of the regional lymph nodes, has not been described in bovine OSCC.

Contributing Factors

Host Factors

The highest risk candidate to develop bovine OSCC is a female Hereford from seven to nine years of age. Although other breeds of cattle have been known to develop the disease, the Hereford is generally agreed to be the most susceptible.[2] The incidence of tumor increases with advancing age but its prevalence decreases in very old animals. This has usually been interpreted to mean that susceptible animals will have developed the carcinoma and died before old age, leaving only the more resistant cattle.[5] Although the length of exposure to a carcinogen may be a factor, the peak incidence of tumor in older animals may also reflect biochemical or immunological defects.

Hereford and Angus cattle were shown not to have an enzymatic defect in the repair syntheses of DNA damaged by ultraviolet light. This reparative defect is present in humans with xerodema pigmentosum, a disease in which ocular squamous cell carcinoma occurs.[7] Although there was no evidence of impaired cell-mediated immunity in Hereford cattle when measured by phytohaemagglutinin stimulation of lymphocytes, Jennings et al. did find that (1) lymphocytes from Herefords differed from control cattle in being more susceptible to ultraviolet light and in being less able to replicate following ultraviolet irradiation and (2) the ability of the host's lymphocytes to respond to phytohaemagglutinin was significantly reduced once ocular carcinomas grew in excess of 2 cm.[8,9] The preference for females may be only apparent, since female cattle are commonly maintained, whereas male cattle are slaughtered for food.

Pigmentation of the animal is also a factor. In general, tumors do not develop on fully pigmented eyelids or on portions of the eyelids that are partially pigmented. If a tumor is growing on an unpigmented section of eyelid, it may encroach on pigmented areas and continue to grow.[2] The inhibitory effect of corneoscleral pigment on the occurrence of limbal tumors is not as clear cut, because there may be a delay in its development for several years of the animal's life. However, breed resistance seems to be related to the presence of corneoscleral pigment.[10,11]

Genetic predisposition to the development of bovine OSCC, especially the Hereford breed, is an important factor, but an accurate interpretation of studies is difficult because protective pigmentation is highly heritable but distinct from other forms of resistance. In order to decrease the frequency of occurrence within a purebred herd, the strategy of culling the offspring of affected animals and discarding bulls with a history of that tumor has been suggested.[4,12] These suggestions are often not practical.

Environmental Factors

Actinic radiation and nutritional plane have been correlated to the occurrence of bovine OSCC. Anderson studied 5000 animals and found that the age-adjusted incidence of disease increased with (1) an increase in average annual hours of sunlight, (2) a decrease in average latitude, and (3) an increase in average altitude.[13] Thus, geography and pigmentation interplay with the amount of ultraviolet radiation received by susceptible animals.[14] Interestingly, the higher the plane of nutrition, the higher the frequency of the tumor occurrence. Anderson postulated that the animals with better nutrition reached physiologic age more rapidly than animals on lower feeding levels. His observations over a 20 year period conclusively demonstrated that at higher feeding levels there are greater numbers of animals with more lesions of an advanced and severe nature.[15]

Infectious Agents

One intriguing possibility is that a transmissible agent is responsible for bovine OSCC. This possibility would be compatible with the high incidence of the neoplasm in multiple and bilateral forms. It would also be compatible with tumor progression from benign lesions to carcinomas and with predisposition of age and breed. Most studies on infective agents have been concerned with viruses. Herpesviruses have been demonstrated most frequently, in particular, the herpesvirus of infectious bovine rhinotracheitis (bovine herpesvirus 1).[2,16] Neutralizing antibodies against bovine rhinotracheitis virus are more prevalent in cattle with eye tumors than in control animals,[17] and samples of bovine OSCC have been shown to contain an antigen that is present in a number of herpesviruses.[18] Thus Hereford cattle may be susceptible to the carcinogenic action of an ocular herpesvirus that has been inactivated by exposure to ultraviolet radiation.[19]

In a recent report, Ford et al. give the first evidence of virus in a precursor lesion of bovine OSCC.[20] In negatively stained preparations for electron microscopic examination, 8 of 25 precursor lesions showed virions resembling those of papillomaviruses. From this intriguing finding, Ford's study suggests that the carcinomas may be initiated by a papillomavirus in the precursor papilloma. This situation would be analogous to that of the virus-free squamous cell carcinoma of rabbits that develops from the Shope papilloma. Neither virus would persist in the carcinoma in an infectious form, but there should be biochemical or immunological evidence for their presence.[19] Alternatively, multiple etiology involving papillomavirus and prolonged exposure to sunlight could be suggested for the bovine OSCC that develops from ocular papillomas. There are as yet no convincing transmission experiments using cell-free tumor material, either in cattle or in laboratory animals.[2]

The Immune Response

Antibodies

One of the basic assumptions of research in cancer immunology is that cancer cells are distinguished from normal cells by the presence of distinctive cell-surface antigens. This postulate forms the basis of the explanation for specific immunotherapy. Several investigators have been unable to demonstrate or induce specific antibody production against bovine OSCC, even though affected animals respond to immunotherapy.[2] However, the total amounts of serum immunoglobulins are significantly higher in Hereford cattle with ocular carcinomas or precursor lesions than in age-matched Hereford cattle without eye lesions.[21] In a recent serologic study of cattle at various stages of disease using radioiodine-labelled protein A, Atluru et al.[22] found that all the sera tested had antibodies at a high level to autologous cells and that surface reactivity was not observed in these sera in tests for reactivity with normal epithelial cells. Their work using reactive sera, analyzed by absorption tests with autologous and allogeneic cells, indicates that there may be a shared antigen among the cells from precarcinoma and carcinoma lesions.

Cell-Mediated Immunity

There are several studies investigating the functional competence of cell-mediated immune mechanisms in OSCC-bearing cattle.[2] Using a microadaptation of the leucocyte adherence inhibition test, several workers demonstrated antigen recognition in affected versus nonaffected cattle. Affected cattle have populations of lymphocytes that are specifically reactive with saline extracts of OSCC. Intradermal injection of tumor-bearing cattle with saline phenol extracts of OSCC showed delayed hypersensitivity responses. Using histologic and immunofluorescent techniques in bovine OSCC, Hamir, Ladds, and Boland[23] showed the presence of many cells coated with immunoglobulin G (IgG) in all precancerous and carcinomatous lesions. Neither normal bovine tissues nor parotid lymph nodes from affected animals showed this IgG coating. Histologically, however, the prevalence, size, and mitotic activity of lymphoid follicles were each significantly greater in the parotid lymph node of the tumor affected side than in the contralateral parotid lymph node.

Diagnosis and Treatment

Although clinical diagnosis of large ocular carcinomas presents few problems, it is difficult to distinguish between small carcinomas derived from benign precursor plaques and papillomas from other benign proliferative lesions of the bovine eye. Histopathologic examination provides a definitive diagnosis, and superficial eye lesions are accessible to biopsy. The problem of differential diagnosis is becoming more important as bovine OSCC is now known to be highly susceptible to several forms of immunotherapy. The exfoliative cytology technique can be used to avoid excision of the lesions for experimental observation and to prevent unwanted antigenic stimulus in experimental studies or clinical diagnosis of bovine OSCC. Distinguishing characteristics of smears of carcinoma cells include condensation of nuclear chromatin, prominent nucleoli, anisnocleosis, bizarre mitoses, multinucleation, and increased nucleo-cytoplasmic ratios.[24]

Surgical excision, cryosurgery, hyperthermia, radiotherapy, electrocautery, and chemotherapy have been used to treat bovine OSCC with variable success.[2,25-28] The goal of immunotherapy is to increase the resistance of the host by augmenting the immune response directed against malignant cells. Immunotherapy may use immunopotentiating agents such as BCG[29] or it may employ antigenic components of a tumor to induce specific antibody or cell-mediated responses using saline phenol extracts of tumors.[30]

Current Research—Application to Human Disease

The main value of comparative medicine is not that it produces results that can be applied directly to a human disease but rather that it provides opportunities to investigate basic disease mechanisms.[31,32] It is of particular interest because it is economically important and can serve as a model for some human neoplasms. This spontaneous tumor provides a better biological model than the viral and chemically induced tumors of inbred rodents because the tumor in cattle is a potentially metastatic, autochthonous carcinoma occurring naturally in a large outbred species. Additional advantages of this animal model are that (1) the large body size of cattle enables adequately large samples of tissues and blood to be collected; (2) adequate follow-up observations are possible because of the long natural life span of cattle; (3) exfoliative cytological examination can be performed without surgery; and (4) the expense of keeping the animal during carcinogenesis is not borne by the investigator.

The controlled study of this spontaneous tumor is enhanced by the recent success in autografting and allografting the tumor[33] and the highly successful maintenance of continuous cultures of epithelial cancer cells derived from the bovine neoplasm.[2,34] In addition, this tumor is the first instance of a naturally occurring cancer in which the curative effect of immunotherapy is often remarkable.[2,29,30] Continuation of basic studies on the immunopathology, the induced regression, and the viral induction of bovine OSCC will increase our understanding of carcinogenesis and will lead to new methods for the therapy of human tumors.

REFERENCES

1. Russell, W. O., Wynne, E. S., and Loquvam, G. S.: Studies on bovine ocular squamous cell carcinoma (cancer eye). 1. Pathological anatomy and historical review. *Cancer,* 9:1–52, 1956.
2. Spradbrow, P. B., and Hoffman, D.: Bovine ocular squamous cell carcinoma. *Vet Bulletin,* 50:449–459, 1980.
3. Jun Moo Hyung: Bovine ocular squamous cell carcinoma: a review. *Korean J Vet Pub Hlth,* 5:31–47, 1981.
4. Cordy, D. R.: Tumors of the nervous system and eye. In *Tumors in Domestic Animals.* Berkeley, University of California Press, 1978, pp. 430–455.
5. Russell, W. C., Brinks, J. S., and Kainer, R. A.: Incidence and heritability of ocular squamous cell tumors in Hereford cattle. *J Anim Sci,* 43:1156–1162, 1976.
6. Monlux, A. W., Anderson, W. A., and Davis, C. L.: The diagnosis of squamous cell carcinoma of the eye ("cancer eye") in cattle. *Am J Vet Res,* 18:5–34, 1957.
7. Cleaver, J. E., Kainer, R. A., and Zelle, M. R.: Ocular squamous cell carcinoma (cancer eye) in Hereford cattle: Radiation repair processes and a comparison of cultured cells with xeroderma pigmentosum in man. *Am J Vet Res,* 33:1131–1136, 1972.
8. Jennings, P. A., Lavin, M. F., Hughes, D. J., and Spradbrow, P. B.: Bovine ocular squamous cell carcinoma: lymphocyte response to phytohaemagglutinin and tumor antigen. *Br J Cancer,* 40:608–614, 1979.
9. Jennings, P. A., Hughes, D. J., and Lavin, M. L.: An animal model relating UV sensitivity and reduced DNA repair to increased incidence of carcinoma. *Proc Aust Biochem Soc,* 12:81, 1979.
10. Anderson, D. E.: Effects of pigment on bovine ocular squamous carcinoma. *Ann NY Acad Sci,* 100:436–446, 1963.
11. Anderson, D. E.: Genetic aspects of cancer with special reference to cancer of the eye in the bovine. *Ann NY Acad Sci,* 100:948–962, 1963.
12. Woodward, R. R., and Knapp, B.: The hereditary aspect of eye cancer in Hereford cattle. *J Anim Sci,* 9:578–581, 1950.
13. Anderson, D. E., and Skinner, P. E.: Studies on bovine ocular squamous carcinoma ("cancer eye") XI. Effects of sunlight. *J Anim Sci,* 20:474–477, 1961.
14. Kopeohy, K. E., Pugh, G. W., Hughes, D. E., Booth, G. D., and Cheville, N. F.: Biological effect of ultraviolet radiation on cattle: Bovine ocular squamous cell carcinoma. *Am J Vet Res,* 40:1783–1788, 1979.
15. Anderson, D. E., Pope, L. S., and Stephens, D.: Nutrition and eye cancer in cattle. *J Natl Cancer Inst,* 45:697–707, 1970.
16. Gibbs, E. P. J., and Rweyemamu, M. M.: Bovine herpesvirus. Part I. Bovine herpesvirus 1. *Vet Bulletin,* 47:317–343, 1977.
17. Taylor, R. L., and Hanks, M. A.: Viral isolations from bovine eye tumors. *Am J Vet Res,* 30:1885–1886, 1969.
18. Evans, D. L., Barnett, J. W., and Dmochowski, L.: Common antigens in herpesvirus from

divergent species of animals. *Tex Rep Biol Med*, 31:755-770, 1973.
19. Spradbrow, P. B., and Francis, J.: Ox eyes and immuno-surveillance. *Lancet, ii*, 356, 1977.
20. Ford, J. N., Jennings, P. A., Spradbrow, P. B., and Francis, J.: Evidence for papillomaviris in ocular lesions in cattle. *Res Vet Sci*, 32:257-259, 1982.
21. Hoffman, D.: Studies on bovine ocular squamous cell carcinoma. *PhD Thesis*, Univ. Queensland, 1978.
22. Atluru, D., Kleinschuster, S. J., Zupancic, M. L., and Muscoplat, C. C.: Detection of cell surface antigens of bovine ocular squamous cell carcinoma. *J Am Vet Med Assoc*, 43:1156-1159, 1982.
23. Hamir, A. N. J., Ladds, P. W., and Boland, P. H.: An immunopathological study of bovine ocular squamous cell carcinoma. *J Comp Pathol*, 90-535-549, 1980.
24. Hoffman, D., Spradbrow, P. B., and Wilson, B. E.: An evaluation of exfoliative cytology in the diagnosis of bovine ocular squamous cell carcinoma. *J Comp Pathol*, 88:497-504, 1978.
25. Bier, J., Bleinschuster, S. J., and Corbett, R.: Radical surgery of bovine ocular squamous cell carcinoma (cancer eye): A new procedure. *Vet Sci Commun*, 3:221-230, 1979.
26. Farris, H. E.: Cryosurgical treatment of bovine ocular squamous cell carcinoma. *Vet Clin North Am (Small Anim Pract)*, 10:861-867, 1980.
27. Kainer, R. A., Stringer, J. M., and Lueker, D. C.: Hyperthermia for treatment of ocular squamous cell tumore in cattle. *J Am Vet Med Assoc*, 176:356-360, 1980.
28. Hofmeyer, C. F. B.: Radioactive gold in the treatment of bovine ophthalmic squamous cell carcinoma. In *Reports and Summaries. XI International Congress on Diseases of Cattle*. Tel-Aviv, 1980, Vol. II, pp. 1467-1172.
29. Kleinschuster, S. J., Rapp, H. J., Green, S. B., Bier, J., and VanKampen, K.: Efficacy of intratumorally administered mycobacterial cell walls in the treatment of cattle with ocular carcinoma. *J Natl Cancer Inst*, 67:1165-1169, 1981.
30. Hoffman, D., Jennings, P. A., and Spradbrow, P. B.: Immunotherapy of bovine ocular squamous cell carcinomas with phenol-saline extracts of allogeneic carcinomas. *Aust Vet J*, 57:159-162, 1981.
31. Beveridge, W. I. B.: Ox eyes and immunosurveillance. *Lancet, ii*, 356. 1977.
32. Kleinschuster, S. J., Rapp, H. J., Lueker, D. C., and Kainer, R. A.: Regression of bovine ocular carcinoma by treatment with a mycobacterial vaccine. *J Natl Cancer Inst*, 58:1807-1814, 1977.
33. Hoffman, D., Jennings, P. A., Spradbrow, P. B., and Wilson, B. E.: Autografting and allografting of bovine ocular squamous cell carcinoma. *Res Vet Sci*, 31:48-53, 1981.
34. Klenschuster, S. J., Rapp, H. J., Bier, J., VanKampen, K. R., Spendlove, R. S., Johnston, A. V., and Elsner, V.: Epithelial cells cultured from bovine ocular carcinoma. *Vet Sci Commun*, 3:65-71, 1979.

SECTION III
METABOLIC AND MISCELLANEOUS DISORDERS

Chapter 18

OVAL CORNEAL OPACITIES IN BEAGLES
An Animal Model of Schnyder's Crystalline Dystrophy

ALAN M. ROTH, M.D.; MARILYN B. EKINS, M.D.; GEORGE O. WARING, III, M.D.;
LATA M. GUPTA, M.S.; LEON S. ROSENBLATT, PH.D.

Corneal dystrophies and degenerations have rarely been described in dogs.[1] Although sporadic cases have been reported, none has resembled the oval stromal corneal opacities we previously described in 128 eyes of 75 purebred beagles from a colony of 497 dogs.[2] These anterior stromal opacities were oval, about 3 by 5 mm, located at the junction of the middle and inferior thirds of the avascular cornea, and were usually bilaterally symmetrical. We observed three morphologic types: nebular, with a homogenous gray appearance (Fig. 18-1); racetrack, with a gray oval surrounding a slightly depressed, brownish center (Fig. 18-2); and white arc, with subepithelial, dense, white plaques of granular or spicule-shaped material (Fig. 18-3). These three patterns represent different stages in the natural history of the disorder, progressing from the nebular (least severe) to the white arc (most advanced).[3] Because the colony was outbred,[4] we could not establish a hereditary pattern. We have also seen similar corneal opacities in beagles that were not part of this colony (Fig. 18-4).

When we initially described the clinical appearance of oval stromal corneal opacities in beagles,[2] we did not know what material composed these lesions. Negative findings with standard histochemical stains and the presence of vacuoles and crystals in transmission electron micrographs led us to search for lipids. Although we recognized that lipid histochemistry is an imprecise art and that only a few techniques define lipids with certainty, we decided to perform a large battery of techniques to give the most comprehensive data. These may then be interpreted in light of the limitations of such testing and correlated with more precise biochemical analysis. We report here the histopathologic findings and histochemical demonstration of lipids in these

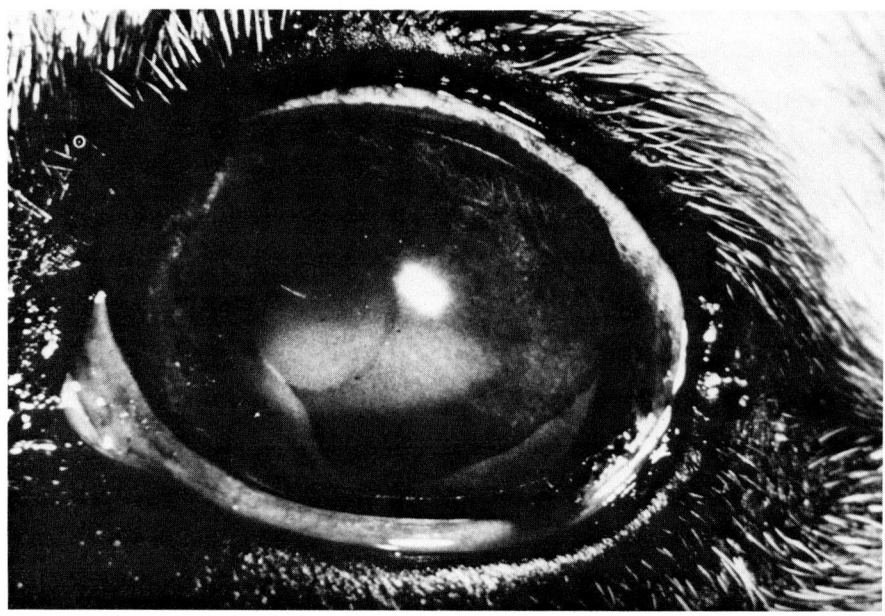

Figure 18-1. Nebular oval corneal opacity has homogeneous gray appearance with indistinct margins. (From *Investigative Ophthalmology and Visual Science, 21*:95–106, 1981. Reproduced with permission.)

opacities and show that serum lipid levels and thyroid hormone assays are similar in both affected beagles and age- and sex-matched controls.

Materials and Methods

All beagles came from a colony involved in lifelong radionuclide toxicity studies at the Radiobiology Laboratory, University of California, Davis.[5,6] As each dog was scheduled for sacrifice, we reviewed our previous records to determine the type of corneal opacity present. After the dog was anesthetized with intravenous sodium pentobarbital, we verified the type of corneal opacity by inspection with a penlight and enucleated the eyes. We immediately removed a corneoscleral shell by cutting into the epichoroidal space 4 mm posterior to the limbus, excising the shell with scissors, and disinserting the ciliary body from the scleral spur. The cornea was placed epithelial side down on a silicone block and trisected through the oval opacity; one-third was fixed in cold 2% glutaraldehyde in Millonig's buffer for electron microscopy, one-third was frozen in liquid nitrogen for biochemical determinations, and one-third was fixed in Baker's formol-calcium solution[7] for light microscopy.

We recorded the nutritional and medical history of each dog. An experienced veterinary pathologist performed a complete autopsy.

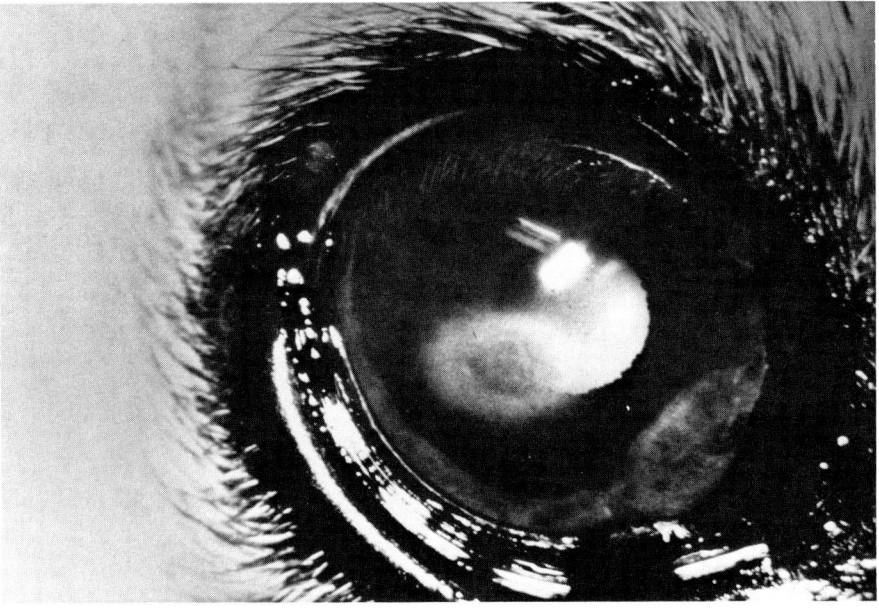

Figure 18-2. Racetrack oval opacity has slightly depressed, brownish center. (From *Investigative Ophthalmology and Visual Science, 21*:95–106, 1981. Reproduced with permission.)

Histochemistry.

We studied 29 corneas from 16 affected beagles that had the nebular type opacity and two corneas from two unaffected beagles. Three specimens from two dogs were blocked in paraffin only. Because routine histochemical stains of sections cut from these blocks revealed no abnormal substances, because the ultrastructural studies on these specimens showed intracellular vacuoles and crystals, suggestive of lipids (Spangler, Waring and Morrin, unpublished data), and because the clinical appearance was compatible with lipid deposits, we divided the formol-calcium-fixed tissue from each of the remaining 26 corneas into two pieces. We embedded one of these in paraffin and stained sections with hematoxylin and eosin, Masson's trichrome method, the periodic acid-Schiff reaction, and Alcian blue at pH 2.5. The other piece was frozen, and sections were cut 10 to 15 μm thick and stained by 16 histochemical methods for demonstrating lipids (Table 18-I). We stained sections of brain known to contain the different lipids with each corneal specimen as a control. Sections being analyzed for cholesterol were examined within 15 minutes of staining because of rapid oxidation of the reaction and because the sections were destroyed by the technique. Paraffin and frozen sections were also examined under plane-polarized light for birefringence.

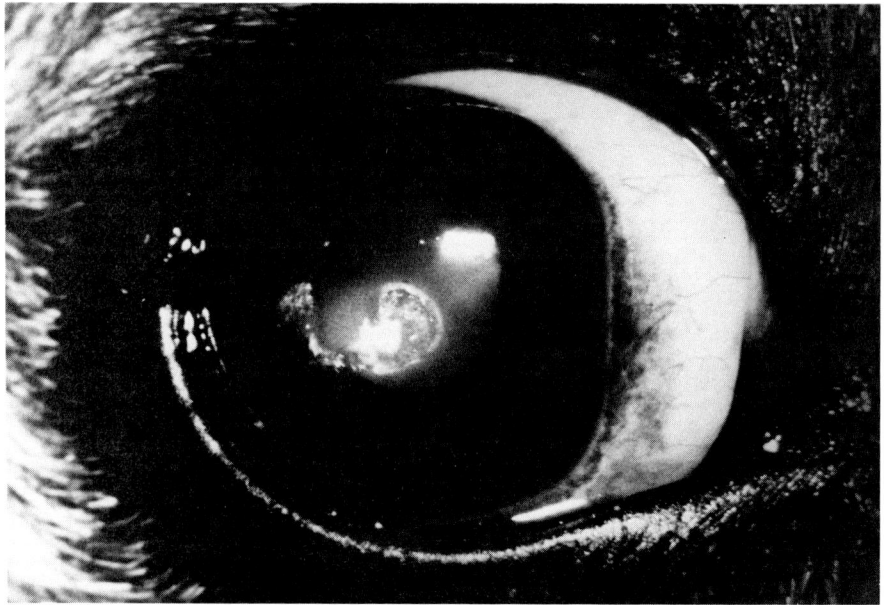

Figure 18-3. White arc oval opacity is densely white, granular subepithelial deposit. (From *Investigative Ophthalmology and Visual Science*, 21:95–106, 1981. Reproduced with permission.)

Serum Lipid Measurements.

We measured serum cholesterol and triglycerides in affected beagles and in age- and sex-matched control beagles on two occasions, one year apart. In December 1977, we paired each of 48 affected beagles (28 males, 20 females) with an unaffected beagle of the same age and sex (27 males, 21 females) in the same radiation group (^{90}Sr, ^{226}Ra, or not radiated). Some of the affected and control dogs were littermates. In January 1979, we reexamined the 29 surviving affected beagles (18 male, 11 female) and the 40 surviving controls (24 male, 16 female). The mean ages of the control and affected dogs were comparable for both sexes (male 12.5 years, female 12.6 years). After the dogs had fasted six hours, we collected 10 ml of clotted blood with a 20-gauge needle from the left jugular vein. The samples were immediately centrifuged at 3000 rpm at 4°C; the serum was removed and stored at 4°C. We measured total cholesterol by the Technicon AutoAnalyzer II (Clinical Method No. 24/preliminary March 1972) for the first determination and by the enzymatic method of Patsch[8] for the second. The high-density-lipoprotein cholesterol (C_{HDL}, α cholesterol) was determined by NIH protocol,[9] and triglycerides by Fletcher's technique.[10] The combined low-density and very-low-density lipoprotein cholesterol (C_{LDL} and C_{VLDL}, β and pre-β cholesterol)

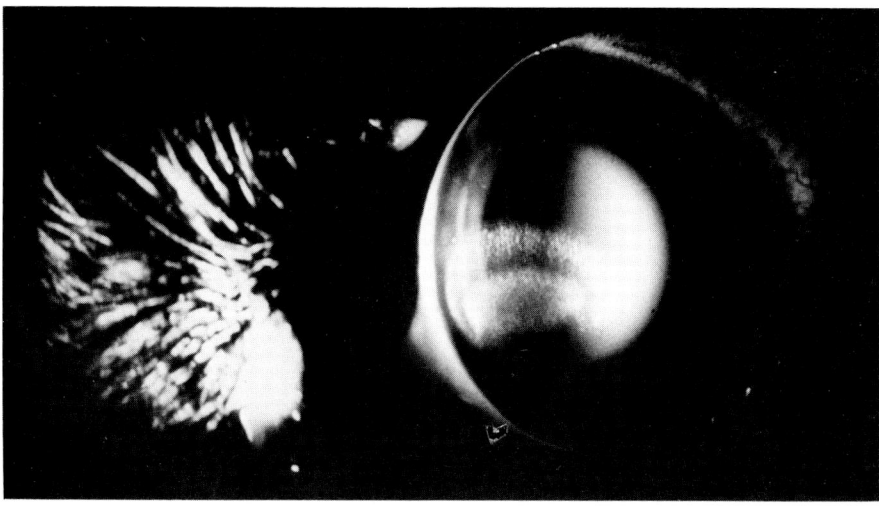
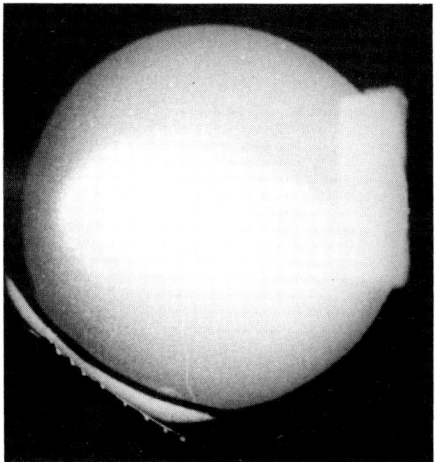

Figure 18-4. Oval opacity in beagle from outside the colony studied shows double row of gray crystalloid deposits (*above*), which stand out prominently in retroillumination (*below*). (From *Investigative Ophthalmology and Visual Science*, 21:95–106, 1981. Reproduced with permission.)

was then calculated by subtracting the C_{HDL} from the total cholesterol.[9] All solvents used were reagent grade. To confirm the accuracy of our serum lipid measurements, we employed standards of known lipid concentration and also sent random beagle serum samples to an independent laboratory that used the same methods.

We employed analysis of variance and regression analysis to compare serum lipid measurements from the total number of affected and control dogs, to compare each of the three affected subgroups (nebular, racetrack, and white arc) to each other and to the controls, and to compare sexes and

TABLE 18-I
HISTOCHEMICAL STAINS DONE FOR LIPID

	Reference	Type of reaction	Lipid demonstrated	Specificity
Oil red O	7	Lipid-soluble dye	Neutral fat	High
Sudan black B	30	Lipid-soluble dye	Neutral fat especially phospholipid	Moderate
Baker	28	Acid hematein with pyridine extraction	Phospholipid	Low
Pearse	31	Copper phthalocyanin	Phospholipid	Low
Menschik	32	Nile blue sulfate	Phospholipid	Low
Landing et al.	33	Phosphomolybdic acid	Choline-containing phospholipid	Low
Fischler	27	Cupric soap-lithium hematoxylin	Fatty acid	Moderate
Holczinger	27	Cupric soap-rubeanic acid	Fatty acid	High
Schultz	27	Acetic-sulfuric acid	Cholesterol	Moderate
Adams	34	Perchloric acid-naphthoquinone	Cholesterol	High
Okamoto	27	Sulfuric-iodide	Cholesterol	Moderate
Bromine-Sudan black B	35	Bromination unmasking	Unmasked cholesterol	Low
Mukherji	27	Bromine-silver	Unsaturated lipid	Moderate
Norton	36	Bromine-silver	Unsaturated lipid	Moderate
Osmium tetroxide	28	Lipid-soluble reagent	Unsaturated lipid	Low
Seligman-Ashbel	7	Naphthoic hydrazide	Active carbonyl lipids	Low

From *Investigative Ophthalmology and Visual Science*, 21:95–106, 1981. Reproduced with permission.

ages. We used data only from beagles whose serum lipids were measured twice. Each of the affected dogs was classed according to the lesion of its more severely affected eye. Between the first and second lipid determination, the opacities in some of the affected dogs progressed; thus the same dog may be in one affected subgroup in 1977 and in another in 1979.

Thyroid Hormone Assays.

We tested thyrometabolic function in 24 affected beagles and in 39 age- and sex-matched control beagles. Blood was collected from the jugular vein and the serum was immediately separated as described above. The samples were stored at 4°C for no longer than 48 hours before analysis. Thyroxine (T_4) levels were measured by the Quantimune T-4 Radioimmunoassay technique (Bio-Rad Laboratories Bulletin 4202, October 1978), and the binding capacity of thyroid hormone carrier proteins was assayed by the Quanta-Count T_3 resin uptake method (Bio-Rad Bulletin 4212, March 1977). The free thyroid index (T_7) was calculated by multiplying the T_4 level and the T_3 percent resin uptake (%RU).

We employed chi-square analysis to compare the results between control and affected dogs, between control dogs and those in each affected subgroup (nebular, racetrack, and white arc), and between dogs in each subgroup. Statistical review was performed by Dr. Rosenblatt.

Results

Complete autopsies on all dogs revealed no changes suggestive of a systemic lipid metabolic disorder.

Histology and General Histochemistry.

Paraffin sections stained with hematoxylin and eosin and with Masson's trichrome method demonstrated that the epithelium and its basal lamina generally were intact with occasional focal acanthosis (facet formation). Although Bowman's layer is not normally present in beagle corneas (Morrin, Waring, Spangler, unpublished data), the normal anterior stroma is hypocellular, with interlacing collagen bundles. The major abnormality in the affected corneas was in this area, with disruption of collagen architecture, focal areas of collagen fibril fragmentation, stromal vacuole formation, and scattered enlarged vacuolated keratocytes. No blood vessels were seen.

Periodic acid-Schiff and Alcian blue reactions revealed no gross abnormalities in glycosaminoglycans. Plane-polarized light showed no birefringence in sections from paraffin blocks. Frozen sections, however, contained many doubly refractile crystals, primarily within keratocytes, but occasionally in the extracellular stroma. The posterior stroma, Descemet's membrane, and endothelium were normal.

Lipid Histochemistry.

Table 18-II shows the results of the histochemical reactions for lipids in 26 affected corneas. The right and left corneas from each dog usually stained similarly. All stains were positive on the known control tissue and showed no reaction in the two unaffected control corneas. The majority of positive stains were intracellular with many having extracellular staining as well. No case showed only extracellular stain, although a few had such dense overall reaction that we could not ascertain its location.

Stains for neutral fats (oil red O and Sudan black B) were positive in all corneas, primarily in the anterior half. In general, the intracellular stain was in large globules, whereas the stromal stain was in finer granules (Fig. 18-5). At least one of the methods for demonstrating cholesterol (Schultz, Okamoto, and Adams) was positive in each cornea (Fig. 18-6). The majority were positive by all three techniques. All corneas demonstrated phospholipids with at least one of four reactions for phospholipid (Baker, Pearse, Landing, and Menschik), and 12 of the 26 corneas demonstrated fatty acids by at least one of the tests (Fischler, Holczinger). The remainder of the histochemical reactions were negative, although sporadic intracellular staining was sometimes present.

TABLE 18-II.
RESULTS OF HISTOCHEMICAL STAINS FOR LIPID

Dog and cornea No.	A		B		C		D		E		F	
	1	2	3	4	5	6	7	8	9	10	11	
Oil red O	+++	+++	+++	+++	+	+	+++	++	++	+++	+++	
Suden black B	+++	+++	+++	+++	++	++	+	++	++	+++	+++	
Bromine-Sudan black B	+++	+++	+++	+++	++	++	++	++	++	+++	+++	
Schultz	+++	+++	++	+++	++	++	−	++	++	++	+++	
Okamoto	+++	+++	+++	++	+	+	++	+	+	+++	+++	
Adams	++	++	+++	+++	++	+	+	++	++	+++	+++	
Baker*	++	+++	+++	+++	++	++	−	+	−	+++	++	
Pearse	+++	++	+++	+++	++	++	+++	++	++	+++	+++	
Landing	+++	+++	+++	+++	+	++	++	++	++	++	++	
Menschik	++	++	+	+	−	−	+	−	−	+	−	
Fischler	+++	+	+	−	−	−	−	++	++	++	++	
Holczinger	*	++	++	−	−	−	−	−	−	+	−	
OsO$_4$	−	−	−	−	−	−	−	−	−	−	−	
Norton	−	−	−	−	−	−	−	−	−	−	−	
Mukherji	−	−	−	−	−	−	−	−	−	−	−	
Seligman-Ashbel	−	++	−	++	−	−	−	−	−	−	−	

From *Investigative Ophthalmology and Visual Science, 21*:95–106, 1981. Reproduced with permission.

− = Negative; + = mildly positive; ++ = moderately positive; +++ = strongly positive.

Dogs D and M supplied only one cornea each.

*With pyridine extraction control

Serum Lipid Measurements.

There was no significant difference between affected and control dogs in either 1977 or 1979 for total cholesterol, C_{HDL}, C_{LDL}, and C_{VLDL}, or triglycerides (Table 18-III). The influence of sex on serum lipids was also negligible except that, in 1979, affected females showed higher triglycerides than affected males. The influence of age on serum lipids was less clear-cut (Table 18-III). In 1977, there was a statistically significant trend for serum cholesterol to rise with age, but this was not confirmed in 1979. When we analyzed total serum cholesterol, C_{HDL}, C_{LDL}, and C_{VLDL} measurements in the three different clinical patterns in 1977, dogs with white arc opacities consistently had higher absolute values, but we could not confirm these differences in 1979 (Table 18-IV).

Thyroid Hormone Assays.

The 39 control dogs had T_3 %RU of 35.2% ± 4.6, T_4 level of 1.37 μg/100 ml ± 0.68, and T_7 of 0.48. Eight beagles with the nebular opacity had T_3 %RU of 34.6% ± 5.4, T_4 level of 1.45 μg/100 ml ± 5.4, and T_7 of 0.51. Eight dogs with the race track lesion showed T_3 %RU of 36.6% ± 5.1, T_4 levels of 1.46 μg/100 ml ± 0.32, and T_7 of 0.55. Six animals with the white arc

G		H		I		J		K		L		M	N	
12	13	14	15	16	17	18	19	20	21	22	23	24	25	26
+++	+++	+	−	+++	++	++	++	++	++	++	++	+	++	+++
+++	+++	++	+	+++	+	++	+	++	++	+	+	+	++	++
+++	+++	++	++	+++	++	++	++	++	++	++	++	++	++	+++
+++	++	−	−	+	−	++	++	++	++	+	+	−	++	+++
++	++	++	++	++	+	+	+	++	++	−	−	−	−	−
+++	+++	−	−	++	++	+	+	++	++	−	−	+	++	++
++	++	−	−	+	−	++	++	−	−	++	++	+	++	+
++	+++	++	++	+++	+	−	−	−	−	++	++	+	++	++
++	++	−	−	++	−	+	++	+	+	++	++	−	++	+
−	−	−	−	−	−	+	+	−	−	−	+	−	−	−
−	+++	−	−	+++	+++	−	−	−	−	−	−	−	+	+
−	−	−	−	−	−	−	−	−	−	−	−	−	−	−
−	+	−	−	−	−	−	−	−	−	−	−	−	−	−
−	−	−	−	−	−	−	−	−	−	−	+	−	−	−
−	−	−	−	−	−	−	−	−	−	−	−	−	−	−
−	−	−	−	−	−	−	−	−	−	−	−	−	−	−

corneal opacity had T_3 %RU of 35.3% ± 4.2, T_4 level of 1.70 μg/100 ml ± 0.70, and T_7 of 0.57. Chi-square analysis showed no significant difference in T_3 %RU, T_4, or T_7 between control and affected dogs, between control dogs and those in each subgroup, or between beagles in each subgroup.

Comment

Relatively little is known about the composition, source, and metabolism of normal corneal lipids. There is no evidence for lipid storage in the normal cornea *in vivo*, and lipids are probably limited to corneal cell membranes in the form of neutral fats (predominantly cholesterol and its esters) and phospholipids (primarily sphingomyelin).[11] These are relatively stable and there appears to be a low lipid turnover rate. Normal corneal stromal cells can synthesize lipids[12,13] and can incorporate labeled phosphorus into phospholipids.[14]

Lipids appear abnormally in the human cornea in a variety of patterns (Table 18-V). Three factors may contribute to these lipid deposits: (1) stromal blood vessels such as those in old scars or in limbal masses, (2) abnormal systemic lipid metabolism such as type II hyperlipoproteinemia or Tangier disease, and (3) primary corneal abnormalities such as central crystalline corneal dystrophy.

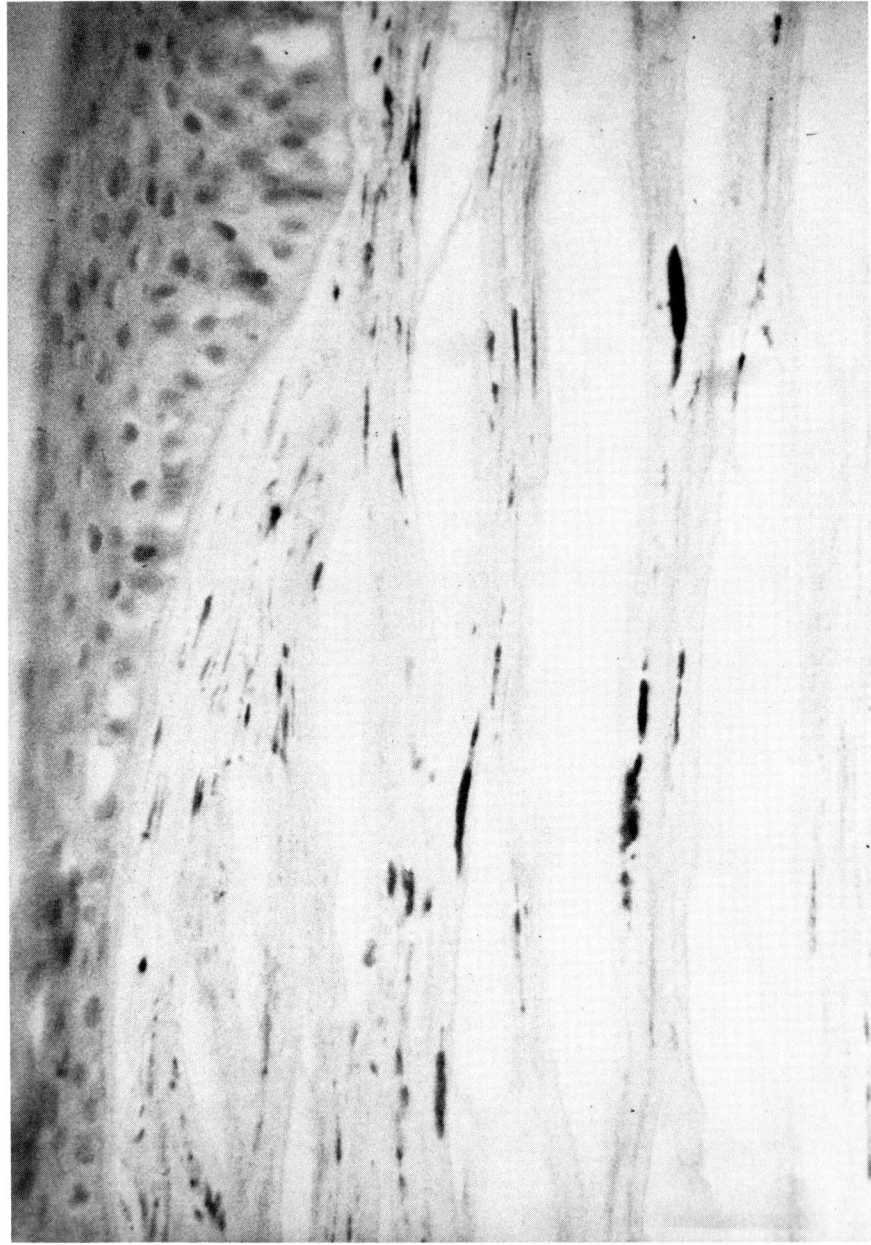

Figure 18-5. Neutral fat appears as large globules in keratocytes, whereas smaller extracellular granules accumulate in anterior stroma. Frozen section, oil red O; ×200. (From *Investigative Ophthalmology and Visual Science, 21*:95–106, 1981. Reproduced with permission.)

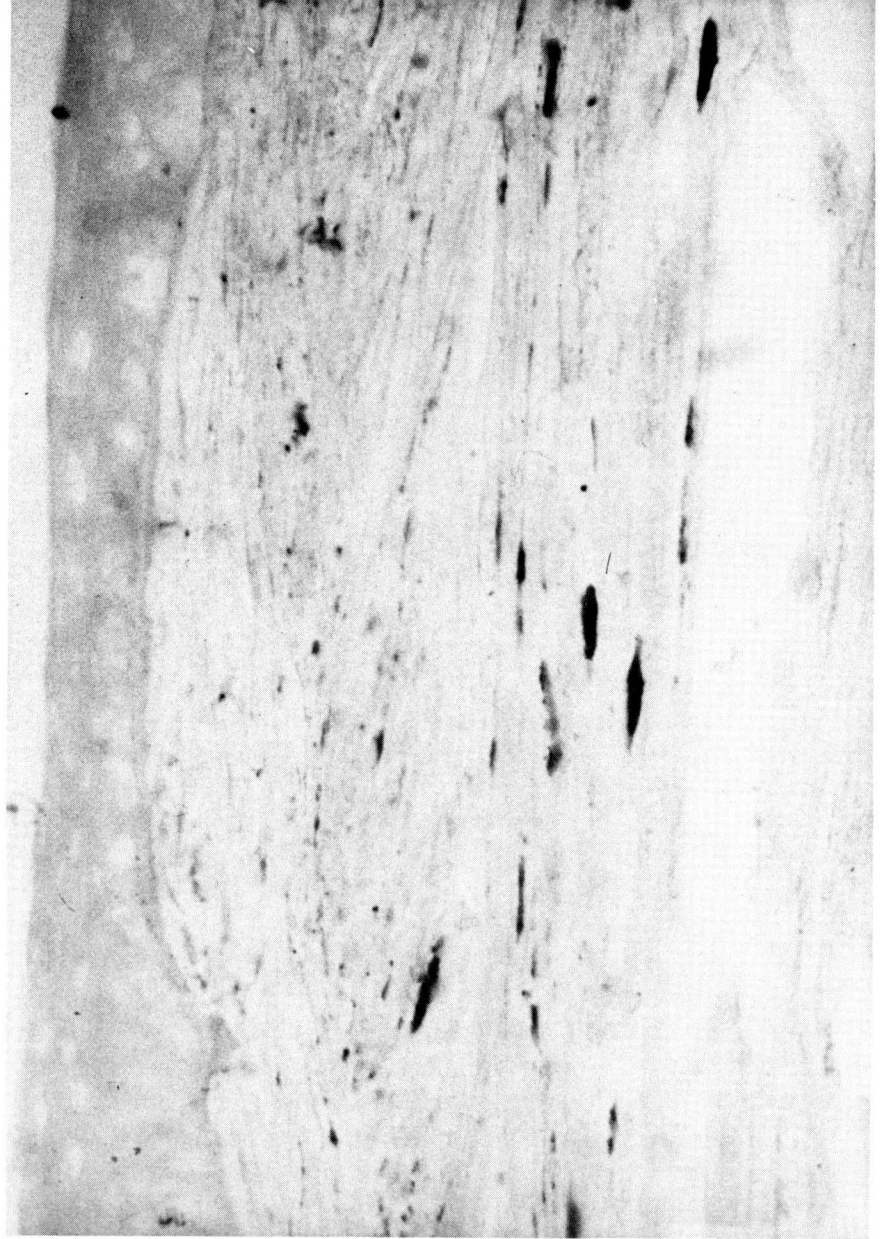

Figure 18-6. Cholesterol accumulates predominantly in keratocytes of anterior stroma. Frozen section, Okamoto's method, ×200. (From *Investigative Ophthalmology and Visual Science, 21*: 95–106, 1981. Reproduced with permission.)

TABLE 18-III

SERUM LIPID MEASUREMENTS (MG/DL) IN BEAGLES WITH OVAL OPACITIES AND UNAFFECTED CONTROLS

	Total cholesterol				C_{HDL}			
	First sample		Second sample		First sample		Second sample	
	Control	Opacity	Control	Opacity	Control	Opacity	Control	Opacity
Male:								
Mean	202.6	222.2	221.3	188.4	163.1	165.8	165.9	142.1
S.D.	43.6	76.2	46.2	39.3	28.7	35.9	32.2	45.0
N	27	28	24	18	27	28	24	18
Female:								
Mean	201.0	220.0	233.0	222.4	160.2	173.0	171.6	170.2
S.D.	56.9	61.1	54.8	79.8	40.6	35.4	31.7	50.2
N	21	20	16	11	21	20	16	11 =
Analysis of variance*:								
By sex	NS		NS		NS		NS	
By group	NS		NS		NS		NS	
By sex and group	NS		NS		NS		NS	
Linear regression against age:								
Male								
r	0.40	0.53	0.32	0.27	0.25	0.40	−0.03	0.10
p(r)	0.04	0.004	NS	NS	NS	0.04	NS	NS
Female								
r	0.57	0.08	0.01	0.03	0.46	0.39	0.05	0.42
p(r)	0.01	NS	NS	NS	0.03	NS	NS	NS

From *Investigative Ophthalmology and Visual Science*, 21:95–106, 1981. Reproduced with permission.

First sample = 1977; second sample = 1979; NS = not significant = $p > 0.05$.

*Normal vs. abnormal; male vs. female.

We searched for these three contributing factors in beagles with oval lipid corneal opacities. The corneas were avascular both clinically and histopathologically. In a few cases, corneal ulceration had occurred in conjunction with the oval opacities, and the corneas vascularized secondarily.

Serum lipid measurements in affected dogs were normal. The environment, nutrition, and medical care of this colony were carefully monitored.[15,16] A complete autopsy on each dog revealed neither atherosclerosis nor excess lipid deposits in parenchymal organs. Our initial analysis of serum cholesterol suggested elevated C_{HDL} in dogs with the racetrack and white arc patterns.[17] Further statistical analysis and a second sampling of affected and control dogs did not reveal statistically significant differences (Table 18-IV). Moreover, corneal opacities have not been described in reports of hyperlipemic beagles.[18,19] Therefore, we concluded that a systemic disorder of lipid metabolism did not contribute to the oval lipid corneal opacities.

However, we did observe consistently higher levels of serum cholesterol in dogs with the white arc type opacity, although the level was not always

C$_{LDL}$ and C$_{VLDL}$				Triglycerides			
First sample		Second sample		First sample		Second sample	
Control	Opacity	Control	Opacity	Control	Opacity	Control	Opacity
39.5	56.5	55.4	46.3	65.6	65.1	108.3	80.4
30.9	51.3	31.5	31.7	30.7	34.3	54.4	32.7
27	28	24	18	27	28	24	18
40.7	47.0	61.6	52.2	66.1	77.7	123.2	170.5
30.7	39.4	32.6	45.6	25.3	66.1	66.4	166.1
21	20	16	11	21	20	16	11
NS		NS		NS		p = 0.02	
NS		NS		NS		NS	
NS		NS		NS		NS	
0.33	0.51	0.50	0.19	0.16	0.06	0.15	0.39
0.01	0.006	0.01	NS	NS	NS	NS	NS
0.43	−0.22	0.13	−0.41	0.16	−0.10	0.46	0.15
0.05	NS	NS	NS	NS	NS	NS	NS

statistically significant and the number of these dogs was small (Table 18-IV). It is possible that these subepithelial white deposits, which we presume are lipids but have not studied histochemically, are related to the elevated serum lipids. On the other hand, although we found clinical progression of these opacities from nebular to racetrack to white arc types, we have not been able to document either a concurrent rise in serum lipids or increased serum lipids with age (Tables 18-III and 18-IV).

In hypothyroidism, serum cholesterol levels may be elevated because of altered metabolism; this metabolic effect has been reported in beagles.[20] Because our pilot study suggested that affected beagles had elevated serum cholesterol levels, we measured thyroxin and thyroglobin binding capacity, calculated T$_7$, and found no significant differences between affected and control dogs or dogs with different subgroups of opacities. Thus, thyroid dysfunction does not play a part in the pathogenesis of the oval opacities.

We think that oval stromal corneal opacities in beagles represent a primary disorder of corneal lipid metabolism. Of the human disorders in which lipid

TABLE 18-IV
TOTAL SERUM CHOLESTEROL MEASUREMENTS IN BEAGLES
WITH NEBULAR, RACE TRACK, AND WHITE ARC OVAL OPACITIES

	First sample				Second sample			
	Control	Nebular	Racetrack	White arc	Control	Nebular	Racetrack	White arc
Male:								
Mean	202.6	210.1	148.0	290.2	221.3	186.0	184.2	204.3
S.D.	43.6	48.9	—	136.8	46.2	30.4	55.0	37.6
N	27	22	1	5	24	9	6	3
Female:								
Mean	201.0	202.3	275.0	296.3	233.2	199.8	202.8	278.7
S.D.	56.9	53.9	—	30.0	54.8	38.8	58.7	133.8
N	21	16	1	3	16	4	4	3
Analysis of variance*								
By sex		NS				NS		
By type		p = 0.001				NS		
By sex and type		NS				NS		

From *Investigative Ophthalmology and Visual Science*, 21:95–106, 1981. Reproduced with permission.
First sample = 1977; second sample = 1979; NS = not significant = p > 0.05.
*Normal vs. abnormal; male vs. female.

is deposited in the cornea, these opacities most closely resemble the central crystalline corneal dystrophy of Schnyder.[21-25] Both occur in avascular, noninflamed corneas, are bilateral, and appear relatively symmetrical. The clinical appearance of both includes a ring-shaped configuration in which a central gray stromal opacity that is most dense superficially is studded with subepithelial white crystals. In advanced cases of both disorders, the opacity may occupy full-thickness stroma. Histochemically, both contain cholesterol and neutral fats,[15,18,19] whereas the beagle corneas also have histochemical evidence of phospholipids and sometimes fatty acids. Both have similar ultrastructure with elongated crystals, extracellular vacuoles and debris, disruption of collagen lamellae, hyperplasia of keratocyte organelles, and stromal cellular degeneration.[26] Hyperlipoproteinemia has been found in some patients with central crystalline dystrophy and in family members of affected individuals.[21,22] Although we did not find hyperlipidemia in affected beagles, the dogs with white arc opacities did have serum cholesterol levels higher than the control population, which may contribute to their clinically more advanced opacity. Bron and colleagues[22] speculated that the stromal keratocytes in central crystalline corneal dystrophy are unable to properly metabolize lipids, so that local lipid deposits occur. Elevated serum lipids then further overload the cells and increase the lipid deposition. In man, the disorder is

TABLE 18-V
CORNEAL STROMAL LIPID DEPOSITS IN MAN

Type	Reference	Clinical appearance
Corneal arcus		Gray pralimbal arc with lucid interval
Normal aging > 40 years	37, 38	
Hyperlipoproteinemia II and II, < 40 years	39	
Secondary (pre-existing stromal vessels)	40	
Vascularized scar		Gray-white, random pattern, spiculated margin
Limbal mass (e.g., dermoid, nevus)		Gray arc, lucid interval
Primary (no known pre-existing corneal pathology)		
Limbal	41	D-shaped, yellow, solid, deep stromal, initially vascular
Central	42	Round, yellow, initially vascular
White ring (of Coats)	40	Small, white, round with gray dots
Central crystalline dystrophy (of Schnyder)	21–26	Central anterior ring of fine, white crystals, hazy gray background, corneal arcus
Systemic disorders		
Tangier disease (decreased C_{HDL} in serum)	43, 44	Diffuse fine gray spots
Lecithin cholesterol acyltranferase deficiency	45–47	Diffuse fine gray spots
Juvenile xanthogranuloma	48	Flat, yellow, vascularized limbal mass

From *Investigative Ophthalmology and Visual Science, 21*:95–106, 1981. Reproduced with permission.

autosomal dominant; it is unfortunate that we cannot determine the hereditary influences in our beagle colony because of the carefully planned outbreeding.[4] Oval corneal lipid opacities in beagles may be an animal model of the human corneal dystrophy of Schnyder.

The demonstration of lipids by histochemical techniques is a tedious process. The methods are not well documented. Many reagents are difficult to obtain, and only after diligent search by laboratory personnel can a meaningful battery of lipid stains be performed (Table 18-I). Even when histochemical methods demonstrate the presence and location of lipids, distinguishing among the classes of lipids is difficult.[27] Many of the reactions are nonspecific for the different types of lipid and can give false-positive and/or false-negative results. The presence of other types of compounds in the tissue may cause capricious staining. Diffusion from the sections can occur and subcellular fractionation has been found.[28] Biochemical analysis of lipids[28,29] is necessary to accurately identify and quantitate the varieties in the oval opacities; we are presently performing these studies on affected beagle corneas.

REFERENCES

1. Vai Nisi, S. J., and Goldberg, M. F.: Animal models of inherited human eye disease. In Goldberg, M. F. (Ed.): *Genetics and Metabolic Eye Disease*. Boston, Little Brown & Co., 1974, pp. 215-236.
2. Waring, G. O., Muggli, F. M., and MacMillan, A.: Oval corneal opacities in beagles. *J Am Anim Hosp Assoc, 13*:204, 1977.
3. Ekins, M. B., Waring, G. O., and Harris, R. R.: Oval lipid corneal opacities in beagles. II. Natural history over four years and study of tear function. *J Am Anim Hosp Assoc, 16*:601, 1980.
4. McKelvie, D. H., Shultz, F. T., Parcher, J. W., et al.: Random selection of beagles to maintain heterogeneity and minimize bias in a life-span experiment. *Lab Anim Care, 16*:337, 1966.
5. Goldman, M., Della Rosa, R. J., and McKelvie, D. H.: Metabolic, dosimetric and pathological consequences in skeletons of beagles fed ^{90}Sr. In Mays, C. W. (Ed.): *Delayed Effects of Bone-Seeking Radionuclides*. Salt Lake City, University of Utah Press, 1969, pp. 61-77.
6. Goldman, M., Dungworth, D. L., Bulgin, M. S., et al.: Radiation-induced neoplasms in beagles after administration of ^{90}Sr and ^{226}Ra. In *Radiation-Induced Cancer*. Vienna, International Atomic Energy Agency, 1969, pp. 345-360.
7. Luna, L. G. (Ed.): *Manual of Histologic Staining Methods of the Armed Forces Institute of Pathology*, ed. 3. New York, McGraw-Hill Book Co., Inc., 1968, pp. 4, 140-152.
8. Patsch, W., Sartor, A., and Braunsteiner, H.: An enzymatic method for the determination of the initial rate of cholesterol esterification in human plasma. *J Lipid Res, 17*:192, 1976.
9. Lipid and lipoprotein analysis. In *Manual of Laboratory Operations*. Lipid Research Clinics Program, Vol. 1. DHEW Publication (NIH) No. 75-628, 1974.
10. Fletcher, M.: A colorimetric method for estimating serum triglycerides. *Clin Chim Acta, 22*:393, 1968.
11. Feldman, G. L.: Human ocular lipids: their analysis and distribution. *Surv Ophthalmol, 12*:207, 1967.
12. Andrews, J. S.: Corneal lipids. I. Sterol and fatty acid synthesis in intact calf cornea. *Invest Ophthalmol, 5*:367, 1966.
13. Culp, T. W., Cunningham, R. D., Tucker, P. W., et al.: In vivo synthesis of lipids in rabbit iris, cornea and lens tissue. *Exp Eye Res, 9*:98, 1970.
14. Broekhuyse, R. M., and Daumen, F. G. M.: The eye. In Snyder, F. (Ed.): *Monographs in Lipid Research: Lipid Metabolism in Mammals*, ed. 2. New York, Plenum Press, 1977, pp. 145-188.
15. Andersen, A. C., and Goldman, M.: Outdoor kennel for dogs. *J Am Vet Med Assoc 137*:129, 1960.
16. Wolf, H. G., Della Rosa, R. J., and Andersen, A. C.: Nutritional management of a large experimental beagle colony. *Lab Anim Care, 16*:309, 1966.
17. Ekins, M. B., Waring, G. O., Roth, A. M., et al.: Oval corneal opacities in hypercholesterolemic beagles. *Invest Ophthalmol Vis Sci*, 18 (ARVO Suppl.):*142*, 1979.
18. Manning, P. J., Corwin, L. A., and Middleton, C. C.: Familial hyperlipoproteinemia and thyroid dysfunction of beagles. *Exp Mol Pathol, 19*:378, 1973.
19. Wada, M., Minamisono, T., Ehrhart, L. A., et al.: Familial hyperlipoproteinemia in beagles. *Life Sci, 20*:999, 1977.
20. Manning, P. J., Corwin, L. A., Jr., and Middleton, C. C.: Familial hyperlipoproteinemia and thyroid dysfunction of beagles. *Exp Mol Pathol, 19*:378, 1973.
21. Delleman, J. W., and Winkelman, J. E.: Degeneratio corneae cristallinea hereditaria.

Ophthalmologica, *155*:409, 1968.
22. Williams, H. P., Bron, A. J., and Tripathi, R. C., et al.: Hereditary crystalline corneal dystrophy with an associated lipid disorder. *Trans Ophthalmol Soc UK, 91*:531, 1971.
23. Bron, A. J., Williams, H. P., and Carruthers, M. E.: Hereditary crystalline dystrophy of Schnyder. I. Clinical features of a family with hyperlipoproteinemia. *Br J Ophthalmol,* *56*:383, 1972.
24. Garner, A., and Tripathi, R. C.: Hereditary crystalline stromal dystrophy of Schnyder. II. Histopathology and ultrastructure. *Br J Ophthalmol, 56*:400, 1972.
25. Eiferman, R. A., Rodrigues, M. M., Laibson, P. R., et al.: Schnyder's crystalline dystrophy associated with amyloid deposition. *Metab Ophthalmol, 3*:15, 1979.
26. Ghosh, M., and McCulloch, C.: Crystalline dystrophy of the cornea; a light and electron microscopic study. *Can J Ophthalmol, 12*:321, 1977.
27. Pearse, A. G. E.: *Histochemistry: Theoretical and Applied,* ed. 3. Boston, Little Brown & Co., 1968, pp. 398–446, 667–704.
28. Adams, C. W. M.: Lipid histochemistry. *Adv Lipid Res, 7*:1, 1969.
29. Baum, J. L.: Cholesterol keratopathy. *Am J Ophthalmol, 67*:372, 1969.

Chapter 19

ANIMAL MODELS OF CORNEAL VASCULARIZATION

JOSEPH A. ELIASON, M.D.

Corneal Vascularization

The growth of new blood vessels in a variety of locations and circumstances has been a topic of research interest for many years. The controlling and stimulating factors involved, as well as the physical processes of growth, are subjects that continue to pose questions. Early work focused on the patterns of vessel growth. Chambers permitting magnified observation of the process were designed for the rabbit ear and the hamster cheek pouch.[1] The chick chorioallantoic membrane was used as an implant site for testing materials and continues to be employed as a model for neovascular growth in current research studies.

The cornea has become a favored location for such studies.[2] It is naturally avascular and transparent and thus permits frequent and detailed observation. Rabbits, rats, and guinea pigs are the animals most frequently selected as experimental animal models of neovascularization. A variety of stimuli have been employed to elicit vascular growth. These have been employed to look at the propensity of the method used to produce vascularization, as well as the mechanics of the growth process itself. The methods used can be grouped into four general categories:

1. Nutritional deficiencies (e.g. riboflavin deficiency) can elicit new vessel growth.
2. The injection of a foreign protein into the stroma to produce an immunologic reaction with subsequent vascularization.
3. The use of a variety of chemical or thermal means to cause a destructive cauterization of the cornea. Alloxan and sodium hydroxide applied topically or injected into the anterior chamber are two examples.[3,4] Thermal burn has been quite useful in producing a discrete lesion that results in a localized vascular response.
4. The direct introduction of a stimulating substance. This has been accomplished by injecting a solution of a biologically active agent or placing a fragment of tissue or impregnated polymer for sustained release into the stroma.[5,6,7]

All of these methods lead to either massive or modest vascularization depending upon the type of stimulus. It has become evident that the cornea will respond with vessel growth to almost any noxious stimulus if sustained for an adequate length of time.

Useful techniques for the induction of corneal vascularization are heat cauterization and a "corneal pocket" method. The latter was first described by Gimbrone.[8] A partial thickness incision is made in the central cornea and a spatula is used to blunt dissect a lamellar pocket toward the limbus. A variety of tissue extracts (dead and living) are placed into this lamellar pocket. In addition, pellets of polymers with adsorbed substances can be placed into this lamellar pouch. The advantage of these polymers is the gradual release of substances over a sustained period of time. This is important since a substance injected intrastromally will be lost to the anterior chamber rapidly if the molecular weight is small, and the limbal vessels will not be exposed long enough for a response to occur. In comparison, the application of a discrete burn to the corneal surface is a simple and relatively reproducible way to create a limited vascularization. The temperature and the location of thermal cauterization determines the extent of corneal vascularization. The severity of the corneal vascularization is directly proportional to the area cauterized and to the proximity of the limbus.

I have developed a system in the rabbit that delivers a constant and precisely known volume of material to the corneal stroma from a point that is small in comparison to the size of the cornea.[9] In a rabbit, an osmotically driven pump (Alza Pharmaceuticals) is placed subcutaneously under the scalp where it maintains from its reservoir a constant 1 μ/hr output. A polyethylene tube runs from the pump through a subcutaneous then subconjunctival tunnel to the superior limbus. It enters the sclera, then passes into the corneal stroma where the tip is positioned at the inferior limbus. The end of the tube is drawn out to a tip diameter of 30–50 microns and placed 2.5–3 mm from the limbal vascular arcade. A single pump will operate for approximately eight days. It can then be replaced at the scalp without disturbing the corneal end of the tube, allowing continuous perfusion of selected substances for an indefinite period.

This system produces an area of stromal edema extending 1–2 mm from the tube tip without disturbing the epithelium or endothelium. If fluorescein is added to the perfusing solution the flow can be directly monitored. There is sufficient space in the scalp for two pumps to work simultaneously, one operating a control solution in one eye, the other delivering test solution to the other eye (Fig. 19-1). Since the cornea tolerates the polyethylene tube very well it can remain in place indefinitely.

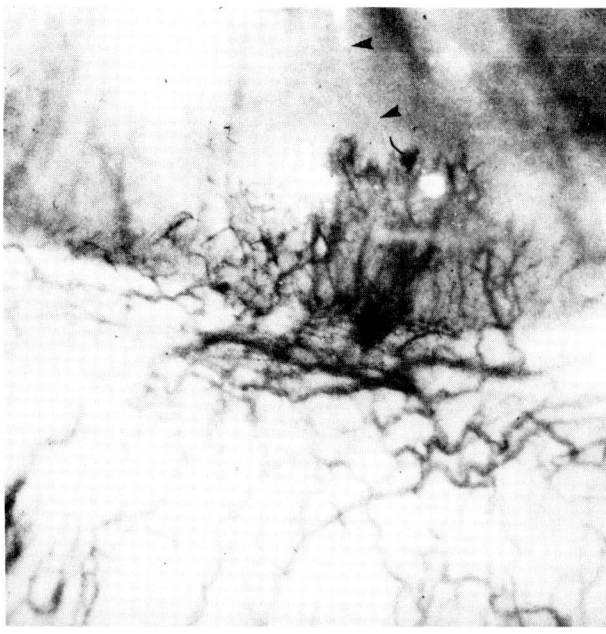

Figure 19-1: Vascularization up to an implanted polyethylene tube perfusing a homogenate of corneal epithelium. (arrows mark tube.)

Vascular Response

The vascular response to a stimulating solution follows a classic pattern. The first changes occur within hours following the application of the stimulant. Dilation and increased tortuosity of the limbal vessels are accompanied by an increased permeability to macromolecules. These changes can be documented by the injection of radioactive tracers or dyes. On an ultrastructural level the increase in permeability can be correlated with the opening of the interendothelial cell junctions. A further and more significant change during this period is the early synthesis of DNA. Tritiated thymidine is incorporated in the vascular endothelial cells as early as 24 hours following stimulation.[10]

The next period of approximately 24–48 hours is characterized by microscopic budding of the capillary endothelial cells with fine cellular processes extending into the stroma. The endothelial cells in capillary and postcapillary venous channels are the most active in these changes. Endothelial cells begin to push into the adjacent stroma while maintaining contact with the vessel wall. A lumen is soon formed within this cellular process in which blood elements are found despite the lack of an active circulation.

These vascular "sprouts" are elicited from the limbal vascular arcades in abundance commensurate with the potency of the stimulus.

At approximately 72 hours these fine sprouts are visible at slit-lamp magnifications. Adjacent ones soon connect to form a complete loop in which circulation can be established. This step is accompanied by an enlargement in the channel in which blood is flowing and a regression of nearby sprouts that have failed to link up into a loop. The process then continues by repeating the pattern starting with new sprout formation from the most advanced margin of the loop followed by linkage of sprouts into new loops.

The sprouts and loops progress toward the source of the stimulus. Once the source is reached, operating loops undergo continued enlargement and maturation, with regression of other elements until the blood circulation is established. With removal of the stimulus, regression of all vascular channels will result until only ghost vessels are left. This process involves both fragmentation of the extended cells as well as retraction into connecting vessels.[7] The rate of progression of corneal vascularization depends on the nature of the stimulus employed. The relationship between stimulus and response is complex.

Evaluation of Models of Corneal Vascularization

The use of these corneal vascularization models requires evaluation of both the nature of the stimulus and the pattern of vascular growth. It is important to recognize that conclusions reached in an animal model cannot be extrapolated to the human conditions. This is particularly true for the rabbit's cornea, which seems to undergo vascularization more readily than the human cornea.

There are many variables in corneal vascularization. Some of these can be controlled to some degree in the various models. The distance separating the stimulus and the responding vessels is critical. Campbell and Michaelson[11] showed it to be a limiting factor and Ausprunk et al.[10] noted that the tumors they implanted in the stroma need to be within 2 mm of the limbal vessels in order for vascularization to occur. With the perfusion model, I have found that vessel growth is poor when the tube tip is positioned at distances greater than 3 mm. Maurice et al.[12] have described the diffusion of a substance in the corneal stroma. They have found that up to a fairly large size the spread of a molecule through the cornea is relatively free. The distance a substance will be found in quantity from its source is determined primarily by the rate of loss across the permeable corneal endothelial cell layer. Movement from the aqueous pool back across the endothelium will produce a low but uniform level in the entire corneal stroma. Thus, the concentration profile of a substance will be determined by the dynamics of its diffusion in the stroma, and its endothelial permeability. Both this "concentration profile" as well as the starting concentration will define the maximum distance at which a stimulating threshold will be obtained. Related factors of duration and frequency of exposure of the limbal vessels to the stimulus will also affect the response. Most work has confirmed the impression that a constant or frequently repeated stimulus is necessary to sustain vessel growth.

The variety of systems that may be acting indirectly as stimuli for vascularization is another major concern. Evidence is mounting that polymorphonuclear neutrophils and possibly lymphocytes are able to produce an angiogenic stimulus.[6] The kinin system leads to dilation and increased permeability of vessels; vascularization has been reported when bradykinin was introduced into the stroma.[5] Prostaglandins have been similarly implicated.[13] Several components of the complement system (C3a C5a) are chemotactic for white blood cells and may also be chemotactic for vascular endothelial cells. Plasminogen activator has also been suggested as a vasostimulating factor.[14] Maurice and Watson have described the normal profile of albumin present in the cornea deriving from passive diffusion from the limbal vessels.[12] It is reasonable to assume that several of the serum macromolecules of diffusible size may establish their individual profiles in the peripheral stroma. Many such macromolecules have been positively identified.[15] It is also safe to assume that the various elements of the inflammatory process are readily available in the corneal stroma and may contribute to vascularization. Attempts to control such factors have been limited to efforts to produce a leucopenia with radiation and/or chemotherapeutic agents.[16,17] Efforts to modulate the inflammatory response involved in corneal vascularization is important in the healing process of many infectious diseases of the cornea caused by viruses or bacteria.

Various means have been employed to evaluate the vascular response: direct biomicroscopic determination, measurements from clinical photographs, or determinations from histologic preparations. These have been translated into terms of length of vascular invasion or growth rates. Many other methods have relied upon subjective clinical judgments. Since DNS synthesis, mitosis, and directed migration are quite rare events in normal capillary endothelium,[10] the presence of such phenomenon in an experimental situation, even to a very limited extent, may be of significance. It can be contended that vascularization is an all-or-none phenomenon and that even a modest invasion of the peripheral cornea by vessels is in a sense comparable to a much larger vascular growth several millimeters into the stroma.

The cornea will surely remain a popular site to study vascularization. This is true both for processes and substances quite foreign to the tissue, such as Tumor Angiogenic Factor and retinal derived materials, as well as native processes such as inflammatory cells, or local tissue extracts. The complex and uncontrollable factors of such animal model systems, however, will require the use of adjunctive *in vitro* methods such as vascular endothelial cell cultures in order to understand certain aspects of corneal vascularization.

REFERENCES

1. Clark, E. R., and Clark, E. L.: Microscopic observations on the growth of blood capillaries in the living mammal. *Am J Anat, 64*:251–301, 1938.
2. [For a complete list of models for corneal vascularization see] Klintworth, G. K.: The cornea—structure and macromolecules in health and disease: a review. *Am J Path, 89*:743–744, 1977.
3. Langham, M.: Observation on the growth of blood vessels into the cornea. Application of a new experimental technique. *Br J Ophthalmol, 37*:210–222, 1953.
4. Cogan, D. G.: Vascularization of the cornea. *Arch Ophthalmol, 41*:406–416, 1949.
5. Zauberman, H., Michaelson, I. C., Bergmann, F., and Maurice, D. M.: Stimulation of neovascularization of the cornea by biogenic amines. *Exp Eye Res, 8*:77–83, 1969.
6. Fromer, C. H., and Klintworth, G. K.: An evaluation of the role of leukocytes in the pathogenesis of experimentally induced corneal vascularization. *Am J Pathol, 82*:157–170, 1976.
7. Ausprunk, D. D., Flaterman, K., and Folkman, J.: The sequence of events in the regression of corneal capillaries. *Lab Invest, 38*:284–294, 1978.
8. Gimbrone, M. D., Jr., Cotran, R. S., Leapman, S. B, and Folkman, J.: Tumor growth and neovascularization: An experimental model using the rabbit cornea. *J Natl Cancer Inst, 52*:413–427.
9. Eliason, J. A., and Maurice, D. M.: An ocular perfusion system. *Invest Ophthalmol Vis Sci, 19*:102–105, 1980.
10. Ausprunk, D. H., and Folkman, J.: Migration and proliferation of endothelial cells in preformed and newly formed blood vessels during tumor angiogenesis. *Microvas Res, 14*:53–65, 1977.
11. Campbell, F. W., and Michaelson, I. C.: Blood-vessel formation in the cornea. *Br J Ophthalmol, 33*:248–255, 1949.
12. Maurice, D. M., and Watson, P. G.: The distribution and movement of serum albumin in the cornea. *Exp Eye Res, 4*:355–363, 1965.
13. BenEzra, D.: Neovasculogenesis. Triggering factors and possible mechanisms. *Surv Ophthalmol, 24*:167–176, 1979.
14. Berman, M., Winthrop, S., Ausprunk, D., Rose, J., Langer, R., and Gage, J.: Plasminogen activator causes neovascularization of the cornea. *Invest Ophthalmol Vis Sci, 20*:172a, 1981.
15. Allansmith, M. R., and McClellan, B. H.: Immunoglobulins in the human cornea. *Am J Ophthalmol, 80*:123–132, 1975.
16. Eliason, J. A.: Leukocytes and experimental corneal vascularization. *Invest Ophthalmol Vis Sci, 17*:1087–1095, 1978.
17. Sholley, M. M., Gimbrone, M. A., and Cotran, R. S.: The effects of leukocyte depletion on corneal neovascularization. *Lab Invest, 38*:32–40, 1978.

Chapter 20

TYROSINEMIA IN MINK

DAVID FUERST, M.D.

Introduction

Abnormalities of tyrosine metabolism in man include neonatal tyrosinemia, the tyrosinosis of Medes, hereditary tyrosinemia (tyrosinemia I), and the Richner-Hanhart syndrome (tyrosinemia II).[1] Hepatic tyrosine aminotransferase deficiency with resultant tyrosinemia and tyrosyluria occurs in the Richner-Hanhart syndrome,[2] a clinical triad of keratitis, hyperkeratosis of the palms and soles, and mental retardation.[3,4] Two animal models have been used to study the pathogenesis of this disease entity. Rats fed a diet high in tyrosine develop a disease resembling the Richner-Hanhart syndrome.[5] An autosomal recessive disease of mink, pseudodistemper, represents a naturally occurring disorder with an enzyme deficiency analagous to that in the human disease.[6–9]

In this chapter I will review the Richner-Hanhart syndrome and the available animal models with emphasis on ocular findings.

The Richner-Hanhart Syndrome

Tyrosinemia type II, the Richner-Hanhart syndrome, is a rare disease that is most likely inherited as an autosomal recessive trait.[2] The complete syndrome is characterized by dendritiform corneal opacities, hyperkeratotic lesions of the distal extremities, and mental retardation.[2–4] The classical syndrome typically begins in the first few months of life with ocular symptoms of tearing, redness, and photophobia. Ophthalmological examination most commonly demonstrates a dendritiform type of keratitis varying from mild epithelial involvement to geographic corneal ulcers associated with stromal clouding.[10–17] Other ocular findings are nystagmus,[10,18] strabismus,[10,11] cataract,[10,19] and thickening of the conjunctiva.[12]

Histopathologic examination of ocular tissues from patients with the Richner-Hanhart syndrome has been limited to a conjunctival biopsy[15] and corneal scrapings.[10,11] The conjunctival biopsy revealed thickened epithelium, keratofibrils in the cytoplasm of basal epithelium, plasma cell infiltration of the subepithelial connective tissue, and inclusion bodies. Some of the inclusion bodies seen in fibrocytes contained fine, needlelike crystalline material.

Corneal scrapings in a different patient[11] disclosed hyperplastic, stratified squamous epithelium infiltrated with occasional polymorphonuclear leukocytes.

The skin lesions in the Richner-Hanhart syndrome are usually seen within one year of birth, with hyperkeratotic papules and lamellar peeling limited to the palms and soles.[2,20,21] These areas are quite painful and occasionally prevent the affected person from walking. Histopathologic examination of the affected skin demonstrates nonspecific findings of acanthosis, parakeratosis, a thickened granular layer, and hyperkeratotis.[2,16,20]

Mental retardation in this disease varies from mild to severe and has been found in most of the reported cases.[10-13,15,18-24]

The complete syndrome of dendritiform keratitis, hyperkeratosis *palmaris et plantaris*, and mental retardation is not seen in all patients with tyrosinemia II. Individuals without eye involvement,[21] without skin findings[10,18] and some with normal intelligence[14,16,17] have been reported. One case of tyrosinemia in a mentally retarded girl without keratitis or dermatologic findings has been reported.[19] Less frequently reported signs associated with tyrosinemia II include seizures,[18,19,25] vertical striations seen on radiologic examination of the distal femur,[11] and multiple congenital anomalies (microcephaly, cleft lip and palate, inguinal hernias, talipes equinovarus, and absence of one kidney).[10]

Tyrosinemia without hepatorenal disease is necessary for the diagnosis of the Richner-Hanhart syndrome; reported serum tyrosine has ranged from about 2.5 to 25 times the normal level.[10-22,24] Urinary tyrosine is also markedly increased, and tyrosine metabolites including *p*-hydroxyphenylpyruvic acid (pHPPA), *p*-hydroxyphenyllactic acid (pHPLA), *p*-hydroxyphenylacetic acid (pHPAA), *n*-acetyl tyrosine, and *p*-tyramine are found in increased concentration in the urine.[2]

Tyrosine aminotransferase (TAT), EC 2.6.1.5, is the enzyme that catalyzes the first step in the metabolism of tyrosine. It is an inducible, cytoplasmic enzyme found most concentrated in liver. TAT converts tyrosine to pHPPA, which is probably the rate-limiting step in the catabolism of tyrosine.[1] TAT activity has been analyzed in the liver biopsies from three patients with the Richner-Hanhart syndrome. In two patients, no soluble TAT activity was detected,[10,22,24] whereas the third patient had detectable but somewhat lower than normal TAT activity.[23] All patients had normal or elevated mitochondrial aspartate aminotransferase, which can also metabolize tyrosine to pHPPA. Normal mitochondria cannot oxidize pHPPA because they lack pHPPA oxidase. The pHPPA that accumulates can be transported to the cytosol and may inhibit cytoplasmic pHPPA oxidase. This presumably accounts for the unusual finding of elevated metabolites both before (tyrosine) and after (pHPPA, pHPLA, pHPAA) the abnormal enzyme (TAT) in the tyrosine pathway.[1,26,27]

The treatment of the Richner-Hanhart syndrome consists of dietary restriction of tyrosine and phenylalanine. The serum tyrosine levels fall rapidly towards the normal range, and the skin and corneal lesions resolve in a few days to several months. Attempts at treatment with corticosteroids, pyridoxine, or ascorbate have been unsuccessful.[16,24]

Tyrosinemia II is thought to be an autosomal recessive condition because several patient families had definite histories of consanguinity.[11,12,15,16] Additionally, most families have had only one child with the disease. One family with consanguineous marriages in three generations had four affected children in a sibship of ten.[21] Attempts at identifying heterozygotes have been unsuccessful. Tyrosine levels in the serum of parents of affected individuals are normal, even after dietary loading with tyrosine.[2]

It is not known why the findings in tyrosinemia II are localized in the eyes, the skin of the extremities, and the central nervous system. It seems most likely that tyrosine has a predilection for crystallizing in these areas, and thereby causes cellular damage.[28] Tyrosine crystals are known lysosome labilizers and could mediate inflammation by this mechanism.[29]

Other Syndromes of Tyrosinemia in Humans

Several other abnormalities of tyrosine metabolism are known to exist in humans. A single case of *p*-hydroxyphenylpyruvic aciduria in a man with myasthenia gravis was reported by Medes,[30] who named this condition "tyrosinosis." Blood tyrosine levels were not determined, and no further cases have been identified. Neonatal tyrosinemia[1] is a common condition that can affect both premature and full-term infants. A deficiency of pHPPA oxidase and a relative deficiency of ascorbic acid (vitamin C) cause tyrosinemia and tyrosyluria. Neonatal tyrosinemia is treated with ascorbic acid and by reducing protein intake for the first few weeks of life. The condition is transient and is not associated with eye or skin involvement, but impaired mental development has been reported in some cases.

Hereditary tyrosinemia (tyrosinemia type I)[1] is transmitted in an autosomal recessive fashion, and usually becomes manifest during the first few months of life. Failure to thrive, vomiting, diarrhea, hepatosplenomegaly, edema, and rickets are seen, and death during the first year is common. Laboratory findings include tyrosinemia, hypermethioninemia, elevated serum pHPPA, tyrosyluria, a generalized amino aciduria, hyperphosphaturia, and increased urinary 5-aminolevulinic acid. The activity of pHPPA ozidase has been found to be severely depressed, but it is not known whether this enzyme deficiency is primary or secondary to the hepatic damage that occurs in hereditary tyrosinemia.

Tyrosinemia in the Rat

An animal model of tyrosinemia has been described in white rats fed a diet high in tyrosine.[5] The characteristic syndrome consists of keratoconjunctivitis, alopecia, cheilitis, brown urine, hyperkeratosis, and inflammation of the toes. There is loss of weight, and life span is shortened. Histopathologic changes in the corneas of tyrosine-fed rats have been studied.[31-34] Corneal epithelial edema develops within 24 hours after starting the high tyrosine diet, and progresses to form "snowflake" opacities. Epithelial lesions, as seen with an electron microscope, demonstrate needle-shaped birefringent crystals that disrupt cellular and nuclear membranes.[34] The crystals have not been biochemically identified, but it seems likely that they are tyrosine. Polymorphonuclear leukocytes invade the anterior corneal stroma and later form endothelial keratic precipitates. Blood vessels grow in from the limbus as the cornea becomes thickened and opaque. Despite the continued dietary tyrosine loading, the corneas generally clear spontaneously within three weeks, probably because of the induction of hepatic tyrosine aminotransferase.[2,32]

Dermatologic lesions in the tyrosinemic rat are found on the bottom of the feet only. Erosions lead to crusting and hyperkeratosis with separation of the nails. Histopathologic examination demonstrates areas of intense polymorphonuclear leukocyte infiltration in the epidermis.[2] The concentration of tyrosine and its metabolites is not increased in affected areas as compared with noninvolved skin.

The findings in the rat tyrosinemia model are similar to the human syndrome of tyrosinemia II, with changes involving the corneas and feet. Disadvantages of this model include the greater amount of inflammation in the rat, and the resolution of disease with continued tyrosine feeding.

Tyrosinemia in Mink

Tyrosinemia in mink has been seen by mink ranchers in the United States and Denmark.[6-9] It occurs in the standard dark mink *Mustela vison*. The syndrome was named "pseudodistemper" because the signs are similar to those seen in canine distemper virus infection in mink.

The mink kits with pseudodistemper appear healthy until about six weeks of age. The first signs are watery eyes and diffuse corneal clouding. A mucoid or seropurulent conjunctivitis occurs together with matting of the eyelids. The foot pads and nose become reddened, and soon there is a necrotizing dermatitis of the feet, nose, and ears. Other signs include a pointed appearance to the face, a soaked abdominal haircoat, and an oily appearance to neck bite wounds (minor bite wounds are not unusual in mink kits).[6] The disease results in the death of all affected kits within two weeks of the onset of clinical disease. The fulminating course of the disease has been attributed to the high protein diet that the kits start eating about one week prior to the onset of clinical signs.[9] Pseudodistemper of mink is inherited in an autosomal recessive pattern. A study of 25 litters in Denmark[7] demonstrated slight inbreeding, a normal sex ratio, and normal litters produced by the parents of affected kits when they were test mated to nonrelated partners.

Affected mink have been shown to have high blood tyrosine levels as well as increased plasma urea and creatinine. Tyrosine concentration in plasma is about 25–90 times higher than the normal range.[7] Hepatic tyrosine aminotransferase activity is significantly decreased with an associated increase in hepatic mitochondrial aspartate aminotransferase.[8] The residual apparent tyrosine aminotransferase activity is not inhibited by an antibody to rat TAT, known to inhibit normal mink liver TAT. This suggests that there is no true TAT activity in the tyrosinemic mink, or that a mutant TAT enzyme exists that does not react with this antibody.[8]

Histopathologic examination of tyrosinemic mink tissue has been performed by Christensen et al.[7] Changes in both eyelid and toe skin include patchy acantholysis, epidermal necrosis, formation of micropustules, sloughing of epithelium, and inflammatory changes in the corium. A fibrinous conjunctivitis with superficial neutrophilic infiltration is present. The kidneys demonstrate superficial necrotic areas accompanied by an acute inflammatory infiltrate as well as a homogeneous material in discrete perivascular or interstitial areas. The corneal findings were not reported.

Tyrosinemia in the mink is thus analagous to tyrosinemia type II in humans, both in its underlying biochemical abnormality and in its clinical expression (Table 20-I). Ocular and dermatologic involvement occurs in both species, associated with a deficiency in hepatic TAT and high blood tyrosine levels. The only noteworthy difference between the human and mink disease is the finding of mental retardation in most affected children and the uniformly fatal outcome in kits. Although this difference has been attributed to the availability of a low tyrosine, low phenylalanine diet for affected children, mink fed a controlled artificial diet do not do as well.[9]

The availability of this naturally occurring animal model of tyrosinemia II in man will allow studies of the underlying metabolic defect, histopathology, and heterozygote identification. Disadvantages of the mink tyrosinemia II model include the early death of affected kits, the inability to identify the carrier state, and infrequent breeding. (Mink breed only once each year for two or three years.)[35]

TABLE 20-I

COMPARISON OF MINK TYROSINEMIA AND HUMAN TYROSINEMIA II

	Mink	Human
Keratoconjunctivitis	+	+
Dermatopathy	+	+
Early death	+	
Mental retardation		+
Elevated serum tyrosine	+	+
Hepatic tyrosine aminotransferase deficiency	+	+

Summary

Tyrosinemia II in humans occurs in individuals who have a deficiency of hepatic tyrosine aminotransferase. Pseudodendritic keratitis, hyperkeratosis of the palms and soles, and mental retardation are seen along with an elevated serum tyrosine level. A disease that resembles tyrosinemia II may be produced in rats fed a diet high in tyrosine. A more relevant animal model of tyrosinemia II occurs in the mink; the affected animals have a deficiency of hepatic tyrosine aminotransferase, elevated serum tyrosine levels, and clinical findings similar to those seen in the Richner-Hanhart syndrome.

REFERENCES

1. Scriver, C. R., and Rosenberg, L. E.: *Amino Acid Metabolism and Its Disorders.* Philadelphia, Saunders, 1973, pp. 338–369.
2. Goldsmith, L. A.: Molecular biology and molecular pathology of a newly described molecular disease-Tyrosinemia II (The Richner-Hanhart Syndrome). *Expl Cell Biol,* 46:96–113, 1978.
3. Richner, H.: Hornhautaffektion bei keratoma palmare et plantare hereditarium. *Klin Monatsbl Augenheilkd,* 100:580–588, 1938.
4. Hanhart, E.: Neue sonderformen von keratosis palmo-plantaris, u.a. eine regelmassig-dominante mit systematisierten lipomen, ferner 2 einfach-rezessive mit schwachsinn und Z.T. mit hornhaut-Veranderungen des auges (ektodermalsyndrom). *Dermatologica,* 94:286–308, 1947.
5. Schweizer, W.: Studies on the effect of *l*-tyrosine on the white rat. *J Physiol,* 106:167–176, 1947.
6. Schwartz, T. M., and Shackelford, R. M.: Pseudodistemper is apparently new ailment of mink. *US Fur Rancher,* 52:6, 1973.
7. Christensen, K., Fischer, P., Knudsen, K. E. B., et al.: A syndrome of hereditary tyrosinemia in mink (*Mustela vison* Schreb.). *Can J Comp Med,* 43:333–340, 1979.
8. Goldsmith, L. A., Thorpe, J. M., and Marsh, R. F.: Tyrosine amino-transferase deficiency in mink (*Mustela vison*): A model for human tyrosinemia II. *Biochem Genet,* 19:687–693, 1981.

9. Marsh, R. F., and Goldsmith, L. A.: Tyrosinemia II, Model number 231. In C. C. Capen, D. B. Hackel, T. C. Jones, G. Migaki, (Eds.): *Handbook: Animal Models of Human Disease. Fasc. 10. Registry of Comparative Pathology.* Armed Forces Institute of Pathology, Washington, D.C., 1981.
10. Burns, R. P.: Soluble tyrosine aminotransferase deficiency: an unusual cause of corneal ulcers. *Am J Ophthalmol, 73*:400–402, 1972.
11. Zaleski, W. A., Hill, A., and Murray, R. G.: Corneal erosions in tyrosinosis. *Can J Ophthalmol, 8*:556–559, 1973.
12. Goldsmith, L. A., Kang, E., Bienfang, D. C., et al.: Tyrosinemia with plantar and palmar keratosis and keratitis. *J Pediatr, 83*:798–805, 1973.
13. Billson, F. A., and Danks, D. M.: Corneal and skin changes in Tyrosinaemia. *Aust J Ophthalmol, 3*:112–115, 1975.
14. Sandberg, H. O.: Bilateral keratopathy and tyrosinosis. *Acta Ophthalmologica, 53*:760–764, 1975.
15. Bienfang, D. C., Kuwabara, T., and Pueschel, S. M.: The Richner-Hanhart syndrome. Report of a case with associated tyrosinemia. *Arch Ophthalmol, 94*:1133–1137, 1976.
16. Goldsmith, L. A., and Reed, J.: Tyrosine-induced eye and skin lesions. A treatable genetic disease. *JAMA, 236*:382–384, 1976.
17. Charlton, K. H., Binder, P. S., Wozniak, L., et al.: Pseudodendritic keratitis and systemic tyrosinemia. *Ophthalmology, 88*:355–360, 1981.
18. Holston, J. L., Levy, H. L., Tomlin, G. A., et al.: Tyrosinosis: A patient without liver or renal disease. *Pediatrics, 48*:393–400, 1971.
19. Wadman, S. K., Van Sprang, F. J., Maas, J. W., et al.: An exceptional case of tyrosinosis. *J Ment Defic Res, 12*:269–281, 1968.
20. Zaleski, W. A., Hill, A., and Kushniruk, W.: Skin lesions in tyrosinosis: response to dietary treatment. *Br J Dermatol, 88*:335–340, 1973.
21. Rehak, A., Selim, M. M., and Yadav, G.: Richner-Hanhart syndrome (tyrosinemia-II) (report of four cases without ocular involvement). *Br J Dermatol, 104*:469–475, 1981.
22. Lemonnier, F., Charpentier, C., Odievre, M., et al.: Tyrosine aminotransferase isoenzyme deficiency. *J Pediatr, 94*:931–932, 1979.
23. Goldsmith, L. A., Thorpe, J., and Roe, C. R.: Hepatic enzymes of tyrosine metabolism in tyrosinemia II. *J Invest Dermatol, 73*:530–532, 1979.
24. Kennaway, N. G., and Buist, N. R. M.: Metabolic studies in a patient with hepatic cytosol tyrosine aminotransferase deficiency. *Pediatr Res, 5*:287–297, 1971.
25. deGroot, G. W., Dakshinamurti, K., Allan, L., et al.: Defect in soluble tyrosine aminotransferase in skin fibroblasts of a patient with tyrosinemia. *Pediatr Res, 14*:896–898, 1980.
26. Fellman, J. H., Vanbellinghen, P. J., Jones, R. T., et al.: Soluble and mitochondrial forms of tyrosine aminotransferase. Relationship to human tyrosinemia. *Biochemistry, 8*:615–622, 1969.
27. La Du, B. N., and Zannoni, V. G.: The tyrosine oxidation system of liver. II. Oxidation of p-hydroxyphenylpyruvic acid to homogentisic acid. *J Biol Chem, 217*:777–787, 1955.
28. Goldsmith, L. A.: Haemolysis induced by tyrosine crystals. Modifiers and inhibitors. *Biochem J, 158*:17–22, 1976.
29. Goldsmith, L. A.: Hemolysis and lysosomal activation by solid state tyrosine. *Biochem Biophys Res Comm, 64*:558–565, 1975.
30. Medes, G.: A new error of tyrosine metabolism: tyrosinosis. The intermediary metabolism of tyrosine and phenylalanine. *Biochem J, 26*:917–940, 1932.

31. Rich, L. F., Beard, M. E., and Burns, R. P.: Excess dietary tyrosine and corneal lesions. *Exp Eye Res, 17*:87–97, 1973.
32. Burns, R. P., Beard, M. E., Weimar, V. L., et al.: Modification of tyrosine-induced keratopathy by adrenal corticosteroids. *Invest Ophthalmol, 13*:39–45, 1974.
33. Beard, M. E., Burns, R. P., Rich, L. F., et al.: Histopathology of keratopathy in the tyrosine-fed rat. *Invest Ophthalmol, 13*:1037–1041, 1974.
34. Gipson, I. K., Burns, R. P., and Wolfe-Lande, J. D.: Crystals in corneal epithelial lesions of tyrosine-fed rats. *Invest Ophthalmol, 14*:937–941, 1975.
35. Marsh, R. F.: Personal communication, July, 1982.

Chapter 21

TAURINE DEFICIENCY IN CATS

LEIGH WEST-HYDE, V.M.D.

Introduction

Taurine is a unique sulfonic amino acid that cannot be incorporated into peptides or proteins and thus remains free within cells and tissues. It is found in high concentrations in meat, seafood, and milk, but is essentially absent in vegetable.[1] Taurine is synthesized in mammals by the conversion of the essential amino acid, methionine, to cysteine and finally to taurine during normal amino acid metabolism. Although its conjugation with bile acids in the liver is well known,[2] taurine has many other postulated functions.[3-6] These include (1) anti-seizure activity in the brain, (2) regulation of membrane excitability in the heart, (3) neuromodulation in the brain and retina, (4) various endocrine and reproductive functions, (5) essential dietary constituent for humans and cats, especially during growth, and (6) key agent in maintaining structural integrity of retina and tapetum in the cat.[7-10]

The cat requires dietary taurine because endogenous taurine biosynthesis is inadequate to meet demands for bile acid conjugation and tissue metabolism, especially those of the muscle and central nervous system.[11,12] In all species studied, including the cat, taurine is the predominant free amino acid in the retina with the highest concentrations (40–80 nM) in the outer nuclear layer where photoreceptor cell soma and Müller cell processes are located.[13] The maintenance of adequate taurine concentrations in the retina is essential for the normal structure and function of photoreceptor cells. Deficiency of dietary taurine in cats results in (1) the progressive decrease of taurine concentrations in tissues, (2) reductions in cone and rod amplitude and delays in the temporal aspects of the cone response of the electroretinogram (ERG), (3) the degeneration of the photoreceptors and tapetum lucidum resulting in eventual blindness, and (4) insufficient growth in the newborn kitten.[9,14-20] These findings demonstrate that the cat can be used as a model for studying the role of taurine in the retina and for investigating a slowly developing and ultimately subtle deficiency in the human infant.

Experimental Production of Retinal Degeneration

The experimental feeding of purified casein (taurine-free) diets to cats results in photoreceptor cell malfunction when there is a 20–50 percent reduction in retinal taurine concentration. Photoreceptor cell death occurs when retinal taurine concentrations exceed 50 percent reductions.[16,21]

Biochemical changes

Pronounced reductions (>50% below normal) in retinal taurine and decreases in rod and cone ERG amplitudes can occur as early as 10 weeks or as late as 45 weeks after feeding cats taurine-free diets. Pronounced reductions in retinal taurine concentrations occur only when liver and plasma concentrations of taurine are near zero. The time required to produce significant reductions of retinal taurine varies. This is partially explained because taurine is stored in varying amounts in the bodies of cats before they began receiving taurine-free diets.[21] Taurine-free casein diets supplemented with inorganic sulfate, vitamin B_6, or taurine precursors (methionine or cysteine) fail to prevent taurine deficiency in cats.[21,22] Neither the source of dietary lipid (animal or vegetable) nor the source of protein (soy or casein or tuna) affected plasma taurine in cats on taurine deficient diets; however, below 1.55 percent total sulfur amino acids, the taurine requirement of the cat appears to be a function of the sulfur amino acid content of the diet.[23] Only cats given taurine in the diet retained normal ERG function and normal plasma and retinal taurine concentrations.

Electroretinography

In taurine-deficient cats, reductions in retinal taurine concentrations have been linearly related to reductions in ERG amplitudes even before photoreceptor cell death. The initial change in the ERG is a delay in the cone ERG b-wave implicit time. This delay could be detected by five weeks when there is a selective decrease in plasma (4% of normal) and retinal (60% of normal) taurine levels. By ten weeks on the taurine deficient diet, the cats' ERGs showed reduced cone and rod ERG amplitudes. At ten weeks the taurine levels were 2–4 percent of normal in plasma and 20–30 percent of normal in retina. During this period, retinal DNA content (as a measure of cell viability) and fundus appearance were normal. By 23 weeks, ERGs were nondetectable, retinal DNA content was reduced, and the fundus showed typical changes in the area centralis.[16,21,22] The early receptor potential (ERP) was at first normal in amplitude when the a-wave and b-wave of the ERG were substantially reduced or even nondetectable.[24] The preserved ERP in these taurine-deficient cats in the early stages can be correlated with the histologic finding that their outer segments are relatively intact over 90 percent of the retinal area subtended by the test flash. In taurine-deficient cats, the reductions in the peak-to-peak ERG amplitudes are closely correlated with the reductions in retinal taurine concentration; this suggests that taurine deficiency may have some effect on the fluxes of Na+ and K+, involved in the generation of the ERG a- and b-waves.[25] In addition to Na+ and K+, taurine may also affect the distribution of calcium (CA^{2+}) in the outer segments of photoreceptor cells.

Ophthalmoscopy

Schmidt et al.[26] report that the first ophthalmoscopic evidence of taurine deficiency in cats is detectable within 15–23 weeks after beginning a taurine-deficient diet; however, some workers report longer periods, up to six to seven months, before fundic lesions are visible. Others report no fundic lesions despite the longevity of taurine deficiency.[20,23,27] These variations may reflect a different dietary composition and a difference in the age of animals tested. Fundic changes, when present, are typically bilateral and symmetrical. Changes begin in the area centralis which, in the cat, is temporal to the optic disk and located in the region of the tapetum lucidum devoid of any of the main retinal blood vessels. An abnormal granularity associated with a central, white highly reflective spot is first seen in the area centralis. Between 23 and 72 weeks, the lesion occupies an oval zone in the area centralis bordered by a narrow pattern of the lesion, which corresponds to the zone of highest cone density in the cat retina. The lesion becomes larger and, ultimately, the whole fundus becomes affected with a generalized retinal degeneration and an attenuation of the retinal blood vessels. Blindness eventually results.

Pathology

Although there are pronounced biochemical and functional changes within 15 weeks of initiation of a taurine-free diet, no changes in the photoreceptor cells are detectable with the electron microscope, and retinal DNA and protein content remain normal. Thus, photoreceptor function is altered by retinal taurine deficiency at least ten weeks before photoreceptor cell death. After 23 weeks on the taurine-free diets, the cats show obvious fundic lesions, and there is a significant decrease in retinal DNA concentration and an increase in retinal protein concentration. The retinal degeneration at first involves the outer segments of photoreceptors in the area centralis and progresses peripherally. Electron microscopy shows cone and rod outer segment lamellar discs that are vesiculated, frayed, disoriented, and twisted. The shortening and disappearance of outer segments is followed by the loss of photoreceptor nuclei, primarily in the area centralis but also in the midperipheral retina. Photoreceptor damage is most severe in the area centralis, even though reductions of retinal taurine in central and peripheral retina are similar. By 72 weeks on the deficient diet, the entire photoreceptor cell degenerates and disappears.[15-1,26–28] When dietary casein was replaced by egg albumin in the diets of cats with minimal to moderately advanced degeneration, the degeneration was reversed; rod ERG function and structure returned almost to normal, whereas some abnormalities of the outer segment of cone structure and a delay in the temporal aspects of the cone ERG persisted.[17]

The tapetum lucidum of the cat is a unique type of cell derived from modified choroidal cells. It consists of cellular layers parallel to the surface of the retina between the lamina capillaris and the lamina vasculosa of the choroid.[29] The regular array of the tapetal rods within these cells reflects light back through the retina and thus maximizes retinal sensitivity in situations where light is low. Recent studies on long term (18 month) maintenance of cats on taurine-free diets showed severe disorganization of the lattice arrangement of tapetal rods. High resolution electron microscopy of ultra-thin sections showed that cats depleted of taurine exhibit disruption and disorganization of this membrane. This is probably the first stage of more severe tapetal degeneration. In addition, taurine and zinc localized on the periphery of the tapetal rods were greatly reduced in taurine-depleted cats. Other tapetal changes included reduction in tapetal size (i.e., half the normal surface area) and a reduction of the layers of tapetal cells from 14–16 to 2–3 layers.[18,19]

Application to Human Disease

These studies in the cat establish a biological role for taurine in maintaining photoreceptor viability. The delay in the cone ERG b-wave in the taurine-deficient cat is similar to that seen in the cone ERGs of many patients in the early stages of retinitis pigmentosa.[30] The structural abnormalities of photoreceptors seen in the taurine-deficient cat have also been observed in the cones of a patient with advanced, dominantly inherited retinitis pigmentosa.[26] Although amino acid analyses of plasma from patients with different types of hereditary retinal degenerations did not reveal any significant taurine depression, this does not preclude the possibility that a defect in taurine uptake and/or incorporation into photoreceptors may exist in the retinas of these patients.[31] The taurine-deficient cat provides an excellent, reproducible model for investigating the mechanism of photoreceptor cell malfunction, degeneration, and regeneration.

Another area of interest is the role of taurine in nutrition and growth, especially in human infants. Babies are unable to synthesize adequate amounts of taurine and are dependent on dietary resources of turine.[32] In human and cat milk, taurine comprises over 20 percent of the total free amino acid pool, whereas cow's milk contains almost no taurine. This shows the varying ability of each species to synthesize taurine *de novo*.[33] The widespread use of cow's milk in human infant formulas opens up the very real possibility of taurine deficiency in infants. The growing kitten and adult cat provide an excellent model for the study of the subtle effects of neonatal taurine deficiency on growth and development and on learning behavior.

REFERENCES

1. Roe, D. A., and Weston, M. O.: Potential significance of free taurine in the diet. *Nature, 205*:287–288, 1965.
2. Vessey, D. A.: The biochemical basis for the conjugation of bile acids with either glycine or taurine. *Biochem J, 174*:621–626, 1978.
3. Huxtable, R., and Barbean, A. (Eds.): *Taurine*. Raven Press, New York, 1976.
4. Barbeau, A., and Huxtable, R. (Eds.): *Taurine and Neurological Disorders*. Raven Press, New York, 1978.
5. Huxtable, R. J., and Pasantes-Morales, H. (Eds.): *Taurine in Nutrition and Neurology*. Plenum Press, New York and London, 1982.
6. Schaffer, S. W., Baskin, S. I., and Kocsis, J. J. (Eds.): *The Effects of Taurine on Excitable Tissues*. New York, SP Medical & Scientific Books, Spectrum Publications, Inc., 1981.
7. Hayes, K. D.: A review on the biological function of taurine. *Nutr Rev, 34*:161–165, 1976.
8. Sturman, J. A., Rassin, D. K., and Gaull, G. E.: Mini review: Taurine in development. *Life Sci, 21*:1–22, 1977.
9. Hayes, K. C.: Nutritional problems in cats: Taurine deficiency and vitamin A excess. *Can Vet J, 23*:2–5, 1982.
10. Huxtable, R. J.: Taurine: Epilepsy, inotropy and eyesight. *Trends Pharmacol Sci, 3*:21–25, 1982.
11. Knopf, K., Sturman, J. A., Armstrong, M., and Hayes, K. C.: Taurine: An essential nutrient for the cat. *J Nutr, 108*:773–778, 1978.
12. Rabin, B., Nicolosi, R. J., and Hayes, K. C.: Dietary influence on bile acid conjugation in the cat. *J Nutr, 106*:1241–1246, 1976.
13. Orr, H. T., Cohen, A. I., and Lowry, O. H.: The distribution of taurine in the vertebrate retina. *J Neurochem, 26*:609–611, 1976.
14. Anderson, P. A., Baker, D. H., Corbin, J. E., and Helper, L. C.: Biochemical lesions associated with taurine deficiency in the cat. *J Anim Sci, 49*:1227–1234, 1979.
15. Hayes, K. C., and Carey, R. E.: Retinal degeneration associated with taurine deficiency in the cat. *Science, 188*:949–951, 1975.
16. Schmidt, S. Y., Berson, E. L., and Hayes, K. C.: Retinal degeneration in cats fed casein. I. Taurine deficiency. *Invest Ophthalmol Vis Sci, 15*:47–52, 1976.
17. Hayes, K. C., Rabin, A. R., and Berson, E. L.: An ultrastructural study of nutritionally induced and reversed retinal degeneration in cats. *Am J Pathol, 78*:505–524, 1975.
18. Wen, G. Y., Sturman, J. A., Wisniewski, H. M., Lidsky, A. A., Corwall, A. C., and Hayes, K. C.: Tapetum disorganization in taurine-depleted cats. *Invest Ophthalmol Vis Sci, 18*:1201–1206, 1979.
19. Sturman, J. A., Wen, G. Y., Wisniewski, H. M., and Hayes, K. C.: Histochemical localization of zinc in the feline tapetum—effect of taurine depletion. *Histochemistry, 72*:341–350, 1981.
20. Aquirre, G. D.: Retinal degeneration associated with the feeding of dog food to cats. *J Am Vet Med Assoc, 172*:791–796, 1978.
21. Schmidt, S. Y., Berson, E. L., Watson, G., and Huang, C.: Retinal degeneration in cats fed casein. III. Taurine deficiency and ERG amplitures. *Invest Ophthalmol Vis Sci, 16*:673–678, 1977.

22. Berson, E. L., Hayes, K. C., Rabin, A. R., and Schmidt, S. Y.: Retinal degeneration in cats fed casein. II. Supplementation with methionine, cysteine, or taurine. *Invest Ophthalmol Vis Sci, 15*:52–58, 1976.
23. O'Donnell, J. A., Rogers, Q. R., and Morris, J. G.: Effect of diet on plasma taurine in the cat. *J Nutr, 111*:1111–1116, 1981.
24. Berson, E. L., Watson, G., Grasse, K. L., and Szamier, R. B.: Retinal degeneration in cats fed caseine. IV. The early receptor potential. *Invest Ophthalmol Vis Sci, 21*:345–350, 1981.
25. Schmidt, S. Y.: Biochemical and functional abnormalities in retinas of taurine-deficient cat (lecture). *Fed Proc, 39*:2706–2708, 1980.
26. Schmidt, K. C., Berson, E. L., and Hayes, K. C.: Retinal degeneration in the taurine-deficient cat. *Trans Am Acad Ophthalmol, 81*-687–693, 1976.
27. Barnett, K. C., and Burger, I. H.: Taurine deficiency retinopathy in the cat. *J Small Anim Pract, 21*:521–534, 1980.
28. Rabin, A. R., Hayes, K. C., and Berson, E. L.: Cone and rod responses in nutritionally induced retinal degeneration in the cat. *Invest Ophthalmol Vis Sci, 12*:694–704, 1973.
29. Vogel, M.: Postnatal development of the cats retina. *Adv Anat Embryol Cell Biol, 54*:1–64, 1978.
30. Berson, E. L.: Retinitis pigmentosa and allied retinal diseases: Electrophysiologic findings. *Trans Am Acad Ophthalmol, 76*:659–666, 1976.
31. Berson, E. L., Schmidt, S. Y., and Rabin, A. R.: Plasma amino acids in hereditary retinal disease. Orithine, lysine and taurine. *Br J Ophthalmol, 60*:142–147, 1976.
32. Rigo, J., and Senterre, J.: Is taurine essential for the neonates? *Biol Neonate, 32*:73–76, 1977.
33. Rassin, D. K., Sutrman, J. A., and Gaull, G. E.: Taurine and other free amino acids in milk of man and other mammals. *Early Hum Dev, 211*:1–13, 1978.

Chapter 22

ANIMAL MODELS OF BAND KERATOPATHY

J. Fraser Muirhead, M.D., F.R.C.S.(C); Laura Tomazzoli-Gerosa, M.D.

Introduction

Band keratopathy (Band KP) is a subepithelial corneal calcification that may occur from local ocular disease or systemic abnormalities of calcium and phosphate metabolism. Several animal models of Band KP resemble the human disease in their clinical appearance, histochemical findings, and electron microscopic changes. We shall discuss animal models of Band KP and describe the pathogenesis of this disease.

Human Band Keratopathy

Although Beers' and Demours' early nineteenth century atlases contain drawings that closely resemble Band KP, the disease was not described until 1849 when Bowman[1] published Dixon's case along with a chemical analysis of corneal scrapings. The illustrations of Demours, Beers, and Bowman clearly show the clinical picture of established disease: interpalpebral location of the deposits with sparing of the juxtalimbal area. Other notable features include the appearance of the earliest deposits near the limbus and clear spaces around corneal nerves.

Histochemical studies show calcium deposited just under the epithelium in the basement membrane and in Bowman's membrane, in close proximity to the epithelium. Electron microscopy shows needlelike electron-dense material ("spicules") arranged in "granules" or "spherules" (Fig. 22-1).[2,3,4] Spherules are at first more dense at the periphery but the density later increases centrally. They appear first along the epithelial basal lamina, frequently abutting onto the plasma membrane of the basal cells. They occasionally appear to be traversed by collagen fibrils. Later they fuse into masses forming "conglomerates," which may be found in the superficial corneal stroma. X-ray diffraction of the material shows a pattern compatible with hydroxyapatite[5] (Fig. 22-2).

Animal Models of Band Keratopathy: Classification

Experimental band keratopathy may be grouped by method of induction: (1) those associated with altered vitamin D metabolism, either an excess or

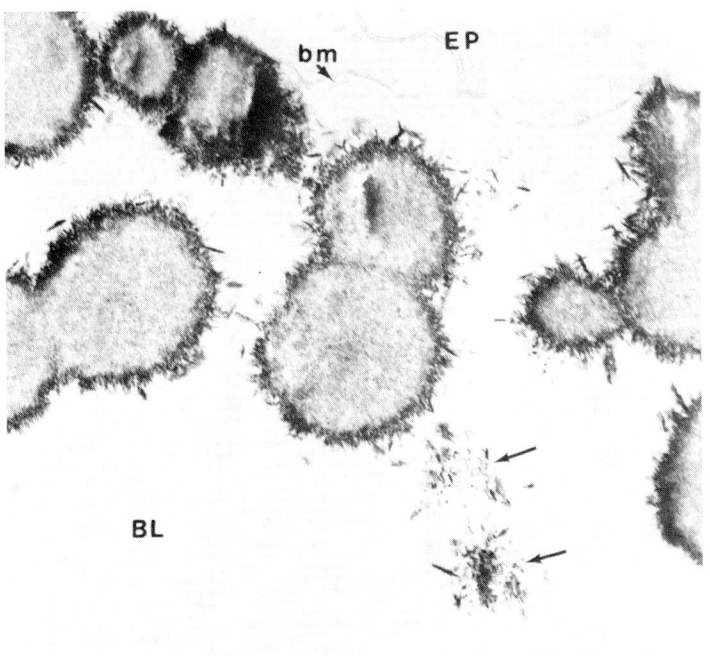

Figure 22-1. Calcific spherules in Bowman's layer (BL) next to basalepithelial cells (EP). (×13,000). Published with permission from *The American Journal of Ophthalmology* 82:395–404, 1976. Copyright by The Ophthalmic Publishing Company.

deficiency; (2) those following laser treatment of the anterior segment; (3) those produced by an overdose of morphine sulfate; and (4) those of genetic origin.

Vitamin D Excess Models

Immunogenic Uveitis.

Doughman and coworkers[6] induced Band KP in rabbits (100% of the time) by injecting 1 mg of ovalbumin intravitreally and 12–14 days later by administering large intramuscular doses of claciferol (600,000–900,000 units). Band KP appeared a few days after the vitamin D injection.

The band was seen subepithelially and there was juxtalimbal sparing in the interpalpebral space. Sewing the eyelids together prevented the development of Band KP but keeping the animals in total darkness did not. Serum Ca levels remained normal. Corneal edema did not develop. Neither the uveitis alone nor vitamin D intoxication alone induced Band KP.

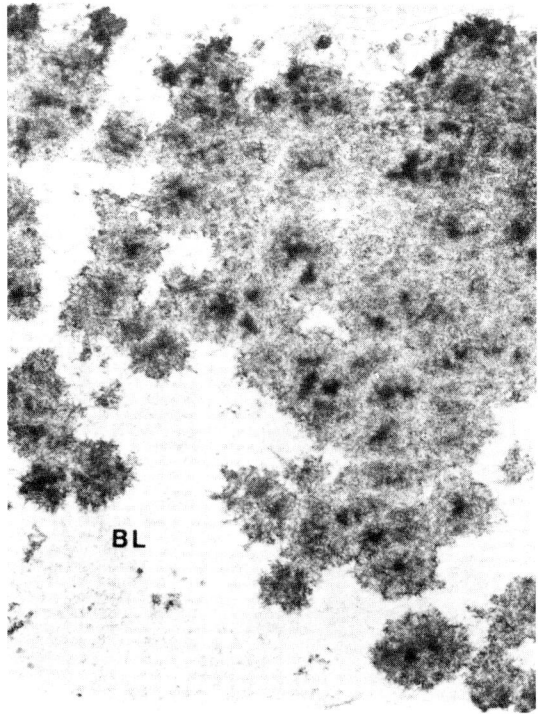

Figure 22-2. Later stage when conglomerates composed of spherules with electron dense centers have formed. Published with permission from *The American Journal of Ophthalmology* 82:395–404, 1976. Copyright by The Ophthalmic Publishing Company.

Corneal Edema.

Obenberger and co-workers[7] induced Band KP in both rats and rabbits by combination treatment with dihydrotachysterol (DHT) and various corneal injuries that produced corneal edema. Both edema and DHT were necessary to induce Band KP. In rabbits, freezing of the cornea produced the most consistent and predictable calcification (94%). $KMnO_4$ perfusion of the anterior chamber was not quite as effective (84%). Still less effective was posterior corneal abrasion (82%). The dose of DHT was 1 mg per kg body weight. In rats the most effective method was central corneal deepithelialization (100%). Less effective were whole corneal deepithelialization (81%) and freezing (73%). The dose of DHT was 1 mg per 100 g body weight.

Vitamin D Depletion Model

Doughman et al.[6] found that 35 percent of rabbits placed on a vitamin D deficient diet for four months and injected intravitreally with polyethylene sulfonic acid developed Band KP in the injected eye 15–90 days after the injection while still on a vitamin D deficient diet.

Laser Models

Without Uveitis

Fine and co-workers[8] produced corneal calcification by mild irradiation with a carbon dioxide laser. Rabbits exposed to CO_2 laser irradiation of approximately 0.35 watt/cm^2 for ten minutes developed superficial calcification typical of Band KP in 12 days. At a stronger power (0.48 watt/cm^2) for seven minutes, a more dense opacification developed. Uveitis was not observed.

With Uveitis

Leibowitz and Berkow[9] used an argon laser to produce corneal edema and uveitis, which was associated with Band KP.

Morphine Sulfate-Exposure Model

Fabian and co-workers[10] noted that rats given doses of morphine sulfate large enough to cause them to lie stuporous with their corneas exposed developed Band KP 45–82 percent of the time. Moistening the corneas with warm saline decreased the percentage of Band KP eyes and suturing the lids closed prevented the disease.

Genetic

The K–K strain of diabetic mice spontaneously develops Band KP.[11]

Morphology of Experimental Band KP

Experimental Band KP may have a clinical appearance very much like human Band KP (Fig. 22-3). Fine et al.[8] described the "typical clinical appearance of Band KP . . . both by gross inspection and biomicroscopy." Doughman et al.[6] noted bands that varied from diffuse gray white plaques to discrete geographic opacities. Obenberger et al.[7] wrote of horizontal, irregularly shaped opacities and meshes composed of tiny subepithelial whitish deposits. Fabian et al.[10] reported that their rats showed "grey clouding to faint grey stippling and distinct opaque areas which in most cases had well defined borders." Liebowitz and Berkow[9] noted "lesions closely resembling Band KP on clinical examination."

Histology

The vitamin D uveitis, vitamin D-corneal edema, and the CO_2 laser without uveitis models all histochemically show deposits of calcium in the

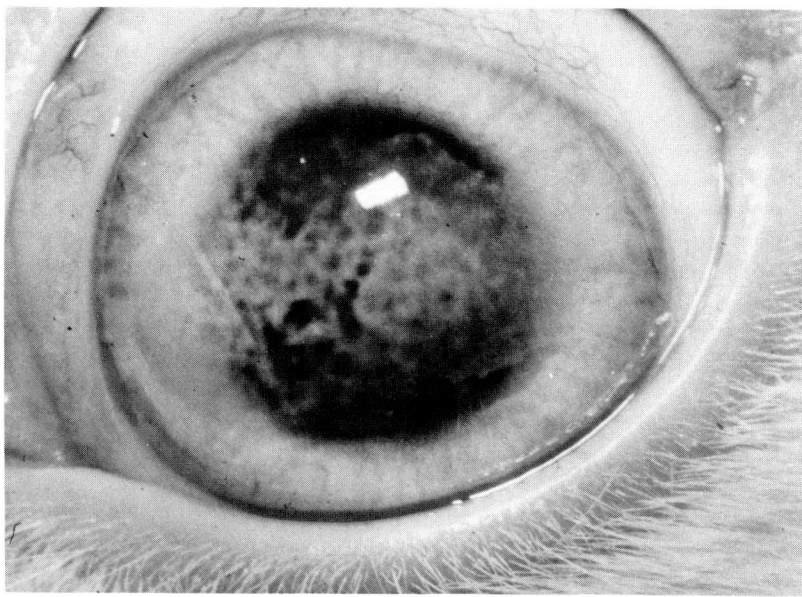

Figure 22-3. Band keratopathy in rabbit produced by the immunogenic iritis Vit. D excess model of Doughman et al., *Arch Ophthalmol*, 81:264–271, 1969. Copyright 1969, American Medical Association.

subepithelial stroma in the early phases. Calcium may later migrate into the deeper stroma and be phagocytosed by keratocytes. Calcium appears in the epithelium and endothelium in later stages of the vitamin D-uveitis model.[6]

Electron Microscopy

Electron microscopy reveals electron dense "spherules" (Fig. 22-4).[8,12] At first these lie close to the basal lamina of the epithelium and to the plasma membrane of the basal cells of the epithelium. Later "conglomerates" of presumably fused spherules are seen in the stroma, often adjacent to and inside keratocytes. The spherules' morphology varies. There are usually one or more concentric rings of varying size and density. The spaces separating the rings may be clear or partially filled with electron-dense material. A single ring with or without a dense central "nucleus" may be seen. The rings exhibit considerable variation in density, extending even to gaps or having a "signet ring-like" appearance. The margins may be quite irregular, flattened, or otherwise distorted. Electron probe analysis of the deposits in the vitamin D-uveitis model showed a 25–100-fold increase in calcium concentration in the subepithelial layers.[13]

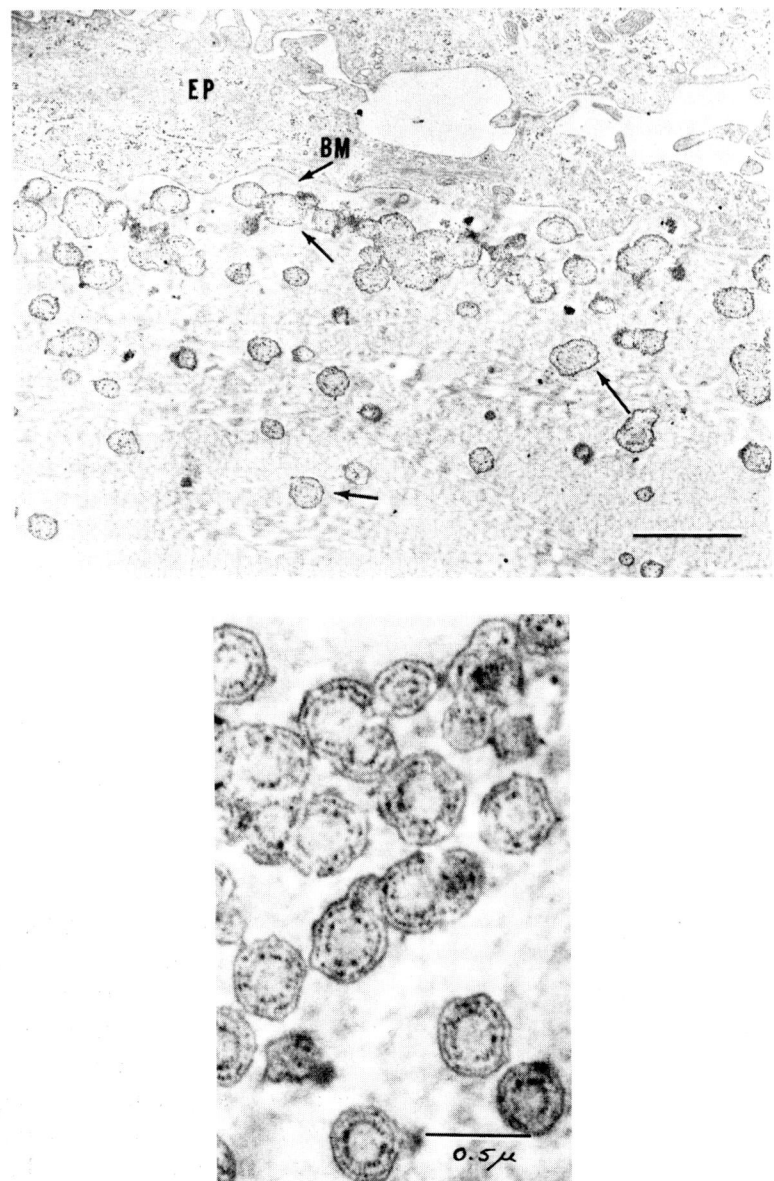

Figure 22-4. *A.* Calcific spherules in Bowman's layer (arrows) and close to the basement membrane (BM) of the basal epthelial cells (EP) (×16,500). *B.* Detailed view of the spherules (×33,000) showing their laminated structure. From B. S. Fine, J. W. Berkow, and S. Fine, *Science*, 162:129–130, 1968. Copyright 1968 by the American Association for the Advancement of Science.

Pathogenesis of Band Keratopathy

The Process of Calcification

Calcification is the deposition of crystals of inorganic calcium compounds in the extracellular matrix. Rapid advances in our knowledge of the process of a calcification have recently been summarized in several excellent review articles.[14,15,16] The present concept of the process involves both changes in the macromolecules of the matrix and in the cells of calcifying tissue.

Crystallization of any compound is influenced not only by the concentration of the involved ionic species but also by the ionic strength of the medium, the pH, the temperature, and the presence or absence of crystallization inhibitors and/or of nucleation sites. The crystal in bone, cartilage, and pathologic calcification is hydroxyapatite (HAP), whose chemical formula is $CA_{10}(PO_4)_6(OH)_2$.

Extracellular fluid is metastable with regard to HAP. Thus, even if the ion product of Ca and PO exceeds the solubility of HAP, crystallization does not occur spontaneously unless nucleating sites are present. These may be either HAP crystals (homogenous) or some other material that resembles HAP well enough to serve as "seed crystal" (heterogenous).

According to present theory, initial calcification takes place at special sites where the micro environment can be altered to permit HAP to crystallize. *Matrix vesicles,* described independently by Anderson[17] and Bonucci[18] in 1967, serve this function in bone, cartilage, and in some pathologic calcification.[14] In other pathologic calcifications, mitochondria serve instead.

Matrix vesicles (MVS) are extracellular structures, generally round and of varying size (diameter 500–3000 Å) (Fig. 22-5). They are membrane invested and osmiophyllic. It is uncertain if they are formed by cells or if they appear as a result of cellular degeneration. Initial calcification is revealed as deposits of HAP crystals in close apposition to the inner leaflet of the MVs. Later, radial clusters of mineral appear at their surface.

Several characteristics enable MVs to serve as the initial site of calcification. Their investing lipid membranes permit control of their interior environment. Ionic strength, pH, and Ca and PO_4 concentration can therefore be optimally set for crystallization of HAP. Certain compounds found in their interiors, such as the acidic phospholipids, phosphatidyl serine and phosphatidyl inositiol, certain phosphoproteins, and proteins containing gamma-carboxyglutamic acid (GCA proteins), may serve as heterogenous nucleating sites. These compounds may also increase the internal Ca concentration by Ca binding. Matrix vesicles contain high concentrations of various phosphatases, including alkaline phosphatase, ATPase and pyrophosphatase. Alkaline phosphatase concentration in MVs is 20 times greater than in whole

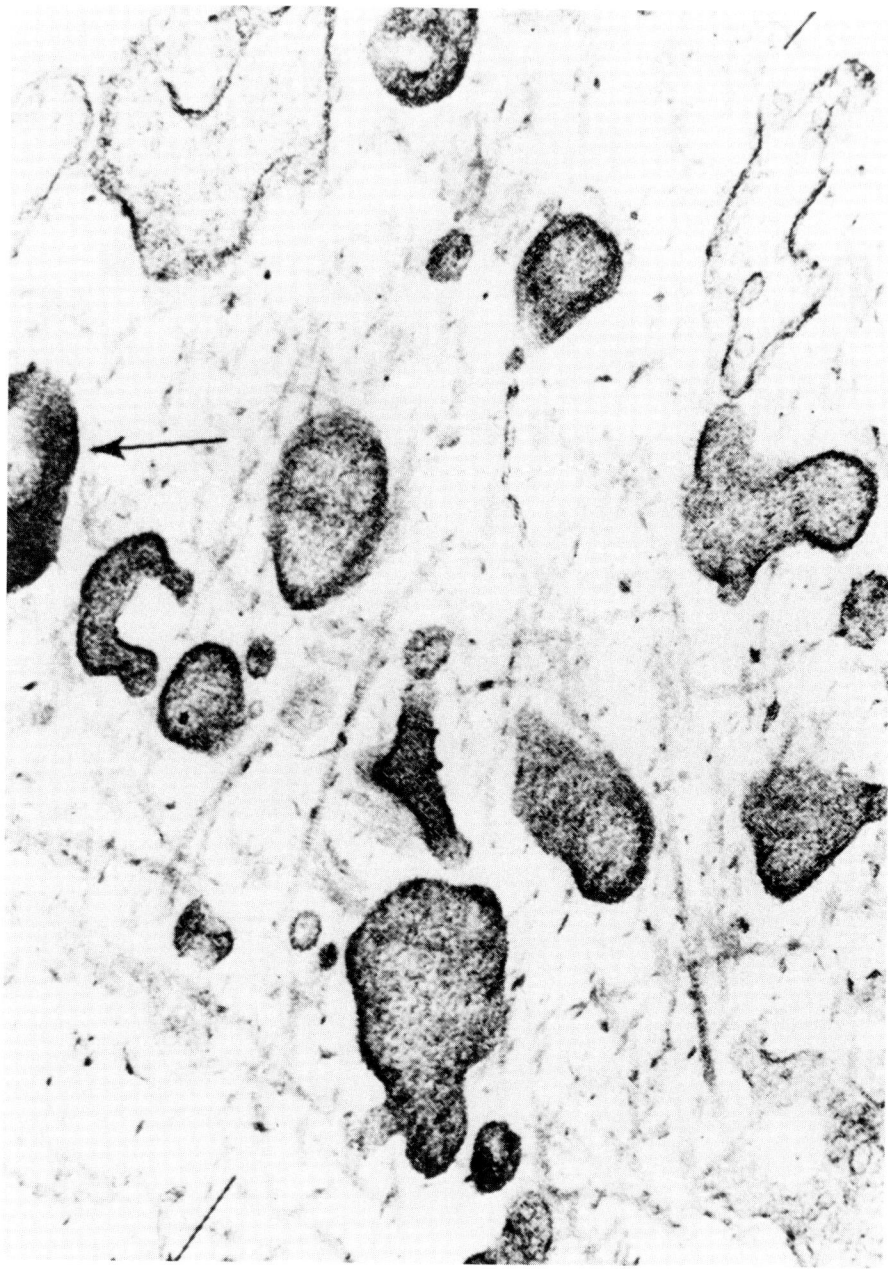

Figure 22-5. Matrix vesicles in hypertrophic cartilage (×36,000). Reproduced from *The Journal of Cell Biology*, 1967, vol. 35 81–101 by copyright permission of The Rockefeller University Press.

cells. The phosphatases may increase the PO_4 concentration and decrease the concentrations of pyrophosphate and ATP, major inhibitors of crystallization of HAP. The ATPase may help produce energy for a membrane Ca pump.

Pathological Calcification

Pathological calcification has been divided into two types: (1) metastatic, in which there is an abnormality of calcium and phosphorus metabolism such as that induced by hyperparathyroidism, vitamin D intoxication, chronic renal disease, metastatic carcinoma, or sarcoid, and (2) dystrophic, in which local tissue injury is the precipitating factor.

The Doughman and Obenberger models require vitamin D intoxication together with some sort of injury. The laser models and the rat-morphine sulfate exposure models are strictly dystrophic.

Theories of Pathogenesis of Band Keratopathy

O'Connor[19] summarized the physicochemical factors that play a role in the pathogenesis of Band KP. These may be classified by the characteristics that result from them.

Distribution of Deposits in the Interpalpebral Space.

This has been thought to result from the evaporation of water from the exposed part of the cornea. This is a very old idea, as Stocker in his discussion of O'Connor's paper points out. Evaporation increases the concentration of the ions and also increases the ionic strength. Both changes favor crystallization. Exposure of the cornea also lowers the temperature, another change that favors crystallization.

Subepithelial Localization of HPA.

O'Connor mentioned several factors that might be responsible for this. Anaerobic glycolysis in the deep corneal stroma would increase lactic acid concentration and lower the pH there. This would inhibit crystallization in those layers. Conversely, the diffusion of the CO_2 from the epithelium would raise the pH in the superficial layers and favor crystallization at that level.

O'Connor also hypothesized that the collagen lattice in the subepithelial stroma or the epithelial basement membrane might serve as a heterogenous nucleating site for crystallization or serve as a filter for any HAP crystals formed deeper and carried to the anterior by water flow.

O'Connor mentioned the resemblance between the spherules of Fine et al. and the spheroidal granules of Pouliquen et al. and noted the location of these entities close to the epithelial basement membrane. Radnot has published pictures of similar structures produced by the Obenberger technique (Fig. 22-6). Similar spherules are seen in the basal lamina and the superficial laminae of the stroma in Doughman's model (Fig. 22-7). Their laminated structure and their proximity to the basal lamina of the epithelium suggests that these structures may in fact be matrix vesicles. Their presence could be a reaction to laser injury to the basal layer of the epithelium, a result of corneal edema in the Obenberger model, or a "toxic effect" of uveitis (as suggested by Stocker in his discussion of O'Connor's paper) in the Doughman model.

Obenberger's observation that calcium deposits were related to fibroblasts suggests a similarity to calcification of aortic valves, where degenerating fibroblasts serve as the source of the nucleating bodies.[20]

Limbal Sparing.

O'Connor suggested that the limbus was the favored primary site because of the diffusion of Ca from the limbal circulation, although Obenberger and Babicky could not demonstrate any Ca concentration gradient in their ^{45}Ca studies.[21] He felt that limbal sparing resulted from a buffer diffusing from the limbal circulation, which would minimize the pH changes mentioned earlier. Diffusion of a circulating inhibitor of crystallization such as inorganic pyrophosphate into the stroma from the limbus is another possibility.

The strictly physiochemical pathogenetic model of O'Connor and others may be modified by hypothesizing that matrix vesicles (or some other cell-generated structure such as a mitochondria) serve as nucleating sites in the development of Band KP. The suggestion provides an explanation for some of the morphologic features of Band KP (such as the spherules seen on electron microscopy and the subepithelial location of the initial deposits) and suggests a final common pathway for a diverse group of etiologies. This modified model of O'Connor also offers a possible role for vitamin D in pathogenesis, a role otherwise difficult to explain in the face of normocalcemia[6] in the vitamin D-dependent models. Vitamin D may increase the Ca concentration in the vesicles in a manner analogous to its effect on intracellular Ca, as Borle has suggested.[22]

If this suggestion is confirmed by further studies, Band KP will be brought together with a group of pathologic calcifications in which this mechanism has been demonstrated.

Summary

Clinical, histochemical, and electron microscopic findings in animal and human Band KP are presented. Recent advances in the process of calcification are described. The suggestion is made that Band KP is not produced

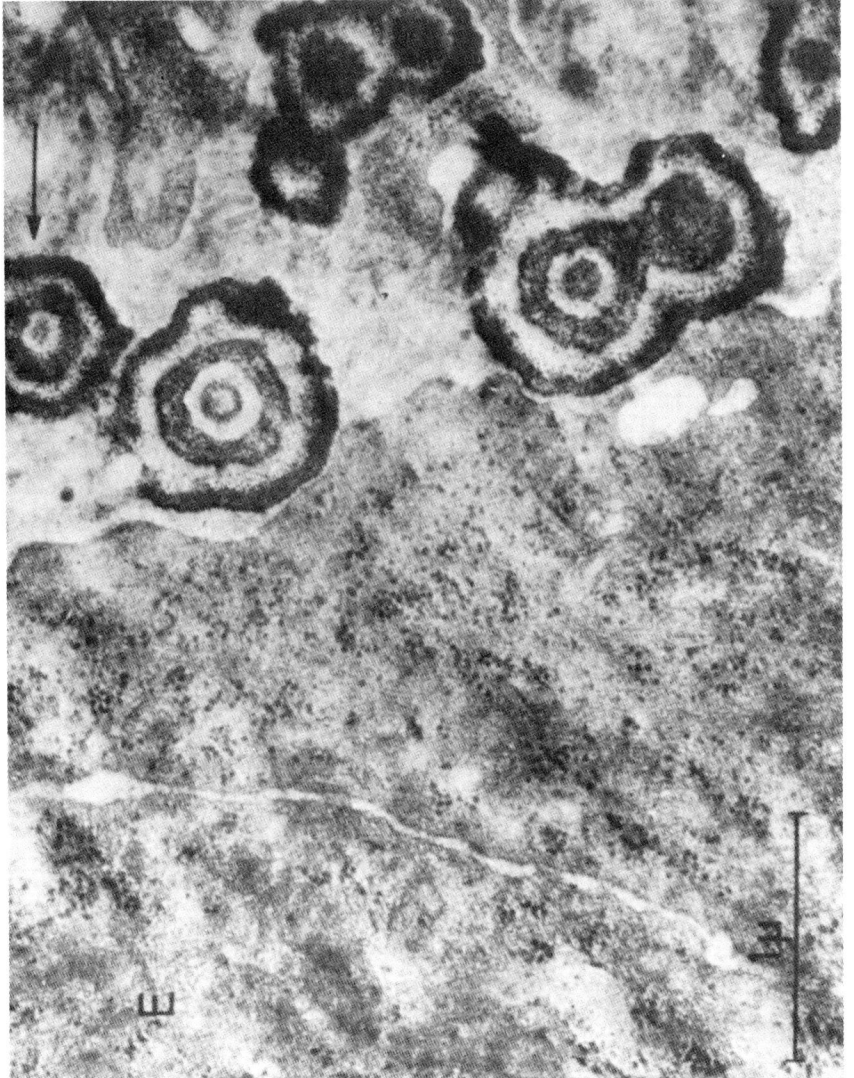

Figure 22-6. Calcific laminated spherules in the Obenberger corneal edema model in rabbit. ×32,000. From M. Radnot et al., *Klin Monatsbl Augenheikd, 157*:225–229, 1970. Courtesy of Ferdinand Enke Verlag, Stuttgart.

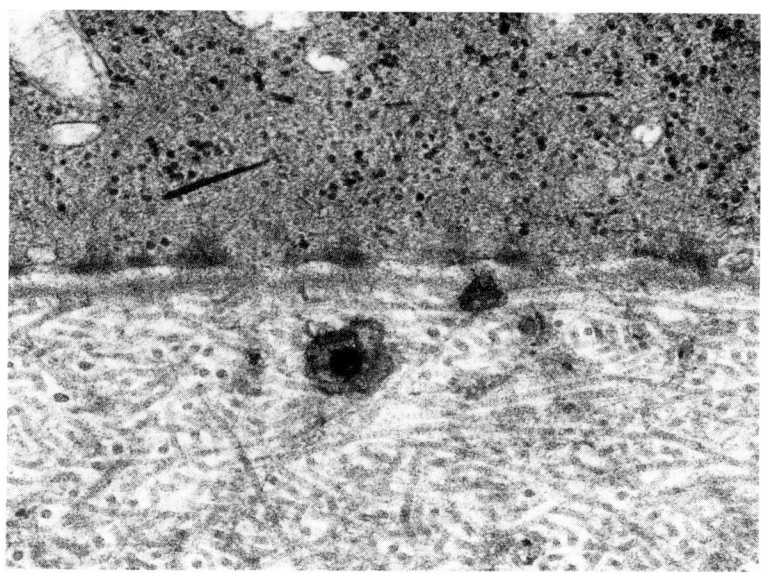

Figure 22-7. Calcific laminated spherules in rabbit cornea (immunogenic uveitis-vitamin D intoxication model). ×32,000. (Courtesy Irmgard Wood.)

solely by the effect of physiochemical factors but through the interaction of those factors with corneal cells, probably epithelial cells. The laminated, spheroidal, electron-dense structures seen in both animal and human Band KP may be matrix vesicles and hence may play an essential role as the initial site of calcification in the disease.

REFERENCES

1. Bowman, W.: Lectures on the Parts Concerned in the Operations on the Eye, and on the Structure of the Retina. Delivered at the Royal London Ophthalmic Hospital, Moorfields, June 1847. To which are added, a Paper on the Vitreous Humor and also a Few Cases of Ophthalmic Disease. London, Longman, Brown, Green, and Longmans, 1849, appendix of cases, pp. 120–121.
2. Pouliquen, Y., Haye, C., Bisson, J., and Offret, G.: Ultrastructure de la kératopathie en bandelette. *Arch Ophthalmol, 27*:149–158, 1967.
3. Edmonds, C., and Iwamoto, T.: Electron microscopy of late interstitial keratitis. *Ann Ophthalmol, 4*:693–711, 1972.
4. Cursino, J. W., and Fine, B. S.: A histologic study of calcific and noncalcific band keratopathies. *Am J Ophthalmol, 82*:395–404, 1976.
5. Barkow, J. W., Fine, B. S., and Zimmerman, L. E.: Unusual ocular calcification in hyperparathyroidism. *Am J Ophthalmol, 66*:812–824, 1968.
6. Doughman, D. J., Olson, G. A., Nolan, S., and Hajny, R. G.: Experimental band keratopathy. *Arch Ophthalmol, 81*:264–271, 1969.

7. Obenberger, J., Ocumpaugh, D. E., and Cubberly, M. G.: Experimental corneal calcification in animals treated with dihydrotachysterol. *Invest Ophthalmol, 8*:467–474, 1969.
8. Fine, B. S., Berkow, J. W., and Fine, S.: Corneal calcification. *Science, 162*:129–130, 1968.
9. Leibowitz, H. M., and Berkow, J. W.: Band keratopathy after ocular exposure to visible laser radiation. *Am J Ophthalmol, 76*:468–471, 1973.
10. Fabian, R. J., Bond, J. M., and Drobeck, H. P.: Induced corneal opacities in the rat. *Br J Ophthalmol, 51*:124–129, 1967.
11. Mittl, R., Galin, M. A., Opperman, W., Camerini-Davalos, R. A., and Spiro, D.: Corneal calcification in spontaneously diabetic mice. *Invest Ophthalmol, 9*:137–145, 1970.
12. Radnot, M., Jobbagyi, P., and Lovas, B.: Die Feins truktur der kalkablagerung in der Hornhaut. *Klin Monatsb d Augenheilkunde, 157*:225–229, 1970.
13. Doughman, D. J., Ingram, M. J., and Bourne, W. M.: Experimental band keratopathy electron microprobe x-ray analysis of aqueous and corneal calcium concentrations. *Invest Ophthalmol, 9*:471–475, 1970.
14. Anderson, H. C.: Calcification processes. *Path Ann, 15*:45–75, 1980.
15. Boskey, A. L.: Current concepts of the physiology and biochemistry of calcification. *Clin Ortho Related Res, 157*:225–257, 1981.
16. Fleisch, H.: Mechanisms of calcification. In Massry, S. G., Ritz, E., and Jahn, H. (Eds.): *Phosphate and Minerals in Health and Disease*. New York, Plenum Press, 1979, pp. 563–577.
17. Anderson, H. C.: Electron microscopic studies of induced cartilage development and calcification. *J Cell Biol, 35*:81–101, 1967.
18. Bonucci, E.: Fine structure of early cartilage calcification. *J Ultrastruct Res, 20*:35–50, 1967.
19. O'Connor, G. R.: Calcific band keratopathy. *Trans Am Ophthalmol Soc, 70*:58–79, 1972.
20. Kim, K. M.: Clacification of matrix vesicles in human aortic valve and aortic media. *Fed Proc, 35*:156–162, 1976.
21. Obenberger, J., and Babbicky, A.: Experimental corneal calcification: A study of transport of ^{45}Ca into the aqueous and cornea. *Ophthalmol Res, 1*:187–192, 1970.
22. Borle, A. B.: Calcium metabolism at the cellular level. *Fed Proc, 32*:1944–1950, 1973.

SECTION IV
IMMUNOLOGIC DISORDERS

Chapter 23

NZB/NZW F₁ HYBRID MICE
An Animal Model of Sjögren's Syndrome

Vincent P. deLuise, M.D.; Khalid F. Tabbara, M.D.

Introduction

The New Zealand Black/New Zealand White F₁ hybrid (NZB/NZW or B/W) mouse develops an autoimmune disease of hemolytic anemia, glomerulonephritis, and arthritis similar to systemic lupus erythematosus.[1] In addition, these mice develop changes in the lacrimal and salivary glands that mimic those seen in patients with Sjögren's syndrome.[2] Kessler first recognized the similarities between the lymphocytic infiltrations in the lacrimal and salivary glands of B/W mice and those seen in patients with keratoconjunctivitis sicca and xerostomia.[3] It was later observed that New Zealand Black (NZB) parents also develop similar autoimmune disease.[4] These mice provide a natural animal model of Sjögren's syndrome. Both salivary and lacrimal glands in the B/W mice show mononuclear cell infiltration beginning in the fourth postnatal month and progressing in severity with age.[4] The early, characteristic lesions seen in the lacrimal glands of both NZB and B/W mice consist of multiple, small, periductal and periarteriolar mononuclear cell infiltrations.

This study presents the longitudinal, chronological changes in the lacrimal glands of NZB, NZW, and B/W mice as observed by histopathological and immunopathological studies.

Material and Methods

Animals:

A colony of New Zealand White (NZW) and New Zealand Black (NZB) mice was used, maintained by brother-sister matings, producing NZB × NZW F₁ hybrid (B/W) mice from this stock. All animals were catalogued as to date of birth, sex, weight at sacrifice, and were raised in cages of four or

---

Supported in part by Grants EY-03436, EY-01597, and EY-07058 from the National Institutes of Health, Bethesda, Maryland.

fewer animals on a diet of regular Purina® chow. No attempt was made in this experiment to alter the diet in any of the mice. A total of 100 mice were catalogued, and divided into five groups, each of which contained three NZB mice, three NZW mice, and fourteen B/W mice. A group of mice was sacrificed at three, six, seven, eight, and nine months after birth. Within each group, all mice were of the same age, with variable numbers of male, female, pregnant, and virgin mice. Each mouse was given a random number and, after ether euthanasia, reexamined as to sex and pregnancy by direct study of the genitalia and incision of the abdomen for inspection of the uterus for fetuses.

Tissue Techniques:

The exorbital lacrimal glands were obtained from both orbits of each mouse with the use of fine jeweler's forceps and Westcott scissors. The lacrimal gland tissue was divided in half. One half was placed in 10% formalin for routine hematoxylin-eosin staining. The other half of each specimen was placed in cold (4°C) Wolman-Bejar solution (19 parts by volume of absolute ethanol to one part glacial acetic acid) and fixed for 24 hours. These tissues were then embedded in paraffin, partially hydrated through xylene, and air-dried. One drop of conjugate was placed on each section and incubated in a moist chamber for one hour at 37°C.

The conjugate was then shaken off, and the sections washed in three changes of 0.15 M phosphate buffered saline, pH 7.2, for three minutes each. Sections were briefly rinsed in distilled water, counterstained with a dilute solution of Evans-Blue for one minute, and rinsed in distilled water. Tissue paper was used to remove excess water. One drop of buffered glycerol (nine parts anhydrous glycerol and one part buffered saline pH 7.00) was placed on a slide and a coverslip placed over that. The fluorescein-stained sections were examined within six hours of processing to ensure an accurate assessment of the immunopathological changes. The specimens were stored horizontally at 0°C.

Histology:

Each specimen was examined by light microscopy with hematoxyline-eosin staining, and by fluorescent-antibody techniques to immunoglobulins G, M, and complement (C'3). The lacrimal glands were graded by lymphocytic infiltrations per 4 mm^2 of tissue as follows: Grade 0 = no lymphocytes (Fig. 23-1); Grade I = few lymphocytes; Grade II = many lymphocytes (less than 50); Grade III = one focus (50 or more) lymphocytes (Fig. 23-2); Grade IV = greater than one focus, nonconfluent or confluent (Fig. 23-3). The immunofluorescent sections were graded by brilliance and intensity of the periductal or periarteriolar staining for immunoglobulins G and M, and separately for complement, as follows: Grade 0 = no staining; Grade 1+ = slight apple green staining around lacrimal ducts; Grade 2+ = moderate apple green staining around lacrimal ducts and vessels; Grade 3+ = intense greenish periductal and perivascular staining, may be confluent.

RESULTS

Three months:

At three months of age, none of the NZW mice had any histopathologic or immunopathologic changes. None of the NZB or B/W mice showed any lymphocytic infiltration or staining by immunofluorescent techniques.

Six months:

At six months none of the NZW mice had any histopathologic or immunopathologic changes. None of the NZB mice had any changes. Three of the 14 B/W mice had occasional lymphocytic infiltration of the periductal tissue (Grade 1). These were two virgin females and one male, one of which had 1+ staining against complement (C'3). There was no staining with immunoglobulin.

Seven months:

At seven months none of the NZW mice had any histopathologic changes. One of the NZW female mice had 1+ staining to complement. There was no correlative staining to the immunoglobulins. Two of the three NZB female mice had confluent foci (Grade IV) changes on histopathology, and 1+ staining to both IgG, IgM, and complement. Four B/W mice showed grade I histopathological staining, two breeding (pregnant) B/W mice showed grade I changes, three B/W virgin females showed grade IV changes by hematoxyline and eosin. Using immunofluorescent techniques, the four male B/W mice showed 1+ to 2+ staining changes to both immunoglobulins and complement, the two breeding B/W females showed 1+ changes, three virgin B/W virgin females showed 3+ staining changes to both complement and immunoglobulins.

Eight months:

At eight months none of the NZW mice showed any positive (Grade III or IV) changes by histopathology. There was no staining of any of the specimens by indirect immunofluorescence techniques to either complement, IgG, or IgM. The NZB females showed grade II to IV changes by histopathological examination. By immunofluorescence, there was grade I to II staining of the specimens to IgG, IgM, and complement. The B/W mice showed grade 0 to II changes by histopathological examination, and no

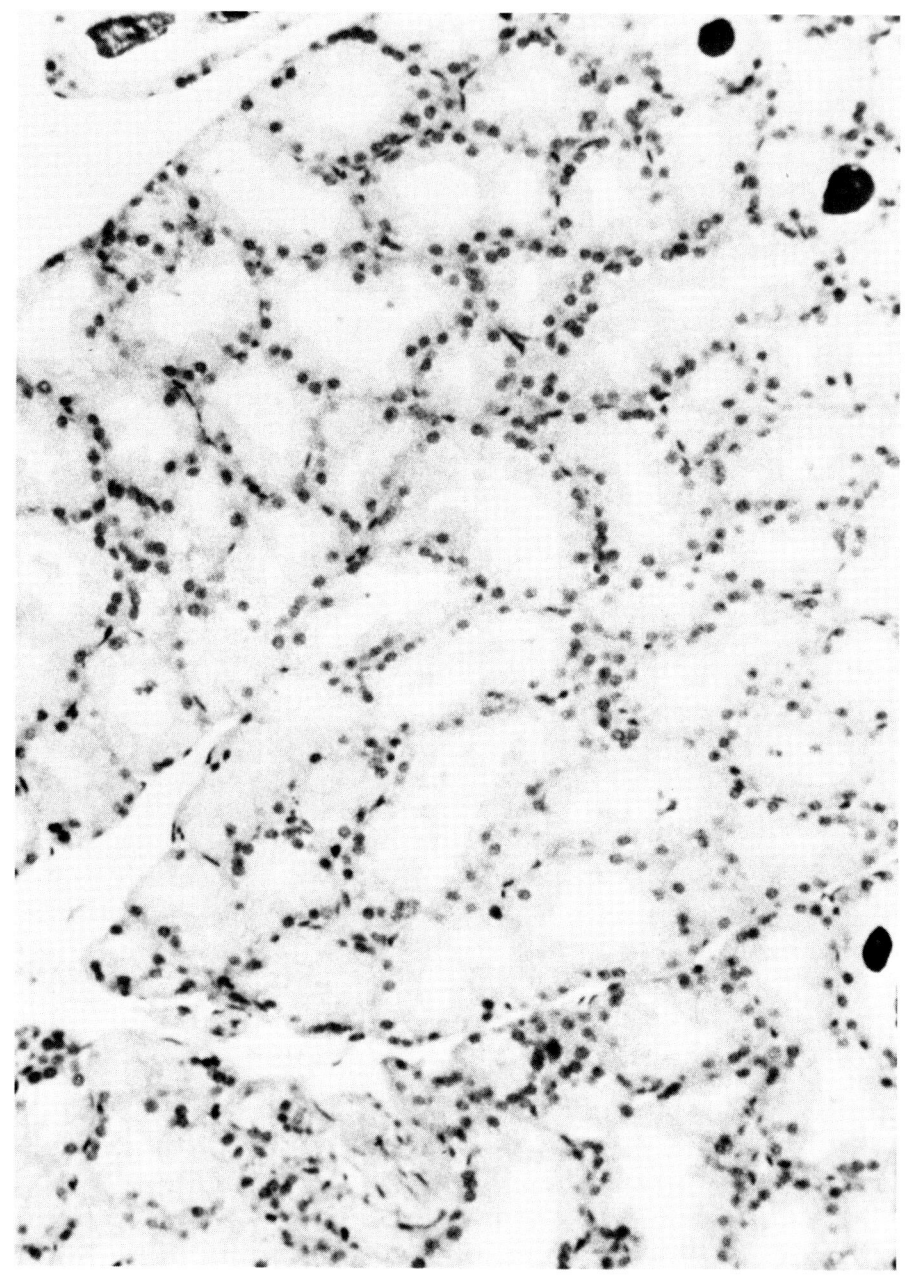

Figure 23-1. Histologic section showing normal lacrimal gland tissue of a three-month-old NZW mouse. ×100.

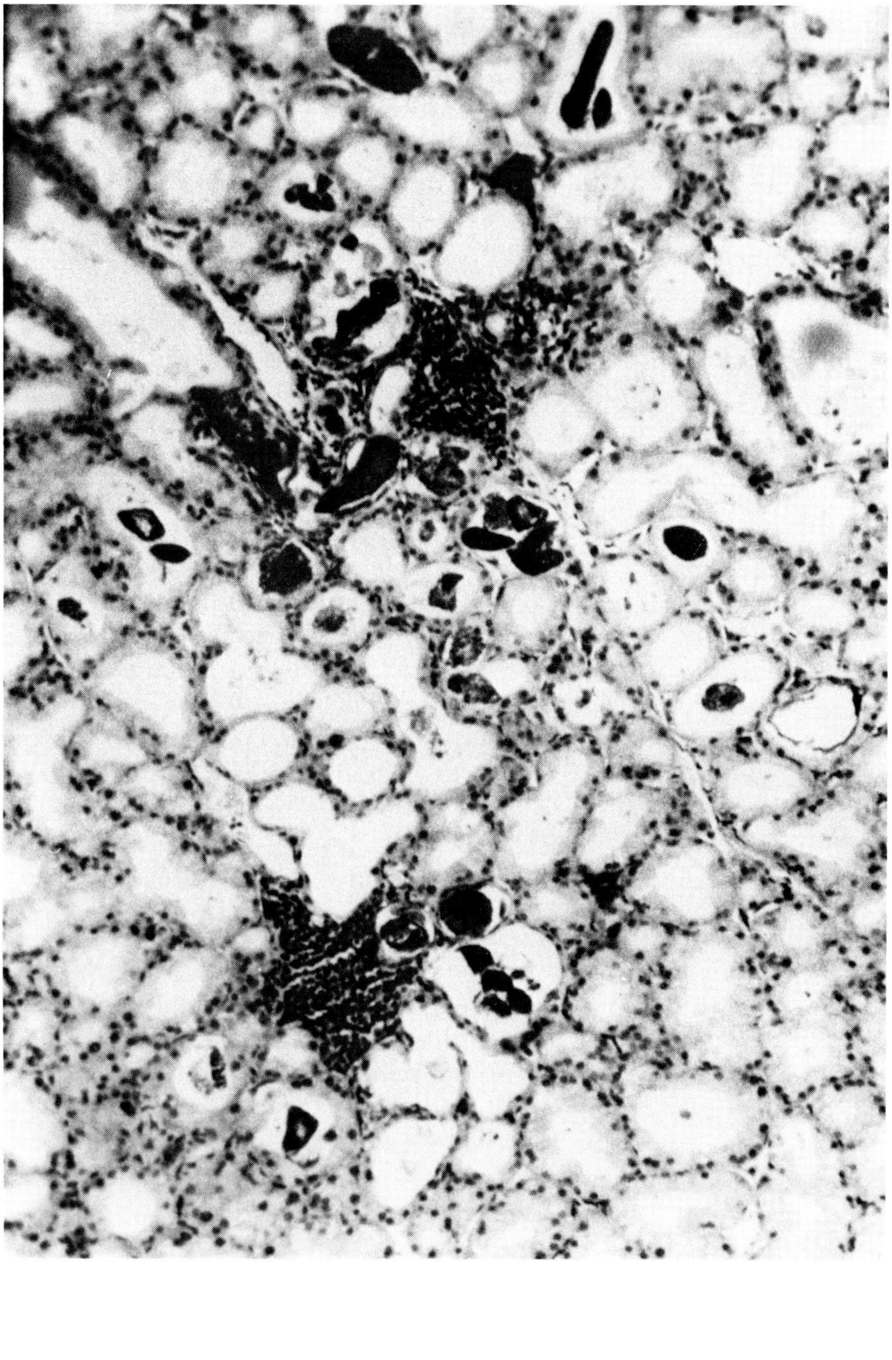

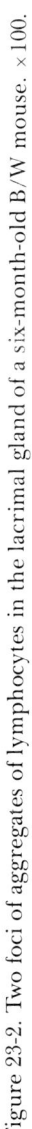

Figure 23-2. Two foci of aggregates of lymphocytes in the lacrimal gland of a six-month-old B/W mouse. ×100.

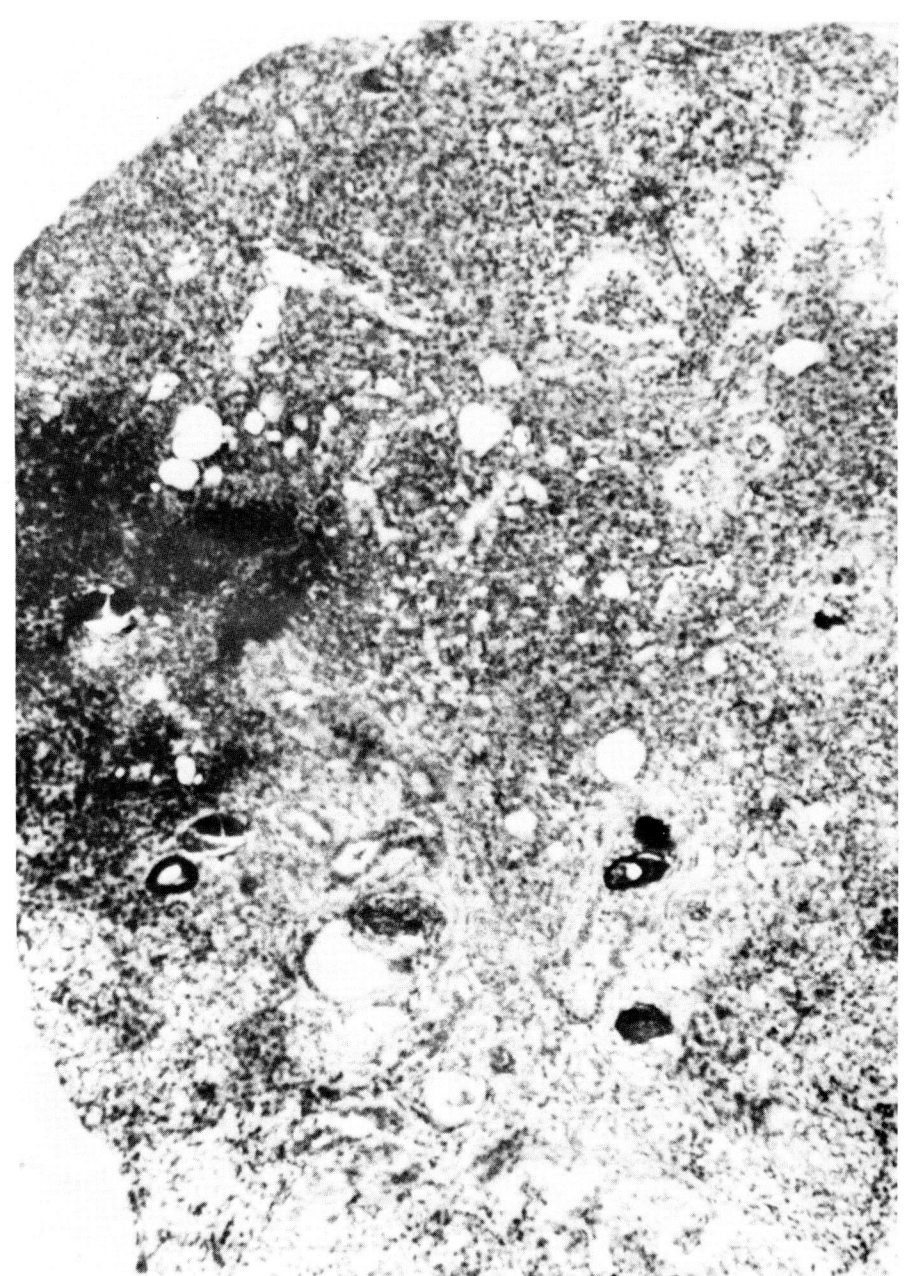

Figure 23-3. Confluent lymphocytic infiltration of the lacrimal gland of a nine-month-old B/W mouse. ×63.

changes by immunofluorescence. The B/W females showed grade II to III changes by histopathology and 1+ to 2+ immunofluorescence changes. The B/W breeding female had grade II histopathological and 1+ immunofluorescent changes.

Nine months:

At nine months of age, none of the NZW mice had any histopathological or immunopathological changes. The NZB females showed a spectrum of change from grade I to IV, and 1+ to 2+ immunofluorescence staining. The B/W males displayed grade I to II histopathological changes and no staining by immunofluorescent techniques. The breeding female showed grade II changes by histopathology and no staining by immunofluorescence. The B/W females uniformly displayed grade II to IV changes by histopathology and 1+ and 3+ immunofluorescence staining.

Graphic illustrations of the histopathologic and immunopathologic changes at three, six, and nine months are shown in Figures 23-4 and 23-5.

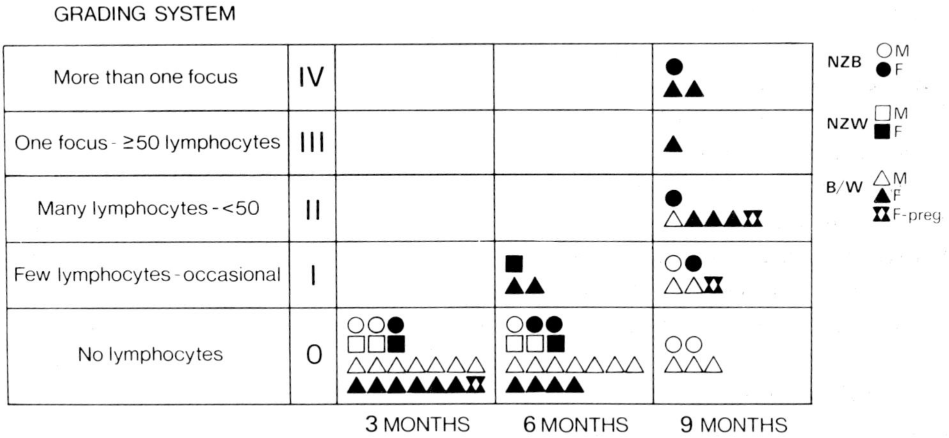

Figure 23-4. Histopathologic changes in the lacrimal glands of NZW, NZB, and B/W mice.

Discussion

Sjögren's syndrome is characterized by keratoconjunctivitis sicca, xerostomia, and connective tissue disease, usually rheumatoid arthritis.[5] Since 1968, an animal model of the New Zealand Black/New Zealand White F_1 hybrid (B/W) mouse has been known to have a course similar to that of patients with Sjögren's syndrome.[3] The underlying pathogenesis of Sjögren's syndrome is an insidious, chronic, progressive infiltration of lacrimal and salivary glands by mononuclear cells and the production of autoantibody

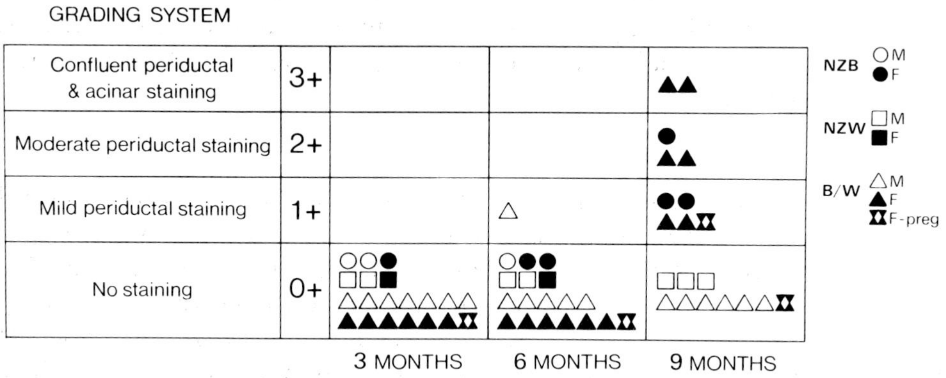

GRADING SYSTEM

		3 MONTHS	6 MONTHS	9 MONTHS	
Confluent periductal & acinar staining	3+			▲▲	NZB ○M ●F
Moderate periductal staining	2+			● ▲▲	NZW □M ■F
Mild periductal staining	1+		△	●● ▲▲✕	B/W △M ▲F ✕F-preg
No staining	0+	○○● □□■ △△△△△△△ ▲▲▲▲▲▲▲✕	○●● □□■ △△△△△ ▲▲▲▲▲▲▲✕	□□□ △△△△△△△✕	

Figure 23-5. Results of immunofluorescent staining for IgG, IgM, and C_3 of the lacrimal glands of NZW, NZB, and B/W mice. (0 = no stain, 1+ = slight staining, 2+ = moderate staining, and 3+ = intense staining.)

against host lacrimal and salivary gland tissue.[3] Because of the occurrence of unusual autoantibodies against cytoplasmic and nuclear components in Sjögren's syndrome, the B/W mouse model becomes important as a marker for the histopathologic and immunopathologic changes in this disease.[4-6]

Kessler showed that profound changes occur in the exorbital lacrimal and salivary glands in parental NZB and B/W mice characterized by periductal and periarteriolar mononuclear cell infiltration and parenchymal degeneration, with retention of the lobular architecture.[4] These changes are sometimes accompanied by preserved areas of normal lacrimal tissue, termed "epimyoepithelial islands." Kessler also found that the ocular pathology was less severe in the parental NZB mice than in the B/W offspring. In addition, there was no change in the NZW parents.[4] These studies formed the basis for our experiment, which further delineated the chronology and severity of the pathologic changes in the lacrimal gland, and we demonstrated the effects of age, sex, and breeding.

This study defined the chronologic changes in the exorbital lacrimal glands of NZB, NZW, and B/W mice. The histopathologic changes in this animal model (B/W) are similar to the changes observed in humans, namely, female preponderance, worsening of the disease with age, the ameliorative effects of pregnancy on the disease, and the fact that females have a poorer prognosis of the disease than males.

The lacrimal gland changes of NZB and B/W F_1 hybrid mice appear to be related to age, sex, and pregnancy. With age, mice develop focal, followed by diffuse, aggregations of lymphocytes, forming periductal and perivascular foci in lacrimal tissue. Within each group of mice, the changes were more profound in virgin, female mice. Pregnant females had fewer changes, and male mice the least. Similar changes were seen in immunofluorescent-stained sections to complement (C'3), IgG, and IgM. The older, virgin female mice displayed more severe and confluent staining to complement and the immunoglobulins.

There is mounting evidence to suggest reciprocal relationships between the neuroendocrine and immune systems in modulating the immune response in both animal models and humans.[7,8] The differences in sex hormonal levels between virgin and breeding females and males may explain the discrepancy in the lacrimal gland infiltration by mononuclear cells and the staining with complement and the immunoglobulins.[8,9] Sjögren's syndrome is seen much more frequently (9:1) in females. Similarly, the B/W virgin females displayed the worst manifestations of the disease in their lacrimal glands. The mean survival time of virgin females is 279.8 days compared to 438.8 days in the male mice. In addition, the pregnant females uniformly displayed fewer, less severe changes both by histopathological and immunofluorescence staining.

A longitudinal analysis of the histopathology and the immunopathology of the lacrimal glands of NZB/NZW and NZB mice provides a means of studying influence of age, sex, and breeding on this animal model of Sjögren's syndrome.

Summary

New Zealand black mice (NZB) and New Zealand black/New Zealand white F_1 hybrid (B/W) mice provide a model for the study of the autoimmune changes of Sjögren's syndrome. One hundred NZB, NZW, and B/W mice of either sex were divided into five groups. Mice were sacrificed at three, six, seven, eight, and nine months after birth. Nine-month old or older NZB and B/W mice had mononuclear cell infiltration of the lacrimal gland, which was more severe in females. The lacrimal glands of female B/W mice showed more severe changes than B/W male mice or NZB mice. Virgin females had more severe changes than pregnant females within each group. Immunofluorescent-stained sections of lacrimal glands showed deposition of IgG, IgM, and complement (C'3) in the ductal epithelial cells, which was more prominent in older, virgin female mice.

REFERENCES

1. Bielschowsky, M., and Bielschowsky, F.: Reaction of the reticular tissue of mice with autoimmune hemolytic anemia to 2-aminofluorene. *Nature*, 194:692, 1962.
2. Howie, J. B., and Helyer, R. J.: Immunology and pathology of NZB mice. *Adv Immunol*, 9:215, 1968.
3. Kessler, H. S.: A laboratory model for Sjögren's syndrome. *Am J Pathol*, 52:671, 1968.

4. Kessler, H. S., Cubberly, M., and Manski, W.: Eye changes in autoimmune NZB and NZB/NZW mice. *Arch Ophthalmol,* 85:211, 1971.
5. Greenspan, J. S., Daniels, T. E., Talal, N., and Sylvester, R. A.: The histopathology of Sjögren's syndrome in labial salivary gland biopsies. *Oral Surg,* 37:217, 1974.
6. Keyes, G. G., Vickers, R. A., and Kersey, J. H.: Immunopathology of Sjögren-like disease in NZB/NZW mice. *J Oral Pathol,* 6:288, 1977.
7. Talal, N.: Autoimmunity and the immunologic network. *Arthritis Rheum,* 21:853, 1978.
8. Besedovsky, H., and Sorkin, E.: Network of immune-neuroendocrine interactions. *Clin Exp Immunol,* 27:1, 1977.
9. Talal, N.: Immunologic and viral factors in the pathogenesis of systemic lupus erythematosus. *Arthritis Rheum,* 13:887, 1970.

Chapter 24

ENDOTOXIN-INDUCED UVEITIS IN RATS

JAMES T. ROSENBAUM, M.D.

Endotoxin, a lipopolysaccharide, is the major outer cell wall substance of gram-negative bacteria. In rats it induces an acute, anterior uveal inflammation after intravenous, foot pad, or intraperitoneal injection. I wish to review briefly the historical background of endotoxin and the eye, discuss the etiological characteristics of this disease in rats, and speculate on the possible relevance of this model to human disease.

Historical Background

In 1916, A. C. Woods described bacterial "poisons" that could affect the uveal tract.[1] His observations led to the concept of treating uveitis by sterilizing remote and sometimes occult sources of infection such as the maxillary sinus or abscesses in teeth. Paradoxically, fever therapy was also in vogue during this same era for the treatment of uveitis. The pyrogen was usually endotoxin. Thus, bacterial toxins were being implicated in both the cause and the therapy of uveitis.

In 1941, Ayo observed that Shwartzman toxins (endotoxin) induced a toxic ocular reaction in rabbits that included iris hyperemia and aqueous flare.[2] A wide variety of species were susceptible to this response, although rats were specifically noted to be refractory to the ocular effects of endotoxin.[3] A number of investigators, including Howes,[4] Levene,[5] and Bengtsson,[6] have further characterized the rabbit response to endotoxin. Based on antibody-induced depletion, Howes concluded that the platelet is critical to the induction of increased vascular permeability by endotoxin.[4] Pharmacologic studies have implicated prostaglandins,[7] thromboxane,[6] serotonin,[8] and, to a lesser degree, histamine[8] in the endotoxin-induced effect. My colleagues and I have used fluorescein tagged albumin and slit lamp fluorophotometry to quantitate the ocular vascular permeability changes induced by endotoxin.[9] All of the above observations refer to systemic administration of endotoxin

---

The author is the recipient of the New Investigator Research Award from the National Institutes of Health, R23, AM-31076. This work was supported in part by the Kuzell Institute for Arthritis Research, San Francisco, California.

in rabbits. It should also be noted that the eye is exquisitely sensitive to nanogram quantities of endotoxin when it is injected intravitreally.[10]

Characteristics of Endotoxin-Induced Uveitis in Rats

My own interest in endotoxin-induced eye effects arose by accident. I was studying an arthritis model in rats that develops after injection of killed mycobacteria in the foot pad. This disease has many of the stigmata of Reiter's syndrome, including a spondyloarthropathy with eye, skin, and genital lesions.[11] Reiter's syndrome can follow a variety of gram-negative dysenteries. Therefore, we tested the possibility that killed, gram-negative organisms could induce arthritis in rats. Although we did not produce joint lesions, we induced a reproducible, acute anterior uveitis. This form of uveitis could be duplicated by the intravenous or intraperitoneal injection of endotoxin alone.[12]

The disease that we observed was characterized histologically by an anterior uveal infiltrate of polymorphonuclear leukocytes and mononuclear cells within 24 hours of the endotoxin injection (Figs. 24-1 and 24-2). Disease was always bilateral. The cellular infiltration starts to diminish by 48 hours and vanishes by 96 hours. The dose required to produce uveitis in rats was 100 μg of a phenol extract of *E. coli* lipopolysaccharide produced by phenol extraction. This dose is well below the lethal dose and induces no light microscopic changes in other organs including the heart, lung, liver, kidney, and spleen. Lower doses produce ocular changes irregularly while higher doses do not necessarily induce a greater cellular infiltration. Repeated doses of endotoxin produce a phenomenon known as tolerance, that is, the cellular infiltrate is markedly reduced. The ocular changes appear to be largely independent of the strain of rat or the source of the endotoxin. Endotoxin administered to rabbits induces a marked change in vascular permeability and a relatively scant uveal cellular infiltrate, whereas endotoxin given to rats induces a modest change in vascular permeability and marked cellular infiltration.

An analysis of the causes of endotoxin-induced uveitis is complicated by the multiple biological effects of endotoxin, both direct and indirect. These effects include activation of complement,[13] coagulation,[14] and kinin;[15] cascades, platelet aggregation,[16] mast cell degranulation,[17] and prostaglandin synthesis.[18] The unique susceptibility of the eye does not appear to be due to an endotoxin concentrating effect as determined by radiolabelled studies.[19,20] The active moiety of the endotoxin molecule is probably the core lipid A.[12,21]

Pharmacologic studies in the rat have been more limited than those in the rabbit. In both rat and rabbit, prostaglandins and serotonin appear to be involved, based on studies using indomethacin and cyproheptadine (Cousins,

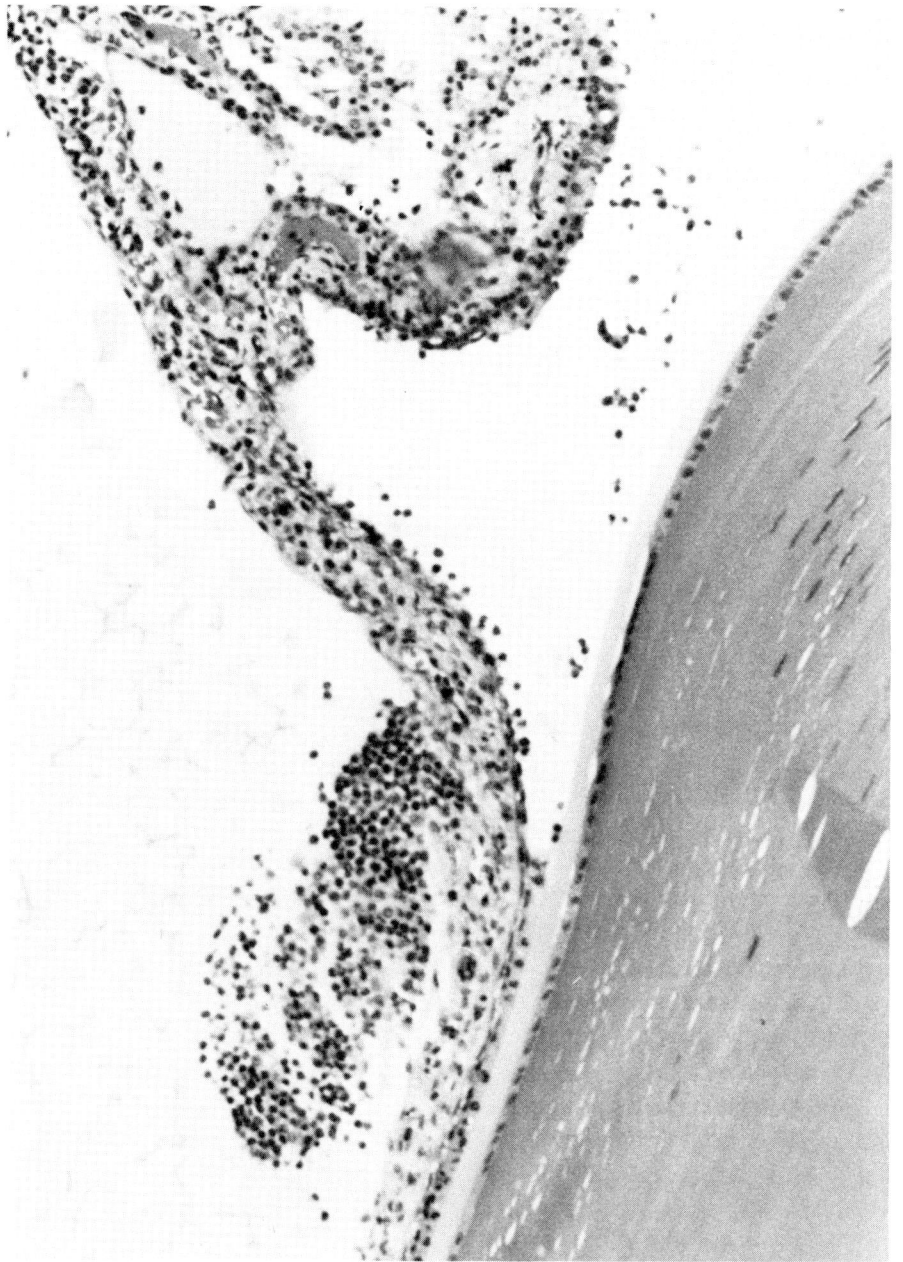

Figure 24-1. Low power view of the anterior uveal tract of a rat 24 hours after systemic administration of 100 μg of endotoxin. A cellular infiltrate is present in and around the iris and ciliary body. A nodule of cells is adjacent to the iris. The lens is at the bottom of the photomicrograph.

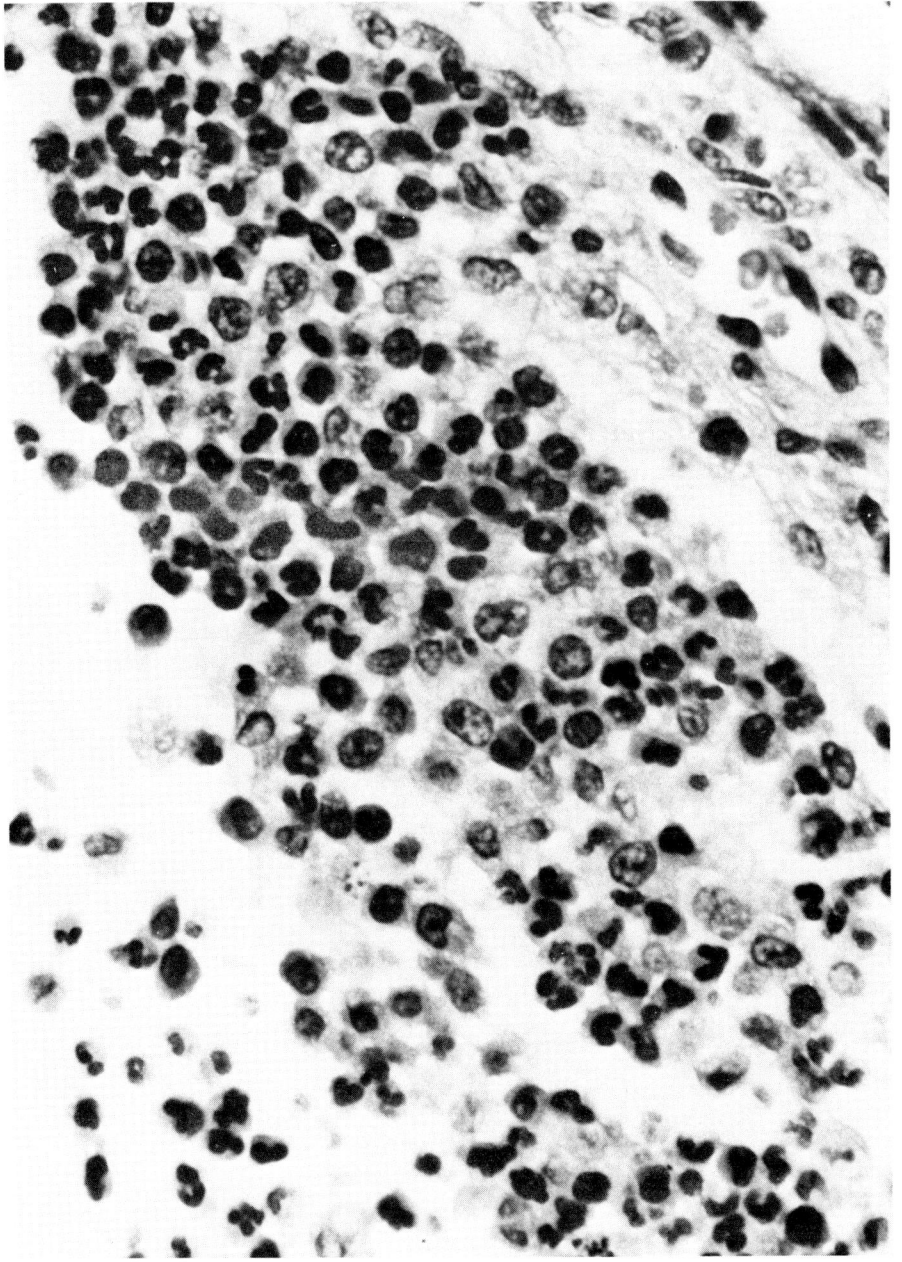

Figure 24-2. A higher power view of the iris nodule seen in Figure 24-1. The cellular infiltrate is a combination of polymorphonuclear leukocytes and mononuclear cells.

Rosenbaum, Guss, Howes, unpublished). The ability of a drug to affect one phase of the response does not necessarily parallel its ability to affect another phase.

Relevance of Endotoxin-Induced Uveitis to Human Disease

Some forms of uveitis have a temporal relationship to bowel diseases that are a possible source of endotoxin.[22] This includes the uveitis associated with inflammatory bowel disease and that which follows the gram-negative dysenteries associated with Reiter's syndrome. A cross reaction between the major histocompatibility antigen HLA B27 and certain isolates of *Klebsiella* has been reported.[23] Bowel colonization with *Klebsiella*, in association with episodes of acute anterior uveitis, has also been observed.[24] However, several observations argue against a direct role for endotoxin-induced uveitis in humans. First, anterior uveitis is not seen in association with gram-negative sepsis or when small doses of endotoxin are given as with typhoid vaccine. Second, the uveitis observed in rats is bilateral and begins within 24 hours after endotoxin injection. The uveitis associated with gram-negative dysentery or Reiter's syndrome occurs from one to four weeks after the diarrhea and is characteristically unilateral. Finally, the B27–*Klebsiella* cross reaction has been difficult for several investigators to reproduce.[25]

As I have mentioned, fever therapy was for many years a standard treatment for uveitis.[26] Often the fever was induced by salmonella endotoxin in the form of typhoid vaccine. Could a substance used for uveitis therapy also be implicated in the pathogenesis of a disease? Anterior uveitis is no more a single disease entity than arthritis. Uveitis represents inflammation that could be the end product of a variety of inciting events. Although endotoxin is unlikely by itself to induce a sustained uveitis in man, circumstantial evidence would at least suggest that in some instances it might contribute to eye inflammation. For example, one hypothesis would be that endotoxin from, say, *Shigella* dysentery induces only a mild, subclinical change in ocular vascular permeability, but that this change is sufficient to allow the deposition of a foreign antigen that eventually becomes the target of a cellular immune response and inflammation.[27] Paralleling the observation that endotoxin in the form of fever therapy can be used to treat uveitis is the recent experimental demonstration that endotoxin can potently inhibit some forms of ocular inflammation.[28] For example, rabbits made tolerant to endotoxin by five daily injections are resistant to the uveal inflammation induced by an ocular reversed passive Arthus reaction.

Circumstantial evidence suggests that endotoxin might contribute to the induction of uveitis in man, and uncontrolled clinical evidence suggests that endotoxin is capable of inhibiting uveal inflammation. Other substances such as prostaglandins are also known to be both inflammatory and anti-inflammatory.[29] Hopefully, endotoxin-induced uveitis in the rat will prove a useful model for resolving the role of endotoxin in human ocular inflammation.

REFERENCES

1. Woods, A. C.: Action of toxins on eye. *Arch Ophthalmol, 45*:451–464, 1916.
2. Ayo, C.: New observations on a primary ocular reaction to Shwartzman toxins. *Proc Soc Exp Biol, 47*:500–501, 1941.
3. Ayo, C. A.: Toxic ocular reaction: I. New property of Shwartzman toxins. *J Immunol, 47*:113–125, 1943.
4. Howes, E. L., McKay, D. G., and Margaretten, W.: The participation of the platelet in the vascular response to endotoxemia in the rabbit eye. *Am J Path, 70*:25–44, 1973.
5. Levene, R. Z., and Breinin, G. M.: Ocular effects of endotoxin. *Arch Ophthalmol, 61*:568–577, 1959.
6. Bengtsson, E.: The effect of imidazole on the disruption of the blood-aqueous barrier in the rabbit eye. *Invest Ophthalmol, 15*:315–320, 1976.
7. Howes, E. L., and McKay, D. G.: The effects of aspirin and indomethacin on the ocular response to circulating bacterial endotoxin in the rabbit. *Invest Ophthalmol Vis Sci, 15*:648–651, 1976.
8. Howes, E. L., and McKay, D. G.: Comparison of the ocular effects of circulating endotoxin and immune complexes. Role of vasoactive amines. *J Immunol, 114*:734–740, 1975.
9. Cousins, S. W., Rosenbaum, J. T., Guss, R. B., and Egbert, P. R.: Ocular albumin fluorophotometric quantitation of endotoxin-induced vascular permeability. *Infect Immun, 36*:730–736, 1982.
10. Bito, L. Z.: Inflammatory effects of endotoxin-like contaminants in commonly used protein preparations. *Science, 196*:83–85, 1977.
11. Pearson, C. M., and Chang, Y. M.: Adjuvant disease: pathology and immune reactivity. *Ann Rheum Dis* (Suppl) *38*:102–109, 1979.
12. Rosenbaum, J. T., McDevitt, H. O., Guss, R. B., and Egbert, P. R.: Endotoxin-induced uveitis in rats as a model for human disease. *Nature, 286*:611–613, 1980.
13. Gilbert, Y. E., and Braude, A. I.: Reduction of serum complement in rabbits after injection of endotoxin. *J Exp Med, 116*:477–490, 1962.
14. Shen, S. M.-C, Rapaport, S. I., and Feinstein, D. I.: Intravascular clotting after endotoxin in rabbits with impaired clotting produced by Factor VIII antibody. *Blood, 42*:523–534, 1973.
15. Erdos, E. G., and Miwa, I.: Effect of endotoxin shock on the plasma kallikrein-kinin system of the rabbit. *Fed Proc, 27*:92–95, 1968.
16. Walker, R. I., Shields, L. J., and Fletcher, J. R.: Platelet aggregation in rabbits made tolerant to endotoxin. *Infect Immun, 19*:919–922, 1978.
17. Hook, W. A., Snyderman, R., and Mergenhagen, S.: Further characterization of a factor from endotoxin treated serum which releases histamine and heparin from mast cells. *Infect Immun, 5*:909–914, 1972.
18. Wahl, L. M., Olsen, C. E., Sandberg, A. L., and Mergenhagen, S. G.: Prostaglandin regulation of macrophage collagenase production. *Proc Natl Acad Sci, 74*:4955–4958, 1977.
19. Rosenbaum, J. T., Hendricks, P. A., Shively, J. E., and McDougall, I. R.: Distribution of radiolabelled endotoxin with particular reference to the eye. Concise communication. *J Nucl Med, 24*:29–33, 1983.

20. Howes, E. L., Hoffman, M. A., Ulevitch, R. J., and Morrison, D. C.: Ocular localization of circulating lipopolysaccharide in the rabbit. *Invest Ophthalmol* (Suppl), *20*:101, 1981 (Abstract).
21. Howes, E. L., and Morrison, D. C.: Lipid A dependence of the ocular response to circulating endotoxin in rabbits. *Infect Immun, 30*:786–790, 1980.
22. Aoki, B.: A study of endotoxemia in ulcerative colitis and Crohn's disease. I, Clinical Study. *Acta Med Okayama, 32*:147–158, 1978.
23. Seager, K., Bashir, H. V., Geczy, A. F., Edmonds, J., and De Vere-Tyndall, A: Evidence for a specific B27-associated cell surface marker on lymphocytes of patients with ankylosing spondylitis. *Nature, 277*:68–70, 1977.
24. Ebringer, R., Cawdell, D., and Ebringer, A.: Klebsiella pneumoniae and acute anterior uveitis in ankylosing spondylitis. *Br Med J, 1*:383, 1979.
25. Archer, J. R.: Search for cross-reactivity between HLA B27 and *Klebsiella* pneumoniae. *Ann Rheum Dis, 40*:400–403, 1981.
26. Solomon, H. C., and Kopp, I.: Fever therapy. *N Engl J Med, 217*:805–809, 1937.
27. Rosenbaum, J. T., and Cousins, S. W.: Uveitis and arthritis. Experimental models and clinical correlates. *Seminars Arthr Rheum, 11*:383–389, 1982.
28. Howes, E. L., Rosenbaum, J. T., and Goldstein, I. M.: Endotoxin-tolerant rabbits resist an ocular reverse passive Arthus reaction. *Invest Ophthalmol* (Suppl), *22*:210, 1982 (Abstract).
29. Kunkel, S. L., Thrall, R. S., Kunkel, R. G., McCormick, J. R., Ward, P. A., and Zurier, R. B.: Suppression of immune complex vasculitis in rats by prostaglandin. *J Clin Invest, 64*:1525–1529, 1979.

Chapter 25

CANINE SYSTEMIC LUPUS ERYTHEMATOSUS

ROBERT M. WEBB, M.D.

Introduction

Systemic lupus erythematosus (SLE) is a disease of diverse features with clinical and immunological manifestations. The etiology is unknown. An immune complex mediated mechanism[1] is known to be involved in the pathogenesis of certain clinical features of the disease, which occurs spontaneously in three known species: man, dog, and mice. Much information concerning the causes and pathophysiology of the disease in man has been gleaned from the study of murine[2,3] and canine[4] models of naturally occurring systemic lupus erythematosus. In this chapter I shall review the canine model of SLE.

Clinical Manifestation of Canine SLE

Systemic lupus erythematosus as a spontaneously occurring canine disease was first described in a classic paper by Lewis et al.[4] The disease is characterized by autoimmune hemolytic anemia, membranous glomerulonephritis, and idiopathic thrombocytopenic purpura. Symmetrical polyarthritis and vesiculobullous skin disease have since been recognized as common manifestations of the disease process.[5] The disease affects young adults of various breeds—females more commonly than males.[3,6] In addition to these major features, other less frequently encountered clinical findings are recognized.[7]

The course of canine SLE is characterized by remissions and exacerbations that may lead to renal failure secondary to chronic glomerulonephritis. Renal failure is the most common cause of death.[6,8] High dose systemic corticosteroids is the treatment of choice, although other immunosuppressive drugs and salicylates may be helpful in certain cases.[9] The corticosteroids are effective in combating the autoimmune hemolytic anemia and idiopathic thrombocytopenic purpura, but they do not prevent or improve the glomerular lesions.[6] Appropriate analgesics are given for pain; concurrent infections are given antibiotics, and digitalis and low salt diets are prescribed for the cardiovascular disease. Transfusions may be performed to correct the anemia.[7]

Laboratory Features of Canine SLE

Multiple serologic abnormalities are characteristic of canine SLE. The most important of these is the LE cell phenomenon, which is highly specific for SLE in dogs[10] and is the most reliable indicator of the disease.[11] The LE cell is a polymorphonuclear leukocyte that has in its cytoplasma a large basophillic inclusion body composed of IgG (antinuclear antibody of ANA) and nuclear material. The cytoplasma becomes distended with this material, so that the normal nucleus of the cell is compressed against the cytoplasmic membrane.[7,12,13] The LE cell test thus represents an indirect test for antinuclear antibody.[4] The ANA test is frequently positive as well in SLE, although it is said to be less specific for the disease than the LE cell test.[14]

The most specific indicator of the disease is an antibody to DNA found in the serum of patients with SLE. This antibody is unique to SLE.[14,15] Other, less specific, findings indicative of the autoimmune nature of the disease are the presence of antithyroid antibody, erythrocyte autoantibody, anti-platelet antibody, and rheumatoid factor.[6,11,16,17]

An autoantibody that has recently been described as occurring in 75–90 percent of dogs with SLE is natural lymphocytotoxic antibody (NLA).[5] This autoantibody may serve as a marker for the disease years before it becomes manifest clinically and can be responsible for the systematic destruction of both T and B lymphocytes. Circulating immune complexes have also been found in a majority of dogs with SLE and can also be present in the serum before clinical signs develop.[5]

As a result of these multiple autoantibodies, a polyclonal hypergammaglobulinemia is found in patients with SLE.[18]

TABLE 25-I
CLINICAL AND LABORATORY FINDINGS OF CANINE SLE

	Clinical	Laboratory
Most Common	Autoimmune hemolytic anemia	LE cell
	Membranous glomerulonephritis	Antinuclear antibody (ANA)
	Idopathic thrombocytopenic purpura	Anti-DNA antibody
	Symmetrical polyarthritis	Natural lymphocytotoxic antibody (NLA)
	Vessiculobullous skin disease	Circulating immune complexes
		Polyclonal hypergammaglobulinemia
Least Common	Lymphadenopathy	Antithryoid antibody
	Polymyositic	Erythrocyte autoantibody
	Peripheral neuritis	Antiplatelet antibody
	Pleuritis	Rheumatoid factor
	Pericarditis	

Histopathologic Features

The pathological lesions are variable and correlate well with the clinical signs[19] but the most distinctive lesions found in canine SLE are those in the blood vessels and lymphoid tissue.[14] The vascular lesions can affect many organs and most frequently involve the small muscular arterioles. These develop a fulminant, necrotizing vasculitis and eventually undergo a chronic, segmental fibrinoid change.[14] This is particularly evident in the kidney, where the characteristic lesion is a chronic proliferative membraneous glomerulonephritis. There is marked thickening of the glomerular basement membrane and focal accumulations of lymphocytes and plasma cells.[10] The glomerular capillaries assume a "wire loop" configuration, and there is hyaline thickening of Bowman's capsule.[6] The end result is glomerulosclerosis and chronic renal failure.

These pathologic changes are mediated by immune complexes, with the deposition of complement and immunoglobulins on the glomerular basement membranes.[5] These complexes are demonstrated by immunofluorescent techniques, which show apple green, granular deposits on the glomerular basement membrane.

Lymph nodes become enlarged in canine SLE, and both the lymph nodes and thymus exhibit active germinal centers with large accumulations of lymphocytes and plasma cells.[10,14] Joint tissues show thickening of the synovial membrane and inflammatory cell infiltration, with eventual periarticular fibrosis.[14,20] The skin lesions also show infiltrations of lymphocytes and plasma cells, with degeneration of basal epithelial cells and hyperkeratosis and parakeratosis.[14] Direct immunofluorescence demonstrates granular accumulations of immunoglobulin and complement in the basement membrane between the dermis and epidermis.[5]

Other changes include extramedullary hematopoiesis, erythrophagocytosis, magakaryocytic hyperplasia, and multifocal hemorrhages.[14]

Etiology

Most of what is known about the etiology of canine SLE has resulted from genetic and viral experiments. Lewis and Schwartz[21] established a large closed inbred colony of dogs to study the possibility of a hereditary role in the pathogenesis of SLE. A positive LE cell test was chosen as the phenotypic marker for the disease. Several experiments using inbred, outbred, and backcrossed progeny were performed.[22] Ninety-five percent of the inbred dogs were LE-cell-test positive by 18 months of age, and a high percentage of the outbred and outcrossed animals were also positive.[14] Many of the animals had antinuclear antibody as well as rheumatoid factor in their serum.[21]

Despite these serologic abnormalities, no clinical disease developed in the progeny, although there was a high incidence of thymic lesions in the inbred progeny.[22] These lesions were typical of those found in animals with overt SLE and consisted of multiple lymphoid follicles with active germinal centers.[22]

The data compiled from the experiments does not conform to any typical or classical mode of inheritance, but it indicates a more complicated genetic mechanism. A theory involving a complex interaction of two classes of unlinked genes has been proposed by Quimby et al.[23] Class I genes are postulated as being involved with immunoregulation, specifically with the interaction between T and B lymphocytes. They impart a general predisposition to an autoimmune disease. The immune response (Ir) genes are in all likelihood members of this class. Class II genes are those that determine the pathological features of the disease (i.e. complement levels, antibody type and concentration, and immune complex size). An individual would need alleles from both of these classes of genes to develop an autoimmune disease.[23]

A viral etiology in canine SLE was suggested by transmission experiments using cell-free filtrates from the spleens and lymph nodes of dogs with positive LE cell tests and ANA from within the breeding colony.[8,22,24] These filtrates were injected into dogs, mice, and rats, and the animals were tested for the serologic markers of SLE. They were also observed for the development of clinical disease. Although overt disease did not develop in the recipients, many of the dogs and mice were seropositive for antinuclear antibody, antibody to native DNA, and the LE cell. The rats did not demonstrate these markers. This suggests an infectious agent in the transmission of SLE, although none was isolated from the filtrates.[25]

The development of lymphomas in 5.9 percent of the murine recipients of the canine filtrates in the above experiments supports the theory that a transmissable agent was present. These lymphomas consisted of three cell types: an atypical reticulum cell tumor, a lymphoblastic lymphoma, and an undifferentiated type that produced a monoclonal immunoglobulin.[24] These tumors are all transplantable, and multiple testing methods showed that the tumors contained murine leukemia viruses.[22,26] In all cases, the tumors followed the development of antinuclear antibody in the recipients, and cell-free filtrates prepared from them induced the formation of ANA in normal newborn puppies and allogenic mice.[8,27]

The tumor that produced the monoclonal protein was found to be a plasmacytoma that produced monoclonal IgA antibody against native DNA. It was designated "SP-104" and underwent extensive investigation.[25,28] When this tumor was grown in tissue culture, the cultivated cells were shown to produce numerous C-type virus particles, as well as monoclonal IgA antibody against native DNA.[29] The virus was identified as a B-tropic virus with an AKR envelope coat, and purified virions are capable of inducing anti-DNA antibodies in 75 percent of murine recipients.[25]

It is conceivable, then, that the canine cell-free filtrates contained a virus that was transmitted to murine cells. In some way, a latent murine leukemia virus was activated and led to the development of anti-DNA antibody, ANA, and malignant lymphomas in the host.[22,25,28]

The lymphocytes of a dog, with serological but without clinical evidence of SLE, were studied using immunofluorescent techniques.[25] They were found to contain an antigen on their cell membrane that reacted positively to antisera prepared to viral antigen. The viral antigen was P-30, a common interspecies C-type viral particle. The animal eventually developed clinical disease and died of the nephrotic syndrome. Immunopathological studies of the kidneys showed deposits of immune complexes on the glomerular basement membranes. Positive immunofluorescence was also found to antisera prepared to the viral antigens P-30 and SP-104. Eluates prepared from the kidney showed antibodies to DNA and to SP-104 by indirect immunofluorescence.[25] These studies imply that viral antigen is deposited in the kidney as part of a circulating immune complex, and that the presence of viral antigen on the surface of lymphocytes serves as a marker for prior or present viral infection.[25]

Studies on the canine led to the investigation of possible human correlates to the canine SLE model. Lewis et al. showed that the serum of a 12-year-old girl with active SLE contained an antibody that reacted with the lymphocytic cell membrane of eight of ten patients with SLE.[30] No reaction was found with lymphocytes from normal patients. When adsorption studies were performed, it was found that this cell membrane antigen shared determinants with C-type virus particles produced by the SP-104 tissue culture.[12,30] Strand and August documented the presence of P-30 antigen in the extracts of spleens from two humans with SLE.[31] Panem et al. found a human C-type viral antigen (HEL-12 virus) deposited as part of an immune complex on the glomerular basement membrane in kidneys from human patients with SLE.[32,33] Mellors and Mellors showed, by indirect immunofluorescence, an antigen related to the P-30 C-type virus in the kidney and spleen of a patient with SLE.[34]

The possibility of SLE transmission between dog and humans was suggested by a study of dogs in the households of two families in which several people had the disease.[35] The dogs both had clinical and serologic abnormalities suggestive of SLE, including high levels of anti-DNA antibody. This important correlation between the human and canine disease needs further support and is fertile area for further study.

It is interesting that ocular findings, a well-recognized entity in human SLE, have not been described in the canine. They occur mostly in patients with overt, active disease.[36] The clinical signs are retinal arteriolar narrowing, retinal hemorrhages, retinal edema, papilledema, cottonwool spots, arteriolar and venous occlusion, retinal perivasculitis, conjunctivitis, scleritis, episcleritis, and anterior uveitis.[36,37] The retinal vasculitis is presumed to be mediated by immune complexes, which have been nicely demonstrated by Aronson et al., who found deposits of immunoglobulins and complement in the vascular layer of choroidal capillaries and on the basement membrane of ciliary processes and bulbar conjunctiva.[37] Thus, the same pathogenesis is implicated in the ocular lesions as that occurring in other organs of the body. It could be that ocular lesions were simply not looked for either clinically or histopathologically in the canine experiments, and thus not recognized.

Conclusion

Systemic lupus erythematosus is a complex multisystem disease with interacting genetic, immunologic, and viral factors. The study of the disease in dogs has led to a greater understanding of its human counterpart. Once again, the dog has proved its immeasurable worth to man.

REFERENCES

1. Agnello, V., Koffler, D., and Kunkel, H. G.: Immune complex systems in the nephritis of systemic lupus erythematosus. *Kid Int, 3*:90–99, 1973.
2. Talal, N.: Disordered immunologic regulation and autoimmunity. *Transpl Rev, 31*:240–263, 1976.
3. Quimby, J. W., and Schwartz, R. S.: The etiopathogenesis of systemic lupus erythematosus. *Pathobiol Annu, 8*:31–65, 1978.
4. Lewis, R. M., Schwartz, R., and Henry, W. B.: Canine systemic lupus erythematosus. *Blood, 25*:143–160, 1965.
5. Lewis, R. M., and Quimby, F.: Systemic lupus erythematosus, model no. 27, supplemental update, 1981. In Capen, C. C., Hackel, D. B., Jones, T. C. and Migaki, G. (Eds.): *Handbook: Animal Models of Human Disease*. Fasc. 10. Registry of Comparative Pathology, Armed Forces Institute of Pathology, Washington, D.C., 1981.
6. Lewis, R. M., Schwartz, R. S., and Gilmore, C. E.: Autoimmune diseases in domestic animals. *Ann NY Acad Sci, 124*:178–200, 1965.
7. Alexander, J. W., George, J. W., and Moffa, J. V.: A case of systemic lupus erythematosus in a dog. *Vet Med Small Anim Clin, 70*:147–154, 1975.
8. Lewis, R. M.: Spontaneous autoimmune diseases of domestic animals. *Int Rev Exp Pathol, 13*:55–82, 1974.
9. Utroska, B.: Autoimmune hemolytic anemia associated with lupus erythematosus. *Vet Med Small Anim Clin, 71*:1247–1249.
10. Lewis, R. M.: Animal model: canine systemic lupus erythematosus. *Am J Pathol, 69*(3):537–540, 1972.
11. Schultz, R. D.: Immunologic disorders in the dog and cat. *Vet Clin North Am [Small Anim Pract], 4(1)*:153–174, 1974.

12. Lewis, R. M.: Clinical evaluation of the lupus erythematosus cell phenomenon in dogs. *J Am Vet Med Assoc, 147*(9):939–943, 1965.
13. Schalm, O. W., and King, C. V.: The LE cell phenomenon in the dog. *Calif Vet, 12*:20–25, 1970.
14. Lewis, R. M.: Systemic lupus erythematosus. In Shifrine, M., and Wilson, F. D. (Eds.): *The Canine as a Biomedical Research Model.* Oak Ridge, Tn, DOE, 1980, pp. 244–262.
15. Lewis, R. M., Stollar, B. D., and Goldberg, E. B.: A rapid sensitive test for the detection of antibodies to DNA. *J Immunol Meth, 3*:365–374, 1973.
16. Lewis, R. M., and Hathaway, J. E.: Canine systemic lupus erythematosus presenting with symmetrical polyarthritis. *J Small Anim Pract, 8*:273–284, 1967.
17. Wilkins, R. J., Hurvitz, A. I., and Dodd-Laffin, W. J.: Immunologically mediated thrombocytopenia in the dog. *J Am Vet Assoc, 163*:277–282, 1973.
18. Quimby, F. W.: Systemic lupus erythematosus. In Andrews, E. J., Ward, B. C., and Altman, N. H. (Eds.): *Spontaneous Animal Models of Human Disease.* New York, Acad Pr, 1979, vol. I, pp. 300–301.
19. Lewis, R. M.: Specific immunologic lesions. In Bernischke, K., Gainer, F. M., and Jones, T. C. (Eds.): *Pathology of Laboratory Animals.* New York, Springer-Verlag, 1978, vol. II, pp. 1953–1978.
20. Pederson, N. C., Weisner, K., Castles, J. J., Ling, G. C., and Weiser, G.: Non-infectious canine arthritis: the inflammatory, nonerosive arthritides. *J Am Vet Med Assoc, 196*:304–310, 1978.
21. Lewis, R. M., and Schwartz, R. S.: Canine systemic lupus erythematosus: genetic analysis of an established breeding colony. *J Exper Med, 134*(2):417–438, 1971.
22. Lewis, R. M., and Schwartz, R. S.: Canine systemic lupus erythematosus: a communicable disease? In Dumorde, D. C. (Ed.): *Infection and Immunology in the Rheumatic Diseases.* Philadelphia, Blackwell Scientific Publ., 1978, pp. 259–263.
23. Quimby, J. W., Jensen, C., Nawrock, D., and Scollin, P.: Selected autoimmune diseases in the dog. *Vet Clin North Am, 8*(4):665–682, 1978.
24. Lewis, R. M., Andre-Schwartz, J. A., Harris, G. S., Hirsch, M. S., Black, P. H., and Schwartz, R. S.: Canine systemic lupus erythematosus—transmission of serologic abnormalities by cell-free filtrates. *J Clin Invest, 52*(7):1893–1907, 1973.
25. Lewis, R. M.: Evidence for a virus in canine systemic lupus erythematosus. In Glynn, L. E. and Schlumberger, H. D. (Eds.): *Experimental Models of Chronic Inflammatory Diseases.* New York, Springer-Verlag, 1977, pp. 71–76.
26. Schwartz, R. S.: Viruses and systemic lupus erythematosus. *N Engl J Med, 293*(3):132–136, 1975.
27. Lewis, R. M.: Lessons learned from man's best friend: canine systemic lupus erythematosus. *Int J Derm, 16*(2):117–119, 1977.
28. Quimby, F. W., Gebert, R., Datta, S., André-Schwartz, J., Tannenberg, W. J., Lewis, R. M., Weinstein, T. B., and Schwartz, R. S.: Characterization of a retinovirus that cross-reacts seriologically with canine and human systemic lupus erythematosus (SLE). *Clin Immun Immunopath, 9*(2):194–210, 1978.
29. Dixon, J. A., Sugar, S., and Talal, N.: An unusual mouse myeloma protein-binding native DNA. *Clin Exp Immunol, 19*:347–354, 1975.
30. Lewis, R. M., Tannenberg, W., Smith, C., and Schwartz, R. S.: C-type viruses in systemic lupus erythematosus. *Nature, 252* (5478):78–79, 1974.
31. Stand, M., and August, J. T.: Type-C RNA virus gene expression in human tissue. *J Virol, 14*(6):1584–1596, 1974.

32. Panem, S., Ordonez, N. G., Kirsten, W. H., Katz, A. I., and Spargo, B. H.: C-type virus expression in systemic lupus erythematosus. *N Engl J Med*, 295(9):470–475, 1976.
33. Panem, S., Ordonez, N. G., Katz, A. I., Spargo, B. H., and Kirsten, W. H.: Viral immune complexes in systemic lupus erythematosus, specificity of C-type viral complexes. *Lab Invest*, 39:412–420, 1978.
34. Mellors, R. C., and Mellors, J. W.: Antigen related to mamallian type-C RNA viral P-30 proteins is located in renal glomeruli in human systemic lupus erythematosus. *Proc Natl Acad Sci USA*, 73(1):233–237, 1978.
35. Beaucher, W. N., Garman, R. H. and Condemic, J. J.: Antibodies to DNA in household dogs. *N Engl J Med*, 296(15):982–984, 1977.
36. Henkind, P., and Fox, L. E.: Ocular involvement in systemic immune disorders. In Garner, A., and Klintworth, G. K. (Eds.): *Pathobiology of Ocular Disease.* New York, Dekker, Marcel, 1982, pp. 203–207.
37. Aronson, A. J., Ordonez, N. G., Diddie, K. R., and Ernest, J. T.: Immune complex deposition in the eye in systemic lupus erythematosus. *Arch Intern Med*, 139:1312–1313, 1979.

Chapter 26

CONTACT HYPERSENSITIVITY IN GUINEA PIGS

MITCHELL H. FRIEDLAENDER, M.D.

Introduction

Immunologists have long been interested in experimental contact sensitivity in the guinea pig as a model of cell-mediated immunity and human allergic contact dermatitis. Jadassohn, in 1895, suggested that a skin reaction of low molecular weight was due to hypersensitivity rather than to toxicity. Since then, contact hypersensitivity has been studied extensively and has been clearly established as an antigen-specific form of delayed hypersensitivity. Once considered a relatively simple model of delayed hypersensitivity, contact sensitivity is now recognized as an extremely complex phenomenon. In this chapter we discuss our current understanding of contact sensitivity in the guinea pig, including the histologic changes we have studied in the skin and in the eye. The eye has been a useful organ in the study of contact sensitivity since its special anatomic features provide a unique setting in which we can observe complex immunologic phenomena.

Contact Sensitivity: Induction and Elicitation

The ability of a contactant to sensitize or elicit sensitivity when applied to the skin is proportional to its ability to couple covalently to protein. Thus, highly reactive compounds, such as the dinitro compounds, are good couplers and good sensitizers. Moderately reactive compounds, which are fair couplers, are weak sensitizers, and nonreactive congeners do not couple and therefore do not sensitize.

When a contact allergen is applied to the skin, it can escape by the hematologic or lymphatic route. Most of the compound leaves the skin site by the hematologic route. A small amount of the compound, however, can be detected in the lymph nodes draining the site of skin application. Whether interaction between the hapten and the lymphocyte takes place at the skin periphery (peripheral sensitization) or in the regional lymph node (afferent sensitization) is not clear. The draining lymph node enlarges, and increased cellular proliferation can be demonstrated. The manner in which the chemical arrives at the lymph node, the steps that take place in processing the

---

Supported in part by National Institutes of Health research grant EY-02502.

antigen, and the mechanisms by which lymphocytes recognize antigen are still unknown even after many years of study.

The efferent limb of the contact sensitivity reaction can be studied by painting the guinea pig's skin with a low concentration of hapten in acetone, alcohol, or olive oil. Delayed reactions develop over a period of 24–72 hours. These reactions are erythematous with a variable amount of induration. Serial dilutions of the hapten can be used to measure the threshold level of sensitivity, as can foot pad or ear swelling in mice, or the production of lymphokines (such as migration inhibition factor).

Histology

Lesions produced by contact sensitivity contain perivascular accumulations of mononuclear cells, similar to the tuberculin reaction. Dvorak[1] and Askenase[2] have noted the accumulation of basophilic leukocytes in contact sensitivity lesions both in guinea pigs and humans. The exact role of these cells is far from clear. However, it has been suggested that they may regulate the permeability of blood vessels through the vasoactive amines contained in their cytoplasmic granules.[3]

Antibody in Contact Sensitivity

It is widely believed that contact sensitivity reactions are dependent on T lymphocytes, and that B lymphocytes and plasma cells do not play a major role. Antibody can, however, be formed during the sensitization process, especially when adjuvants are used. Although no definite role for these antibodies has been elucidated, Askenase has shown that contact sensitivity can sometimes be transferred with serum.[4] Thus, the role of antibody and other serum factors in contact sensitivity may require further study.

Genetic Control of Contact Sensitivity

Successful transfer of contact sensitivity occurs only when donor and recipient animals share common region I genes. It is now clearly established that immune responses are controlled by genes, most of which lie in the major histocompatibility complex (MHC). Activation of most T cell functions requires recognition of antigen in association with certain gene products of the MHC. In general, region I gene products, in association with antigen, control the activation of helper T cells and T cells mediating delayed hypersensitivity, whereas gene products of the K and D region control effector functions of cytotoxic T cells.

Tolerance

Tolerance, or immune unresponsiveness, can be induced by contact sensitizers in several ways. Repeated low-dose applications of a sensitizer will diminish contact sensitivity. Intravenous or oral administration of the sensitizer before cutaneous application will also lower the level of sensitivity. The epicutaneous painting of mice with supraoptimal doses of a hapten will also lead to significantly depressed levels of sensitivity. The mechanism of tolerance is not clear. It is widely believed, however, that certain abnormally high or low dosages of antigen and certain routes of administration lead to an enhanced generation of suppressor cells or factors.

Langerhans Cells

The Langerhans cell, lost in obscurity for nearly a century, has emerged as a possible link in the afferent limb of the contact sensitivity response. Langerhans cells are not avidly phagocytic, but they can take up clinically important contact allergens. Furthermore, after contact sensitivity has been elicited by painting the skin of sensitive animals, Langerhans cells are frequently seen in close apposition to leukocytes at the challenge site.[5] These features suggest that Langerhans cells are antigen-presenting cells similar to macrophages of the lymphoid tissues. The appropriateness of these conclusions was reinforced by the finding that Langerhans cells carry the Ia histocompatibility antigens on their surfaces.

Ocular Contact Sensitivity

Most studies of contact sensitivity have employed the topical cutaneous or intradermal route of sensitization. It is not entirely clear whether contact sensitivity can be induced through the mucous membranes or elicited on the mucous membranes of the conjunctiva or the oral mucosa. In order to study this question, we sensitized guinea pigs systemically with the contact sensitizer oxazolone, by topical skin application and by intradermal injection with complete or incomplete Freund's adjuvant.[6] One to three weeks later, they were challenged with applications of oxazolone to the conjunctiva and skin. All guinea pigs sensitized with oxazolone by any of the three methods of sensitization demonstrated strongly positive skin test reactions upon cutaneous challenge. Inflammation of the external eye was also present in all animals 24 hours after challenge, but it was most intense in animals sensitized with oxazolone incomplete Freund's adjuvant. Reactions developed over a 24-hour period and consisted of erythema and induration of the eyelids, conjunctival injection, and a variable chemosis. Corneas remained clear except that when animals were sensitized with complete Freund's adjuvant, they developed corneal opacification and punctate epithelial defects.

The eyelids, conjunctiva, corneas, and ciliary bodies were diffusely infiltrated by large numbers of inflammatory cells, most of which were mononuclear. The intensity of inflammation was greatest in animals sensitized with oxazolone in CFA. Basophils were commonly observed in eyelid skin, but were generally absent from ocular tissues. In contrast, eosinophils were prominent features of all eye reactions and comprised up to 32 percent of the infiltrating cells.

It is clear from this study that contact sensitivity reactions can be elicited in ocular tissues, and that clinically significant changes can be produced in the conjunctiva and cornea. Conjunctival injection and chemosis as well as punctate corneal staining are especially marked when mycobacterial adjuvants are used during sensitization.

Materials and Methods

Fifty-five Hartley strain guinea pigs weighing 400–600 grams were used. Animals were sensitized with oxazolone (4-ethoxymethylene-2-phenyl oxazolone, BDH Chemicals, Poole, England) by five different routes (Table 26-I).

TABLE 26-I
SENSITIZATION WITH 4% OXAZOLONE ON THREE CONSECUTIVE DAYS

Route of Sensitization	Method of Application	Number of Animals
Conjunctiva	Subconjunctival injection	15
Conjunctiva	Topical	15
Oral mucosa	Topical	5
Nasal mucosa	Topical	5
Skin	Topical	15

A 4% solution of oxazolone was made up in olive oil, and .05 ml were injected subconjunctivally into the right eye of 15 guinea pigs on three consecutive days. Fifteen other animals received .05 ml of 4% oxazolone in olive oil instilled as eye drops into the right eye on three consecutive days. Five animals received a similar schedule of oxazolone application to the oral mucosa, and five animals had oxazolone applied to their nasal mucosa. Fifteen control animals were sensitized by applying .05 ml of 4% oxazolone in olive oil or alcohol to the skin of the right ear on three consecutive days.

Ten days after the first oxazolone application, all sensitized animals were skin tested by applying serial dilutions of oxazolone in alcohol to the shaven skin of the flank. Dilutions ranged from 1% to .05%. The weakest dilution to which an animal reacted with a positive, delayed onset skin reaction was considered the threshold skin reactive dose. The left eye of all guinea pigs was challenged with .05 ml of 1% oxazolone at the time of skin testing.

RESULTS

Animals sensitized by each of the five methods had positive skin reactions ten days after sensitization was begun. Reactions began to develop approximately eight hours after skin testing and reached a maximum 24 hours after testing. Usually lesions were somewhat faded by 48 hours. Reactions were erythematous but nonindurated.

Fifty-two of 55 guinea pigs became sensitive, while only three animals were nonreactive at the highest test dose. The threshold skin reactive dose was determined for each animal. This dose was the lowest concentration of oxazolone to which a sensitive animal responded. The mean threshold skin reactivity was calculated for each group (Table 26-II). There was no statistically significant difference in threshold skin reactivity between any two groups.

TABLE 26-II
SENSITIVITY TO OXAZOLONE

Number of Animals	Route of Sensitization	Mean Dose (% solution) for Threshold Skin Reaction Skin Reaction ± S.D.
15	Subconjunctival	0.39 ± .66
15	Conjunctiva-topical	0.22 ± .23
5	Oral	0.26 ± .22
5	Nasal	0.13 ± .06
15	Skin	0.23 ± .49

The left eyes were examined for evidence of inflammation 24 hours after oxazolone challenge. In those animals sensitized by the cutaneous route, the lids and conjunctiva of the challenged left eye became moderately inflamed within 24 hours after oxazolone application. Those animals sensitized by subconjunctival injections or by direct application to the right eye, or to the oral or nasal mucosa, showed only mild injection and chemosis of the opposite eye. The more inflamed eyes of animals sensitized through the skin contained a moderate number of inflammatory cells consisting mainly of mononuclear cells and eosinophils. The challenged eyes of animals sensitized by the mucosal route showed considerably less inflammation but they displayed a similar cellular composition.

Discussion

This study indicates that contact sensitivity in guinea pigs can be induced through the mucous membranes and that the level of sensitivity, as measured by skin testing, seems to be about the same whether animals are sensitized through the skin or the mucous membranes. Earlier studies held that application of simple chemicals to the conjunctiva and other mucous membranes did not lead to significant levels of sensitization. Indeed, some investigators have claimed application of simple chemicals to the mucous membranes favors the induction of tolerance rather than sensitization. Numerous factors, including the physical and chemical properties of the hapten, and the method of sensitization and challenge, may account for the difference in our results. We have observed patients who appear to develop ocular contact sensitivity by repeated application of drugs to the eye and who present with an allergic conjunctivitis or keratitis. While direct toxicity of a drug may produce similar clinical findings, it is possible that contact allergy induced through the conjunctiva could account for conjunctival and corneal inflammation. The role of the eosinophil in these reactions remains somewhat obscure. These cells seem to have a great affinity for ocular tissues and appear to be a prominent feature of delayed hypersensitivity reactions in the eye and in the skin.

Summary

In summary, contact sensitivity in the guinea pig has led to a better understanding of the mechanisms of cellular immunity, although several questions remain unanswered. The interaction between antigen and cells in the sensitization process requires further clarification. The role of Langerhans cells, while intriguing, has not been definitively studied. The role of the basophil and the eosinophil, prominent cells in cutaneous and ocular contact sensitivity respectively, requires further study that may shed some light on the broader functions of these cells.

REFERENCES

1. Dvorak, H. F., Dvorak, A. M., Simpson, B. A., Richerson, H. B., Leskowitz, S., and Karnovsky, M. J.: Cutaneous basophil hypersensitivity. II. A light and electron description. *J Exp Med,* 132:558, 1970.
2. Askenase, P. W.: Role of basophils, mast cells, and vasoamines in hypersensitivity reactions with a delayed time course. *Prog Allergy,* 23:199, 1977.
3. Friedlaender, M. H., and Dvorak, H. F.: Morphology of delayed-type hypersensitivity reactions in the guinea pig cornea. *J Immunol,* 118:1558, 1977.
4. Askenase, P. W.: Cutaneous basophil hypersensitivity in contact-sensitized guinea pigs. I. Transfer with immune serum *J Exp Med,* 138:1144, 1973.
5. Silberberg, I., Baer, R. L., and Rosenthal, S. A.: The role of Langerhans cells in allergic contact hypersensitivity. A review of findings in man and guinea pigs. *J Invest Dermatol,* 66:210, 1976.
6. Friedlaender M. H., and Cyr, R. J.: Contact sensitivity in the guinea pig eye. *Curr Eye Res,* 1:403, 1981.

Chapter 27

IMMEDIATE CONJUNCTIVAL HYPERSENSITIVITY REACTIONS IN THE GUINEA PIG AFTER SYSTEMIC SENSITIZATION

E. LEE STOCK, M.D.

Interest in immediate hypersensitivity reactions in the guinea pig conjunctiva began when Feinberg[1] noticed ocular inflammation coexisting with genital and pinnal inflammation of the guinea pig. These reactions developed after rabbit serum was injected intradermally for passive cutaneous anaphylaxis experiments. Although Feinberg felt that the reaction was a type of serum sickness, Dwyer and Darougar[2] established that the conjunctival reaction was a type of immediate hypersensitivity. They found that guinea pigs sensitized to low doses of normal rabbit serum developed edema of the conjunctiva shortly after topical ocular challenge. These animals developed both IgG and IgE-like homocytotropic serum antibody to the rabbit serum.[3] Histologic examinations showed that eosinophils, as well as some polymorphonuclear cells, had invaded the conjunctiva. The reactions were limited to the conjunctiva; the cornea was never involved.

Experimental Design

In our study, outbred Hartley female guinea pigs were sensitized. Sensitization consisted of the intradermal injection of 0.1 cc of normal rabbit serum (diluted 1:10 in normal saline) in each flank. The injections were repeated one week later. Three groups of animals were studied two years after sensitization. These animals had been used for pharmacologic experiments and had been challenged in the conjunctiva with normal rabbit serum at weekly intervals intermittently during the two years after sensitization. In the present experiments, one group of animals (Group A) was given 20 microliters of normal rabbit serum with a 30 gauge needle in the central cornea and four days later the same group of animals was skin tested with 0.1 cc of normal rabbit serum diluted 1:10 given intradermally to each animal. Four days after the intradermal challenge (eight days after the corneal challenge), the animals were anesthetized with pentobarbital, bled by cardiac puncture, killed with an overdose of pentobarbital, and the orbit and skin test sites were removed and subjected to histologic evaluation.

Two groups of animals were challenged topically in the conjunctiva with one drop of normal rabbit serum (Groups B and C). At 24 hours they were anesthetized, bled by cardiac puncture, killed with an overdose of pentobarbital, and the orbits were removed and processed for histologic study.

Controls for the corneal injections consisted of animals not previously sensitized, which were given 20 microliters of normal rabbit serum in the central cornea with a 30 gauge needle. They were killed with an overdose of pentobarbital three days later and the orbits removed and processed for histologic examination.

Serum was tested for precipitating antibody on Oucterlony plates against various dilutions of ovalbumin. Serum was tested for IgG homocytotropic antibody and IgE-like homocytotropic antibody by the passive cutaneous anaphylaxic (PCA) test of Ovary. For IgE-like homocytotropic antibody, serum at different dilutions was placed intradermally in neutral guinea pigs. Ten days later the animals were given ovalbumin in Evans Blue dye intravenously. The test sites were read 30 minutes after the intravenous injection. Any bluing of greater than 5 mm was considered positive. IgE-like antibody is heat and 2-mercaptoethanol sensitive. IgG homocytotropic antibody titers were determined by either heating the serum for one hour at 56°C or dialysing it against 2-mercaptoethanol. Dilutions were then placed in neutral guinea pigs and challenged after 24 hours as described above.

Results

The animals injected intracorneally (Group A) showed progressive corneal edema and vascularization. At 30 minutes the cornea was edematous centrally secondary to the injections (Fig. 27-1). In addition, the conjunctiva showed marked hyperemia, an immediate hypersensitivity reaction. At eight hours there was a diffuse ground glass appearance to the cornea and by 24 hours there was diffuse edema with intracorneal hemorrhage. At four days there was severe vascularization and opacification of the cornea, which progressed through the seventh day (Fig. 27-2). Histologic examination revealed a diffuse corneal infiltration, mainly of mononuclear cells, and new vessels in the cornea (Fig. 27-3). Skin tests showed immediate wheal and flare reaction followed by subsequent induration and necrosis (Fig. 27-4).

The two groups (B and C) challenged topically showed conjunctival edema immediately after the topical application of rabbit serum. The edema often persisted for eight hours but not for as long as 24 hours. Histologically, the conjunctiva showed eosinophils and polymorphonuclear cells infiltrating the tissue. There was no corneal damage.

Control animals that were not previously sensitized and that received 20 microliters of normal rabbit serum in the central cornea showed corneal

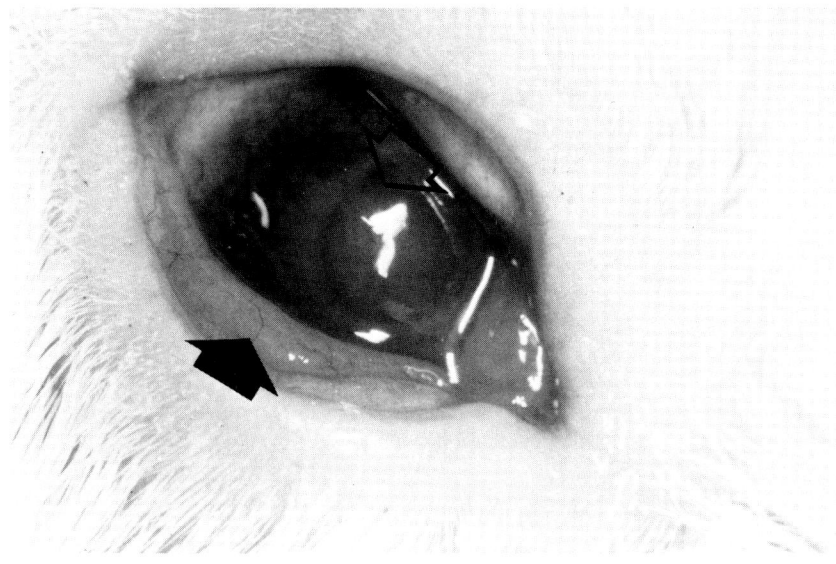

Figure 27-1: Thirty minutes after intracorneal injection of normal rabbit serum in sensitized guinea pigs. Note edematous cornea (white arrow) and conjunctival edema (black arrow).

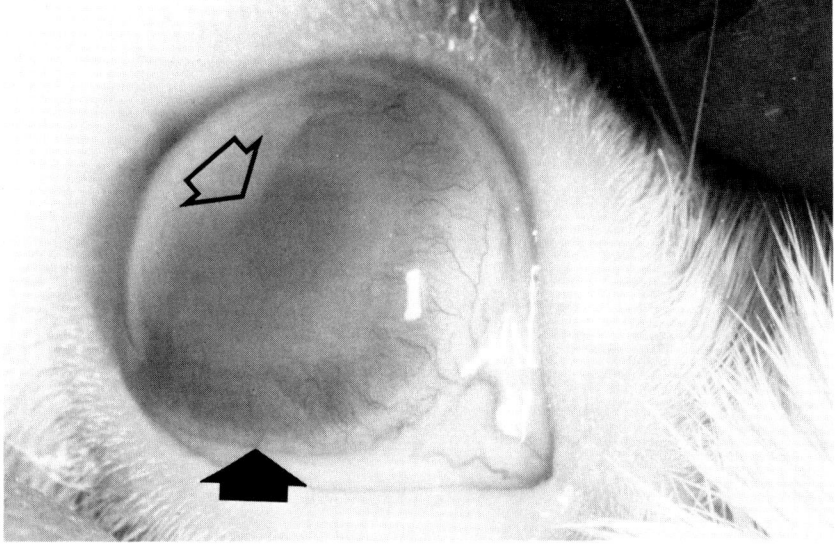

Figure 27-2: Seven days after intracorneal injection. Note opaque cornea (white arrow) and neovascularization (black arrow).

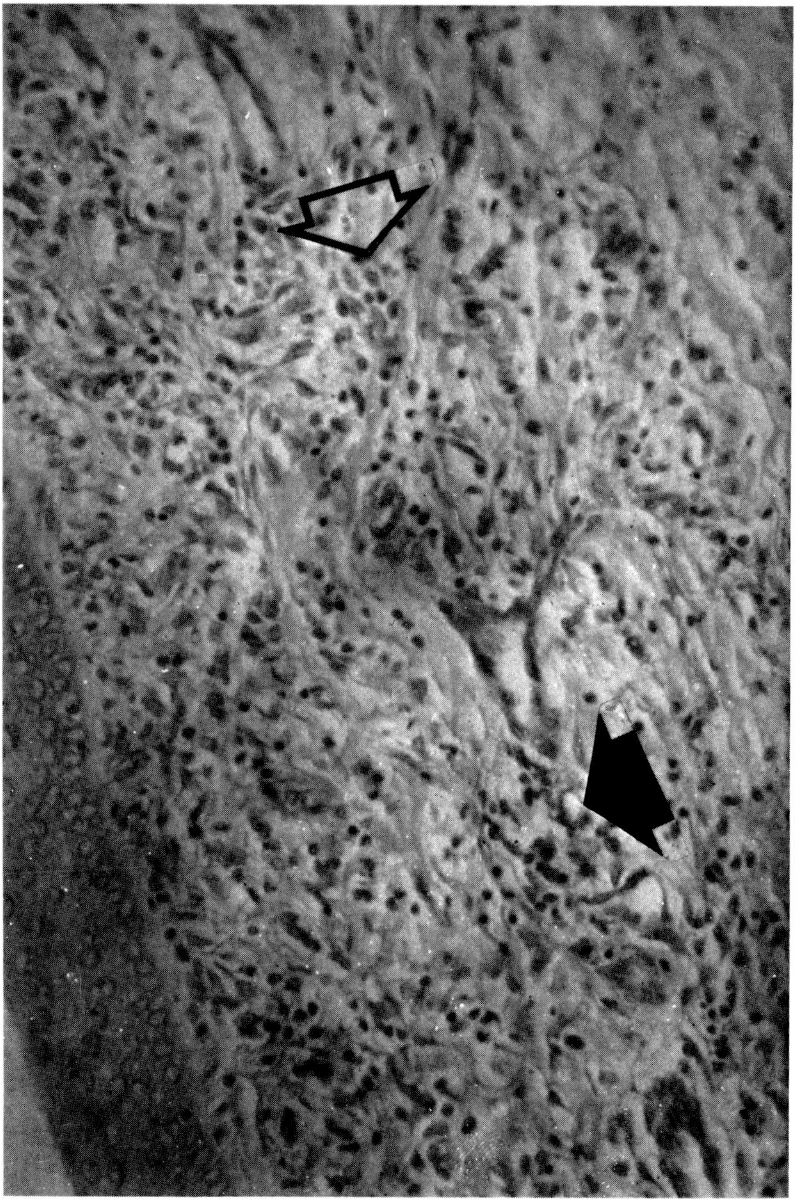

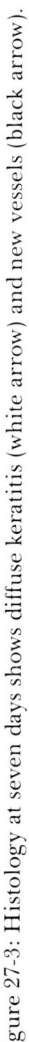

Figure 27-3: Histology at seven days shows diffuse keratitis (white arrow) and new vessels (black arrow).

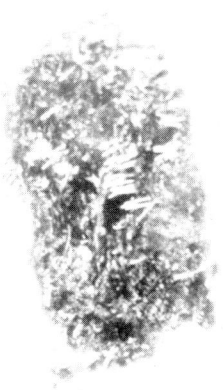

Figure 27-4: Skin necrosis in sensitized animals skin tested with normal rabbit serum.

edema after the injection, but there was no evidence of severe keratitis. Focal scarring, however, could be noted (Fig. 27-5). Serum tested on Ouchterlony plates showed no precipitating antibody. Serum antibody showed IgE-like titers of 1:5000 for Group A and 1:6000 for Groups B and C. Groups B and C did not have cornea or skin challenges and served as controls for Group A. Testing for IgE homocytotropic antibody showed lower titers, suggesting that most of the antibody was IgE-like with some IgG (Fig. 27-6).

Comment

Guinea pigs sensitized to low doses of normal rabbit serum mounted large antibody responses, mostly IgE-like, which could be detected two years after sensitization. They had immediate hypersensitivity responses in the conjunctiva with no conjunctival or corneal complications even after many challenges. However, when the antigen was given intracorneally and intradermally, severe vascularization of the cornea occurred, as well as skin necrosis.

This suggests that the high serum IgE-like titers and topical challenge do not result in permanent corneal or conjunctival structural change, but that

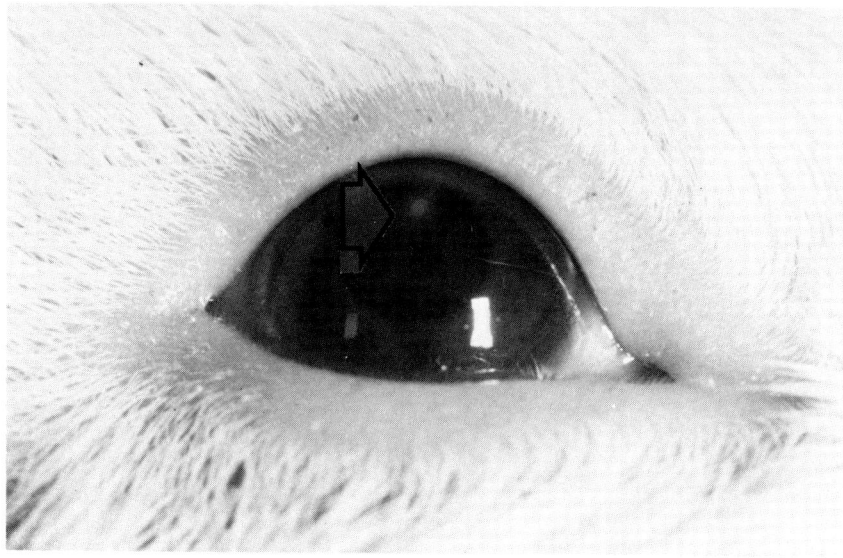

Figure 27-5: Focal scarring (white arrow) of cornea of control animals not previously sensitized, seven days after intracorneal injection of normal rabbit serum.

	Untreated 10 days	Heat treated 24 hours	2 M E treated 24 hours
Group A	5,000	3,000	1,000
B	6,000	2,000	1,000
C	6,000	2,000	1,000

Figure 27-6: Reciprocal PCA titers of the three groups of guinea pigs two years after sensitization.

another mechanism, perhaps a delayed type of hypersensitivity, may be required for corneal changes.

Additional studies were planned using this same model. However, it was found that this type of sensitization did not induce hypersensitivity when additional animals were sensitized. These negative results were demonstrated by the investigators working in London with Professor Barrie Jones' laboratory and by our group. I, therefore, sought other models for immediate conjunctival hypersensitivity.

A short paper by Tuffin and Feinberg[4] suggested that ovalbumin injected intradermally would be satisfactory in sensitizing guinea pigs for immediate conjunctival hypersensitivity. In a paper presented at the Ocular Microbiology and Immunology Group Meeting in 1980,[5] we reported that animals sensitized in this manner did develop immediate conjunctival hypersensitivity with eosinophils in the conjunctiva and serum PCA antibody. However, in a recent group of experiments we found that this hypersensitivity was extremely variable and short lived depending on the group of animals.

Twenty guinea pigs were sensitized in four groups of five animals with 500 micrograms of ovalbumin dissolved between the two flanks. They were challenged with 500 micrograms of ovalbumin dissolved in 20 microliters of normal saline dropped onto the eye. The animals were examined with an operating microscope 30 minutes after challenge and the conjunctival edema was graded on a scale of 0 to 3 in five different areas of the conjunctiva: upper tarsal conjunctiva, upper bulbar conjunctiva, medial conjunctiva near the canthus, inferior bulbar conjunctiva, and inferior tarsal conjunctiva. Scores were averaged, giving a mean edema score per animal. In two groups (Experiments 543 and 539), booster injections were given at 36 or 48 days respectively in an attempt to augment the immune response.

The mean edema score is presented in the graph (Fig. 27-7). The animals

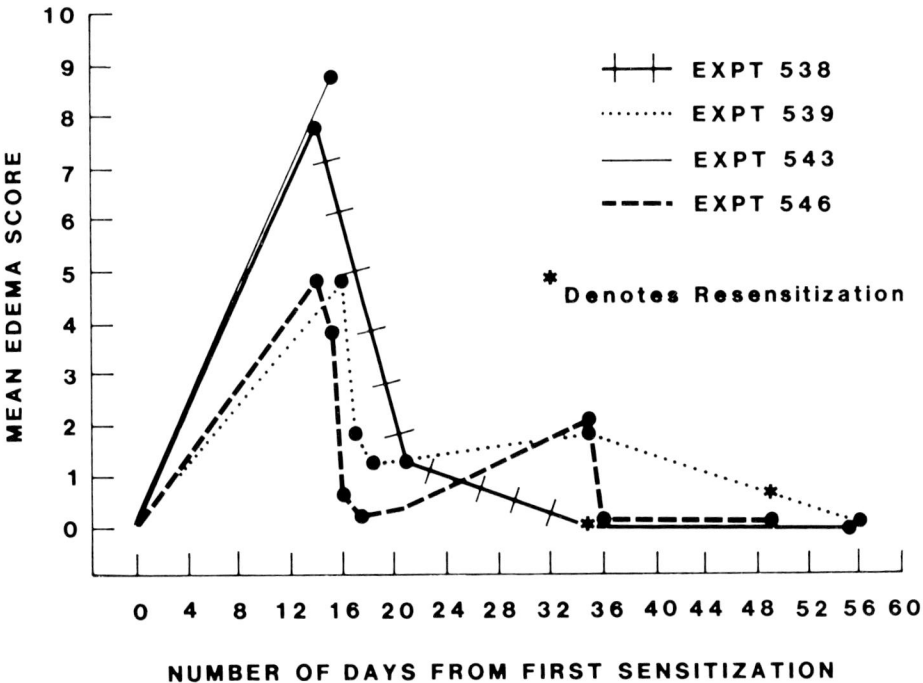

Figure 27-7: Mean conjunctival edema of guinea pigs sensitized to 500 micrograms of ovalbumin intradermally.

were sensitive but sensitivity was short lived and continued for only two weeks. In spite of repeated challenge or attempts at booster sensitization via the intradermal route, these animals apparently lost their sensitivity beyond the two week interval.

We have, therefore, shown that immediate hypersensitivity can be induced in guinea pigs by intradermal injection of ovalbumin. However, the response, using the immediate hypersensitivity of the conjuctiva as a criterion, is variable and in most instances is not long lasting. Future studies will be needed to develop a more reliable method of increased IgE titers in guinea pigs.

REFERENCES

1. Feinberg, J. G., Dewdney, M., and Temple, A.: Serum sickness in guinea pigs. *Int Arch Allergy,* 27:175–192, 1965.
2. Dwyer, R. St. C., and Darouger, S.: Models of immediate and delayed hypersensitivity in the guinea pig conjunctiva. *Trans Ophthal Soc Uk, 1051*: 1971.
3. Dwyer, R. St. C., Turk, J. L., and Darougar, S.: Immediate hypersensitivity in the guinea pig conjunctiva: Characterization of the IgE and IgG_1 antibody involved. *Int Arch Allergy,* 46:910–924, 1974.
4. Tuffin, D. P., and Feinberg, J. G.: Leucocyte infiltration into the conjunctiva following topical challenge with antigen, histamine, or compound 48/80. *Monogr Allergy,* 12:213–215, 1977. (Karger Basel)
5. Stock, E. L., Schwartz, A. E., Watson, S., and Meisler, D. M.: Immediate hypersensitivity in the conjunctiva of guinea pigs sensitized of ovalbumin. Paper presented at the Ocular Microbiology and Immunology Group Meeting, Chicago, Illinois, November 1, 1980.

INDEX

A

Alta California Eye Research Foundation
   purposes of, vii
   seminars sponsored by, vii-viii
Animals
   experiments using
      humane treatment principles for, viii-ix
   inbred strains of, 4
      monitoring of, 4-6
   microbiologically defined, 6
      maintenance of, 6-7
   study of
      environments for (*see* Environments, experimental)
Animal species
   endangered, California, 17
   fully protected, California, 17
   rare, California, 17
   research models of
      information sources for, 17-18
   selection of, 3
      anatomical and physiological characteristics in, 4-7
      costs in, 7
      naturally occurring disease states in, 7
   See also models of Armadillo; Bovine; Canine; Feline; Guinea pig; Hamster; Mink; Monkey; Mouse; Pigeon; Primate; Rabbit; Rat; Swine
Anton's eye test (*see* Listeriosis, ocular)
Armadillo
   characteristics of, 106-107
Armadillo model, Hansen's disease
   advantages of, 107-108
   clinical ocular findings in, 107
   disadvantages of, 108
   experimental lepromatous production in, 105
   inoculation methods in, 105

B

Band keratopathy (Band KP)
   features of, 221
   histochemistry of, 221, *222, 223*
Band keratopathy, animal models of
   calcific laminated spherules in, *231, 232*
   electron microscopy of, 225, *226*
   histology of, 224-225
   induction methods for, 221-222
      genetic, 224
      laser, 224
      morphine sulfate exposure, 224
      vitamin D depletion, 223-224
      vitamin D excess, corneal edema, 223
      vitamin D excess, immunogenic uveitis, 222
   morphology of, 224, *225*
   pathogenesis of
      calcification process in, 227, *228*
      pathological calcification types for, 229
      theories of, 229-230
Beagle model, oval stromal corneal opacities
   contributing factors in, 194-195
   materials for, 184
   methods for, 184
      histochemistry, 185, *188*
      serum lipid measurements, 186-188
      thyroid hormone assays, 188
   morphologic types of
      nebular, 183, *184*
      racetrack, 183, *185*
      white arc, 183, *186*
   relation to human disease of, 195-197
   results in
      histochemistry, general, 189
      histochemistry, lipid, 189, *190-193*
      histology, 189
      serum lipid measurements, 190, *194-196*
      thyroid hormone assays, 190-191
Bovine model, ocular squamous cell carcinoma
   antibodies and, 176
   cell-mediated immunity and, 176

Bovine model (cont'd)
   contributing factors for
      environmental, 175
      host, 174–175
      infectious agents, 175–176
   diagnosis of, 177
   naturally occurring incidence of, 173
   pathogenesis of, 173–174
   pathology of, 173
   relation to human disease of, 177–178
   treatment of, 177

C

Calcification, subepithelial corneal (see Band keratopathy)
California Primate Research Center, 9–10
Canine model, oval stromal corneal opacities (see Beagle model)
Canine model, systemic lupus erthematosus (SLE)
   clinical manifestations of, 255
   etiology of, 257–259
      relation to human disease of, 259
   histopathologic features of, 257
   laboratory features of, 256
   ocular findings in, 259
      relation to human disease of, 260
Chick chorioallantoic membrane model, neovascularization, 201
Chlamydia
   conjunctivitis due to (see Conjunctivitis, chlamydial)
   developmental cycle of, 71
   divisions of, 71
   feline syndrome of (see Chlamydial infection, feline model of)
   genital infections of
      feline, 74
         guinea pig, 80–81
         human, 80
Chlamydial infection, feline model of
   diagnostic verification of, 74
   differential diagnosis of, 72
   disease stages of, 72
   epithelial cell cytoplasm, *73*
   immunization for, 74
   inclusions in, *75*
   multiple infections with, 72
   relation to human disease of, 76
   serological studies of, 74
   transmission of, 74
   zoonotic potential of, 74
Conjunctivitis, chlamydial
   zoonotic, 68

Conjunctivitis, chlamydial, guinea pig model of
   chronic form and, 70
   disease stages of
      experimental, 79
      naturally occurring, 79
   extraocular forms and, 80–81
   immunity studies in, 81–83
   peroxidase enzyme activity in, 83, *84*
   relation to human disease of, 83, 85
   transmission of, 80
   vaccination studies in, 83
Conjunctivitis, chlamydial, primate model of
   inclusion form of
      agent's cultivation for, 67–68
      model's problems in, 65, *66*
      reactivation attempts in, 65–66
   relation to human disease of, 63
   trachoma type of
      agents' cultivation for, 67
      diagnostic features of, 64
      model's problems of, 65
      model's requirements for, 64
      reactivation attempts in, 65–66
Corneal ulcers, bacterial (see Ulcers, bacterial corneal)

D

Dermatitis, allergic contact (see Hypersensitivity)
Dystrophy, corneal (see Opacities)

E

Endophthalmitis, bacterial
   antibiotic studies of
      experimental factors in, 140–142
      experimental design factors for, 138–140
      infection severity measurements in, 141
   intraocular surgery and, 111
      treatment for, 118
   treatment for
      relative efficacy of, 137
Endophthalmitis, bacterial, primate model for
   inflamed vs. noninflamed eye in, 139
   relation to human disease of, 138
Endophthalmitis, bacterial, rabbit model for
   antibiotic injection routes in
      intravitreal vs. periocular with intravenous, 115–116
      retrobulbar vs. subconjunctival, 113
      systemic and subconjunctival, 113–114
   antibiotic intravitreal injection
      efficacy of, inflamed eye, 115
      efficacy of, noninflamed eye, 114–115

Endophthalmitis (cont'd)
  safe levels for, inflamed eye, 115
  safe levels for, noninflamed eye, 114
  vitrectomy vs., 116–117
  antibiotic levels in
    inflamed eye, 112–113
    noninflamed eye, 112
  aphakic vs. phakic eye in, 139
  corticosteroids for, 117–118
  infectious inoculum
    site and size of, 138–139
  inflamed vs. noninflamed eye in, 139
  organism recoverability in, 111
  pathogen virulence in, 139–140
  pigmented vs. albino eye in, 140
  relation to human disease of, 138
Environment, experimental
  domestic, 10
  laboratory
    advantages of, 8
    California Primate Research Center as, 9–10
    disadvantages of, 8
    regional primate centers as, 8
  natural
    advantages of, 10
    disadvantages of, 10
    Natural Land and Water Reserve System as, 11–16

F

Feline model, chlamydial infection
  diagnostic verification of, 74
  differential diagnosis of, 72
  disease stages of, 72
  epithelial cell cytoplasm, 73
  immunization for, 74
  inclusions in, 75
  multiple infections with, 72
  relation to human disease of, 76
  serological studies of, 74
  transmission of, 74
  zoonotic potential of, 74
Feline model, taurine deficiency
  relation to human disease of, 218
  retinal degeneration in, 215–216
    biochemical changes in, 216
    electroretinography in, 216–217
    ophthalmoscopy in, 217
    pathology in, 217–218
Francis I. Proctor Foundation for Research in Ophthalmology
  seminars sponsored by, vii–viii

G

Guinea pig
  Anton's eye test with
    ocular listeriosis and, 126
Guinea pig, immediate conjunctival hypersensitivity in
  antibody titers in, 272, 274
  experimental controls in, 270
    focal scarring in, 273, 274
  experimental design of, 269–270
  experimental results in, 270
    corneal, 271
    histological, 272
    skin necrosis as, 273
    variable, 274–276
Guinea pig model, bacterial corneal ulcers
  pathogens for, 129
  relation to human disease of, 133
  response to therapy in, 132
    cryosurgery and, 133
Guinea pig model, chlamydial conjunctivitis
  chronic form of, 80
  disease stages of
    experimental, 79
    naturally occurring, 79
  extraocular forms and, 80–81
  immunity studies in, 81–83
  peroxidase enzyme activity in, 83, 84
  relation to human disease of, 83, 85
  transmission of, 80
  vaccination studies in, 83
Guinea pig model, contact hypersensitivity
  antibodies in, 264
  elicitation of, 263–264
  experimental materials for, 266
  experimental methods for, 266
  experimental results in
    ocular reactions as, 267
    skin reactions as, 266–267
  genetic control of, 264
  histology of, 264
  induction of, 263
  Langerhans cells in, 265
  ocular reactions in, 265–266
  relation to human disease of, 267–268
  tolerance in, 264–265
Guinea pig model, neovascularization, 201

H

Hamster model, neovascularization, 201
Hamster model, ocular toxoplasmosis, 98–99
  relation to human disease of, 103

Hansen's disease, armadillo model for
  advantages of, 107–108
  clinical ocular findings in, 107
  disadvantages of, 108
  experimental lepromatous production in, 105
  inoculation methods in, 105
Herpes
  historical use of word, 23–24
Herpes simplex retinochoroiditis
  neonatal
    isolates in, 39
    manifestations of, 39
    reported cases of, 40
Herpes simplex retinochoroiditis, neonatal rabbit model of
  experimental materials for, 40
  experimental methods for, 40–42
  experimental results of
    lesion production as, 42, *43–47*
    virologic isolation as, 43–44, *48–49*
    relation to human disease of, 45–47
Herpes simplex retinochoroiditis, rat model of, 45
Herpetic keratitis
  strain virulence and, 33–34
Herpetic keratitis, mouse model for, 33
Herpetic keratitis, rabbit model of
  dendritic form of
    comparison of studies of, 25–26, *26–30*
      inoculation without scarification technique for, 25
      inoculation with scarification technique for, 24–25
    herpes strains and
      histopathology of, 31
      relation to human disease of, 33
    stromal form of, 61
      cell response in, 32
      pathogenesis of, 31–32
      technique to induce, 26, 31
      time course of, 32
Herpetic keratitis, rat model for, 33
Herpetic stromal keratitis, mouse model of
  adoptive spleen cell transfer in
    materials and methods for, 55
    results, athymic mice, 55, *56–58*
    results, normal mice, 56, *59–60*
    results of immunization routes for, 56–57, 59, *60*
  hypothesis for, 53
  immunopathogenesis of, 59, 61–62
  thymus-dependent immune response in, 53–*54*
Hypersensitivity, contact, guinea pig model of
  antibodies in, 264

  elicitation of, 263–264
  experimental materials for, 266
  experimental methods for, 266
  experimental results in
    ocular reactions as, 267
    skin reactions as, 266–267
  genetic control of, 264
  histology of, 264
  induction of, 263
  Langerhans cells in, 265
  ocular reactions in, 265–266
  relation to human disease of, 267–268
  tolerance in, 264–265
Hypersensitivity, immediate conjunctival, guinea pig
  antibody titers in, 273, *274*
  experimental controls in, 270
    focal scarring in, 273, *274*
  experimental design of, 269–270
  experimental results in, 270
    corneal, *271*
    histological, *272*
    skin necrosis as, *273*
    variable responses of, 274–276

I

Institute of Laboratory Animal Resources, 17

J

Jackson Laboratory, 17–18

K

Keratitis, herpetic (*see* Herpetic keratitis)
Keratoconjunctivitis, *Listeria* (*see* Listeriosis, ocular)

L

Leprosy (*see* Hansen's disease)
Lipid deposits, corneal stromal
  beagle (*see* Opacities, oval stromal corneal)
  human, 191, *197*
Listeria monocytogenes
  characteristics of, 121–122
Listeriosis, ocular
  Anton's eye test for, 124
    guinea pigs and, 126
    rabbits and, 124–126, *125*
  human cases of, 122–124
    summaries of, *123*
  therapy for, 126

Listeriosis, ocular (cont'd)
    mouse model and, 126

M

Medical Literature Analysis and Retrieval System (MEDLARS), 18
Melanomas, cutaneous malignant, swine model for
  immunologic studies in, 150–151
  inheritance pattern in, 149
  lesion classification for, 146–147
    relation to human disease of, 148
  naturally occurring incidence of, 145
  necropsy studies in, 148–149
  ocular studies in
    depigmentation with tumor regression, 153–154, *156-158*
    electroretinograms for, 157–159, *162*
    methods for, 153
    normal eye, 153, *154, 155*
    normal eye pigmentation in, 154–155, *158, 159*
    sequential cytotoxicity assays for, 160, 162, *163*
    stages during tumor regression in, 155–156, *157-160*
    system immunologic process of, 163–164
    uveitis, human vs. swine, 164
    variations during tumor regression in, 156–157, *161*
    vitiligo, human vs. swine, 164
  relation to human disease of, 152
Meningitis, rabbit model for
  therapy and, 126
Mink model, tyrosinemia
  characteristics of, 210–211
  disadvantages of, 211
  enzyme levels in, 211
  natural occurrence of, 210
  relation to human disease of, 211, *212*
Monkey model, ocular toxoplasmosis, 100–101
  hypersensitivity studies in, 101–102
  inoculation for, *101*
  relation to human disease of, 101, 103
Mouse model, herpetic keratitis, 33
Mouse model, bacterial corneal ulcers
  bacterial toxins and, 131
  immunocompromised subjects and, 132
  pathogens for, 129
  relation to human disease of, 133
  response to therapy in, 132
  uninjured cornea and, 132
Mouse model, band keratopathy
  genetic origin for, 224

See also Band keratopathy, animal models of
Mouse model, herpetic stromal keratitis
  adoptive spleen cell transfer in
    materials and methods for, 55
    results, athymic mice, 55, *56-58*
    results, normal mice, 56, *59-60*
    results of immunization routs for, 56–57, 59, *60*
  hypothesis for, 53
  immunopathogenesis of, 59, 61–62
  thymus-dependent immune response in, 53–*54*
Mouse model, listeriosis
  therapy and, 126
Mouse model, Sjögren's syndrome
  age-related changes in, 239, 243, *244*
  histology of, 238–239
    Grade IV, *242*
    Grade III, *241*
    Grade 0, *240*
  material for, 237–238
  relation to human disease of, 243–245
  tissue techniques for, 238

N

Natural Land and Water Reserve System, U.C.
  collection of animals on, 16
  mammals present on, 11, 13–15
    rare, endangered, and protected, 17
  map of, *12*
  purpose of, 11
Neovascularization, corneal, 201
Neovascularization, corneal, animal models for
  evaluation techniques for, 205
  indirect stimuli in, 205
  induction techniques for, 202
  maximum stimulating distance in, 204–205
  relation to human condition of, 204
  stimuli methods for, 201
Neovascularization, corneal, rabbit model for
  experimental method for, 202
  stimulating solution in, 202
    vascular response to, *203*–204

O

Ocular conditions (*see specific condition*)
Opacities, oval stromal corneal, beagle model for
  contributing factors in, 194–195
  materials for, 184
  methods for, 184
    histochemistry, 185, *188*
    serum lipid measurements, 186–188
    thyroid hormone assays, 188

Opacities (cont'd)
    morphologic types of
        nebular, 183, *184*
        racetrack, 183, *185*
        white arc, 183, *186*
    relation to human disease of, 195–197
    results in
        histochemistry, general, 189
        histochemistry, lipid, 189, *190–193*
        histology, 189
        serum lipid measurements, 190, *194–196*
        thyroid hormone assays, 190–191

P

Papillomas, immunotherapy for, rabbit model for
    experimental materials in, 167
    experimental methods for, 167–168
    possible complications of, 172
    postapplication tumor regression in, 168, *169–171*
    relation to human disease of, 170–171
    tumor development in, *168, 169*
Pigeon model, ocular toxoplasmosis, 98
    relation to human disease of, 103
Primate centers, regional, 8
Primate model, bacterial endophthalmitis
    inflamed vs. noninflamed eye in, 139
    relation to human disease of, 138
Primate model, chlamydial conjunctivitis
    inclusion conjunctivitis type of
        agents' cultivation for, 67–68
        model's problems in, 65, *66*
        reactivation attempts in, 65–66
    relation to human disease of, 63
    trachoma type of
        agents' cultivation for, 67
        diagnostic features of, 64
        model's problems in, 65
        model's requirements for, 64
        reactivation attempts in, 65–66
Primate model (*see also* Monkey models)

R

Rabbit
    Anton's eye test with
        ocular listeriosis and, 124–126, *125*
Rabbit ear model, neovascularization, 201
Rabbit model, bacterial corneal ulcers
    bacterial toxins and, 131
    nonimmunological cellular responses in, 130
    pathogens for, 129
    polymorphonuclear response in, 130–131
    relation to human disease of, 133
    response to therapy in, 132
        idoxuridine and, 133
Rabbit model, bacterial endophthalmitis
    antibiotic injection routes in
        intravitreal vs. periocular with intravenous, 115–116
        retrobulbar vs. subconjunctival, 113
        systemic and subconjunctival, 113–114
    antibiotic intravitreal injection
        efficacy of, inflamed eye, 115
        efficacy of, noninflamed eye, 114–115
        safe levels for, inflamed eye, 115
        safe levels for, noninflamed eye, 114
        vitrectomy vs. 116–117
    antibiotic levels in
        inflamed eye, 112–113
        noninflamed eye, 112
    aphakic vs. phakic eye in, 139
    corticosteriods for, 117–118
    future investigations for, 118
    infectious inoculum
        site and size of, 138–139
    inflamed vs. noninflamed eye in, 139
    organism recoverability in, 111
    pathogen virulence in, 139–140
    pigmented vs. albino eye in, 140
    relation to human disease of, 138
Rabbit model, band keratopathy
    calcific laminated spherules in, 229–230, *231, 232*
    electron microscopy of, *225, 226*
    histology of, 224–225
    laser induced, 224
    morphology of, 224, *225*
    pathological calcification in, 229
    vitamin D depletion, 223–224
    vitamin D excess
        corneal edema, 223
        immunogenic uveitis, 222
    See also Band keratopathy, animal models of
Rabbit model, endotoxin-induced uveitis, 247
    pharmacologic studies in, 248, 251
Rabbit model, herpetic keratitis
    dendritic form of
        inoculation without scarification for, 25
        inoculation with scarification for, 24–25
        comparison of studies of, 25–26, *26–30*
    herpes strains of
        histopathology of, 31
    relation to human disease of, 33
    stromal form of
        cell response in, 32
        pathogenesis of, 31–32

Rabbit model (cont'd)
    technique to induce, 26, 31
    time course of, 32
Rabbit model, herpetic stromal keratitis, 61
Rabbit model, immunotherapy for papillomas
    experimental materials in, 167
    experimental methods for, 167–168
    possible complications of, 172
    postapplication tumor regression in, 168–169, 170, 171
    relation to human disease of, 170–171
    tumor development in, 168, 169
Rabbit model, meningitis
    therapy and, 126
Rabbit model, neonatal, herpes simplex retinochoroiditis
    experimental materials for, 40
    experimental methods for, 40–42
    experimental results of
        lesion production as, 42, 43–47
        virologic isolation as, 43–44, 48–49
    relation to human disease of, 45–47
Rabbit model, neovascularization, corneal
    experimental method for, 202
    stimulating solution in, 202
    vascular response to, 203–204
Rabbit model, ocular toxoplasmosis, 98, 99–100
    relation to human disease of, 103
Rat model, band keratopathy
    histology of, 224–225
    morphine sulfate exposure, 224
    morphology of, 224
    pathological calcification in, 229
    vitamin D excess
        corneal edema, 223
    See also Band keratopathy, animal models of
Rat model, herpes simplex retinochoroiditis, 45
Rat model, herpetic keratitis, 33
Rat model, neovascularization, 201
Rat model, tyrosinemia
    characteristics of, 210
    disadvantage of, 210
    relation to human disease of, 210
Rats, endotoxin-induced uveitis in
    characteristics of, 248
    endotoxin effects in, 248
    histology of, 248, 249, 250
    historical background for, 247
    pharmacologic studies in, 248, 251
    relation to human diseases of, 251
Registry of Comparative Pathology, 18
    Retinitis pigmentosa
        taurine deficiency and, 218

Retinochoroiditis, herpes simplex (see Herpes simplex retinochoroiditis)
Richner-Hanhart syndrome (see Tyrosinemia)

S

Schnyder's crystalline dystrophy (see Opacities)
Sensitivity, contact (see Hypersensitivity)
Sjögren's syndrome, mouse model for
    age-related changes in, 239, 243, 244
    histology of, 238–239
        Grade IV, 242
        Grade III, 241
        Grade 0, 240
    material for, 237–238
    relation to human disease of, 243–245
    tissue techniques for, 238
Squamous cell carcinoma, ocular, bovine model for
    antibodies and, 176
    cell-mediated immunity and, 176
    contributing factors for
        environmental, 175
        host, 174–175
        infectious agents, 175–176
    diagnosis of, 177
    naturally occurring incidence of, 173
    pathogenesis of, 173–174
    pathology of, 173
    relation to human disease of, 177–178
    treatment of, 177
Swine model, cutaneous malignant melanomas
    immunologic studies in, 150–151
    inheritance pattern in, 149
    lesion classification for, 146–147
        relation to human disease of, 148
    naturally occurring incidence of, 145
    necropsy studies in, 148–149
    ocular studies in
        depigmentation with tumor regression, 153–154, 156–158
        electroretinograms for, 157–159, 162
        methods for, 155
        normal eye, 153, 154, 155
        normal eye pigmentation in, 154–155, 158, 159
        sequential cytotoxicity assays for, 160, 162, 163
        stages during tumor regression in, 155–156, 157–160
        systemic immunologic process of, 163–164
        uveitis, human vs. swine, 164

Swine model (cont'd)
    variations during tumor regression in, 156–157, *161*
    vitiligo, human vs. swine, 164
    relation to human disease of, 152
Systemic lupus erythematosus (SLE), canine model of
    clinical manifestations of, 255
    etiology of, 257–259
        relation to human disease of, 259
    histopathologic features of, 257
    laboratory features of, 256
    ocular findings in, 259
        relation to human disease of, 260

T

Taurine
    functions of
        known, 215
        postulated, 215
    retinal concentrations of, 215
    synthesis of, 215
Taurine deficiency, feline model for
    relation to human disease of, 218
    retinal degeneration in, 215–216
        biochemical changes in, 216
        electroretinography in, 216–217
        ophthalmoscopy in, 217
        pathology in, 217–218
Toxoplasma gondii
    epidemiology of
        congenital infection in, 90
        felines in, 89
        injection in, 89–90
    infection with (*see* Toxoplasmosis)
    life cycle of, 87, *88*, 89
    ocular involvement in (*see* Toxoplasmosis, ocular)
Toxoplasmosis
    asymptomatic, 90–91
    diagnosis of, 92–93
    prevention of, 93
    symptomatic
        acute, 91
        chronic, 91
    symptoms of
        feline, 91
        human, 91
    treatment of, 93–94
Toxoplasmosis, ocular
    signs and symptoms of
        feline, 91–92
        human, 91–92

Toxoplasmosis, ocular, models of
    hamster, 98–99
    ideal, 97
    monkey, 100–101
        hypersensitivity studies in, 101–102
        inoculation technique for, *101*
        relation to human disease of, 101
    pigeon, 98
    rabbit, 98, 99–100
    relation to human disease of, 103
Trachoma (*see* Conjunctivitis, chlamydial)
Tyrosinemia (tyrosine metabolism abnormalities)
    Richner-Hanhart syndrome as
        characteristics of, 207–208
        enzyme levels in, 208
        hereditary pattern in, 209
        treatment of, 209
    types of, 207
        characteristics of, 209
Tyrosinemia, mink model for
    characteristics of, 210–211
    disadvantages of, 211
    enzyme levels in, 211
    natural occurrence of, 210
    relation to human disease of, 211, *212*
Tyrosinemia, rat model for
    characteristics of, 210
    disadvantages of, 210
    relation to human disease of, 210

U

Ulcers, bacterial corneal
    pathogens for, 129, *130*
    test methods for, 130
Ulcers, bacterial corneal, guinea pig model for
    pathogens for, 129
    relation to human disease of, 133
    response to therapy in, 132
        cryosurgery and, 133
Ulcers, bacterial corneal, mouse model for
    bacterial toxins and, 131
    immunocompromised subjects and, 132
    pathogens for, 129
    relation to human disease of, 133
    response to therapy in, 132
    uninjured cornea and, 132
Ulcers, bacterial corneal, rabbit model for
    bacterial toxins and, 131
    nonimmunological cellular responses in, 130
    pathogens for, 129
    polymorphonuclear response in, 130–131
    relation to human disease of, 133
    response to therapy in, 132

Ulcers, bacterial corneal, rabbit model (*cont'd*)
    idoxuridine and, 133
Uveitis
    human vs. swine, 164
Uveitis, endotoxin-induced, rabbit model of, 247
    pharmacologic studies in, 248, 251
Uveitis, endotoxin-induced, rat model of
    characteristics of, 248
    endotoxin effects in, 248
    histology of, 248, *249, 250*
    historical background for, 247
    pharmacologic studies in, 248, 251
    relation to human diseases of, 251

V

Vitiligo
    human vs. swine, 164

DATE DUE